QUICK INVESTIGATION ON ACUPUNTURE POINTS,

Selection of Professor Yang Jiasan

Editor

Guo Changqing

Published by

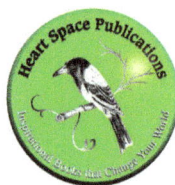

Heart Space Publications
PO Box 1085
Daylesford
Victoria
3460
Australia
Tel +61 450260348
www.heartspacebooks.com
pat@heartspacebooks.com

ISBN 978-0-6489216-1-5

CONTENTS

Preface

Professor Yang Jiasan is one of China's foremost acupuncture and moxibustion scientist. He is the first director, professor, doctoral supervisor and professor of acupuncture and massage at the department of Beijing University of Chinese Medicine (formerly Beijing College of traditional Chinese Medicine). Professor Yang is famous at home and abroad for his exquisite medical skills and unique academic viewpoints.

Professor Yang has devoted himself to the study of acupuncture and moxibustion for his entire professional life, and has made outstanding achievements in clinical, educational, and scientific research. He is recognised as the Chinese authority on acupoint selection, clinical acupoint application, needle injection, needle tonifying, and reducing clinical treatment, etc., especially in acupoints. The "three sides, three middles" acupoint selection method proposed by Yang has the characteristics of accurate acupoint selection, strong acupuncture precision, safe and reliable acupuncture, etc. It has been effectively used in clinical teaching and has a wide range of influence.

Within these pages are the methods of accurately taking the treatment points of acupuncture and moxibustion by Professor Yang Jia-san. With more than 400 clear images, the reader can visually and vividly study the point-taking and apply it to clinical practice. Additionally covered are the methods of point-taking of the fourteen meridians of the body, and nearly 400 extra points.

The book is informative, intuitive, and easy to learn, and is especially suitable for; students of Traditional Chinese Medicine, for acupuncture and moxibustion practitioners, teaching, and research workers. It is also ideal for acupuncture and moxibustion enthusiasts.

In this book, Professor Yang's acupoint selection method is refrenced out and applied, and is clearly presented to readers with exquisite pictures, so that readers can intuitively and vividly learn Professor Yang's acupoint selection, for the application in their practice.

The book is divided into sixteen chapters, each of which introduce the acupoint selection methods of the body's fourteen meridians and the extra points. The appendix offers Professor Yang Jiasan's biography and clinical experience of acupuncture and moxibustion.

Testimonial

Professor Yang is one of my most admired and respect person. By reading this book, it brought the memory of my 5 year college life back. He proposed the "san mian san zhong" acupuncture point allocation method by his rich experience, which will benefit many learners. I hope more Australian Chinese medicine acupuncture lovers will see this book.

Shen Weihong
Australian registered Chinese medical doctor and acupuncturist,
council member of Federation of Chinese Medicine & Acupuncture Societies of Australia Ltd.

CHAPTER 1

Methods of Locating Combination Points

Section 1
Finger-length Measurement

Finger measurement is a method of standard measurement, for the location of the acupuncture point, since the fingers are in proportion with the other parts of the body – that the length and width of the patient's fingers are taken.

1. Four-Finger Measurement

The width of the four fingers (index, middle, ring and little) placed together, taken at the level of the dorsal crease of the proximal interphalangeal joint of the middle finger measures 3 cun. Cun is the term for the measurement relative to the patient (see images below). This method is always used to locate the points in the abdomen, back and lower limbs.

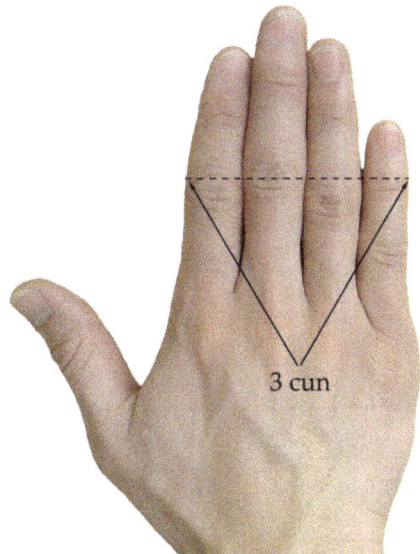

3 cun

2. Thumb Measurement

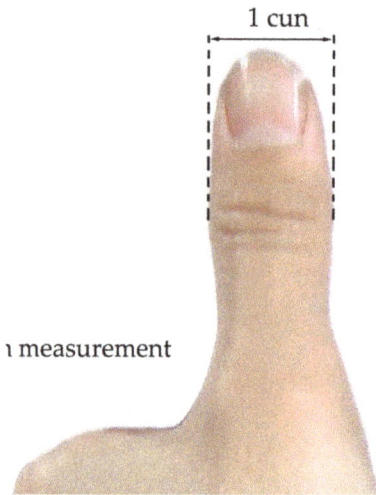

1 cun

Place the thumb straight. The width of the interphalangeal joint of the patient's thumb is 1 cun.

ı measurement

3. Middle Finger Measurement

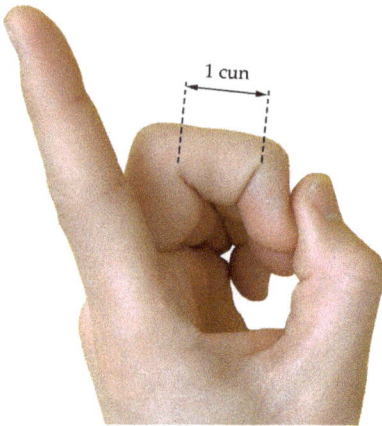

1 cun

When the patient's middle finger is flexed, the index finger is straight, and the end of the middle finger against the belly of the thumb, forming a ring. The width between the two medial ends of the creases of the interphalangeal joints is 1 cun. This method is suitable for limbs and transverse measurement of the dorsal.

Section 2
Bone-Length Measurement

The commonly used modern method of orientation of "bony degree" is based on Ling Shu (superior pivot), and in the long-term medical practice after modification and supplement, see the table below for details.

Standard for Bone-Length Measurement

Body Part	Area between two points on the body	Length in cun
Head	From the midpoint of the anterior hairline to the midpoint of the posterior hairline	12 cun

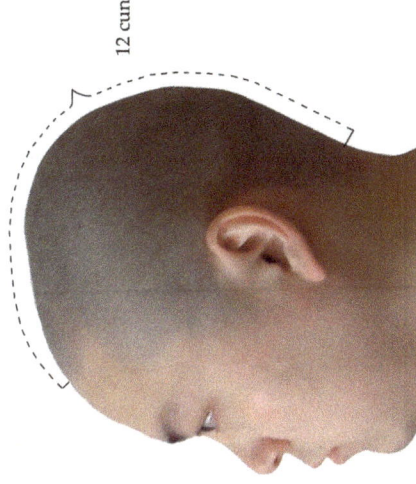

12 cun

Head	Between the corners of the forehead ST 8.	9 cun
Head	Between the two mastoid processes	9 cun
Chest and Abdomen	From the suprasternal fossa to the sternocostal angle	9 cun
	From the sternocostal angle to the center of the umbilicus	8 cun
	From the center of the umbilicus to the upper of symphysis pubis	5 cun
	Between the two nipples	8 cun

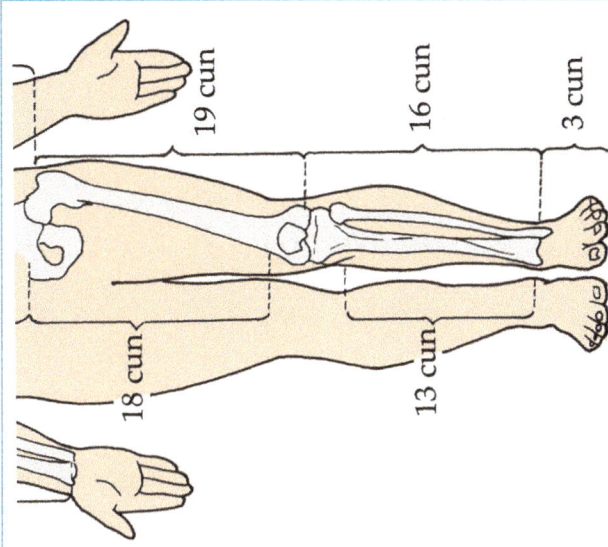

Region	From	Measurement
Lateral side of the trunk	From the tip of the axillary fossa to the tip of the 11th rib.	12 cun
	From the tip of the 11th rib to the prominence of the great trochanter	9 cun
Upper Limbs	From the end of the axillary fold to the transverse cubital crease	9 cun
	From the transverse cubital crease to the transverse wrist crease	12 cun
Lower Limbs	From the level of the border of symphysis pubis to the medial epicondyle of the femur	18 cun
	From the lower border of the medial condyle of tibia to the tip of medial malleolus	13 cun
	From the prominence of the great trochanter to the middle of patella	19 cun
	From the center of patella to the tip of lateral malleolus	16 cun
	From the tip of lateral malleolus to the sole.	3 cun

CHAPTER 2

Lung Channel of Hand Taiyin; LU

There are eleven points on the Lung Channel of Hand Taiyin and twenty-two points in total on both sides. There are two points on the upper part of the chest and nine on the medial side of the upper limb. The first point is LU 1 (Zhōng Fǔ) and the last point is LU 11 (Shào Shāng). The indications for this channel are the diseases which involve the lungs and the symptoms along the course of the channel.

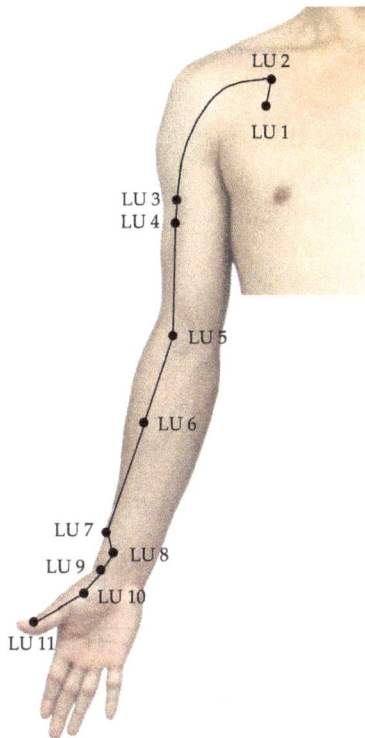

LU 1 – Zhōng Fǔ

[Features]	Front-mu point of the Lung Channel of Hand *Taiyin*.
[Locating]	The point is located in the sitting position with the hand on the hip, first locate LU 2 (Yún Mén) in the center of the tricorner anterior to the deltoid, then locate LU 1 (Zhōng Fǔ) in the first intercostal space approximately 1 cun inferior and slightly lateral to LU 2 (Yún Mén).
[Regional Anatomy]	The needle passes through the subcutaneous tissues and penetrates the m. pectoralis major and m. pectoralis minor.
[Acupuncture and Moxibustion]	① Insert the needle perpendicularly 0.3~0.5 cun deep and stimulate the needle until there is a sore sensation in the local area radiating to the chest or the arm; ② Insert the needle obliquely outward 0.5~0.8 cun deep and stimulate the needle until there is a sensation in the local area. This point can be moxibusted.
[Indications]	Cough, asthma and chest pain.
[Note]	It is not advisable to prick deeply with a straight needle or inwardly to avoid injuring the lungs and causing accidents.

LU 2 – Yún Mén

[Locating]	The point is located in the sitting position with the hand on the hip and elbow turned outward, in the middle of the triangular depression inferior to the lateral segment of the clavicle.
[Regional Anatomy]	The needle passes through the subcutaneous tissues and penetrates the m. triangularis and reaches the coracoid process.
[Acupuncture and Moxibustion]	Insert the needle obliquely outward 0.5~1.0 cun deep and stimulate until there is a sore sensation in the local area radiating to the chest and the upper limbs. This point can be moxibusted.
[Indications]	Cough, asthma, chest and shoulder pain.

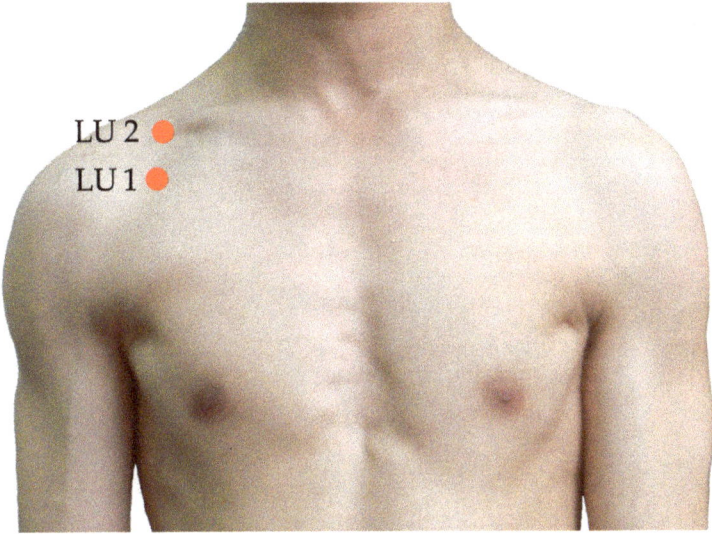

LU 2
LU 1

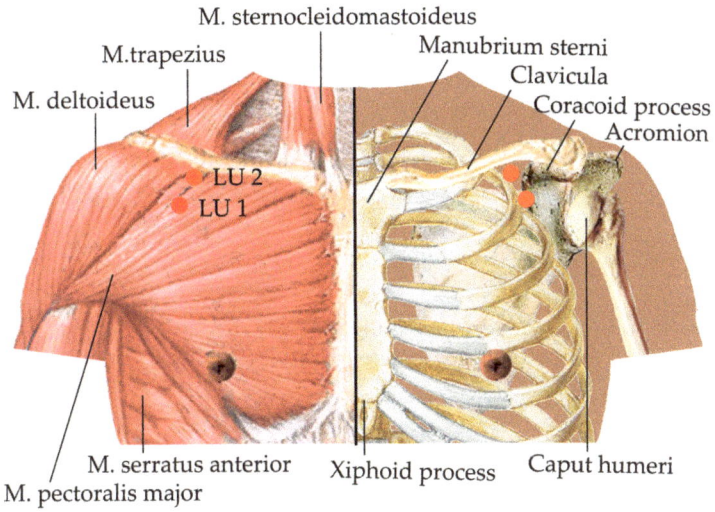

M. sternocleidomastoideus

M.trapezius

Manubrium sterni

M. deltoideus

Clavicula

Coracoid process

Acromion

LU 2
LU 1

M. serratus anterior

Xiphoid process

Caput humeri

M. pectoralis major

LU 3 – Tiān Fǔ

[Locating]	The point is located in the sitting position when the patient raises the arm forward and lowers the head. The point is located where the tip of the nose touches the internal point of the upper arm. Another locating method is in the sitting position when the elbow is bent slightly, on the lateral side of the biceps brachii muscle, 3 cun distal to the anterior end of the axillary fold, and 6 cun superior to the cubital crease.
[Regional Anatomy]	The needle passes through the subcutaneous tissues and reaches the humerus.
[Acupuncture and Moxibustion]	Insert the needle perpendicularly 0.5~1.0 cun deep and stimulate until there is a sore and numbing sensation in the local area radiating to the arm or elbow. This point can be moxibusted.
[Indications]	Cough, asthma.

LU 4 – Xiá Bái

[Locating]	The point is located in the sitting or supine posture, on the medial side of the upper arm, 4 cun distal to the anterior end of the axillary fold and 5 cun proximal to the transverse cubital crease on the radial side of m. biceps brachii.
[Regional Anatomy]	It's same to LU 3 Tiān Fǔ.
[Acupuncture and Moxibustion]	It's same to LU 3 Tiān Fǔ.
[Indications]	Cough, asthma, chest distention, and pain in the medial side of the upper arm.

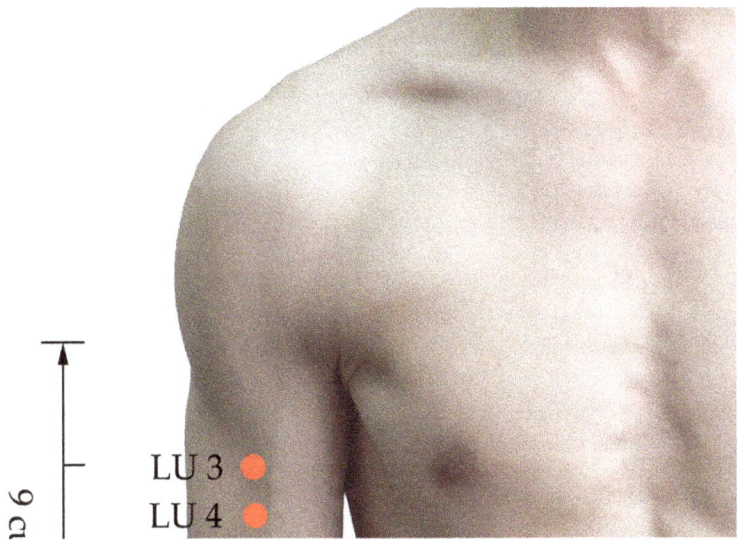

LU 3
LU 4

9 cu

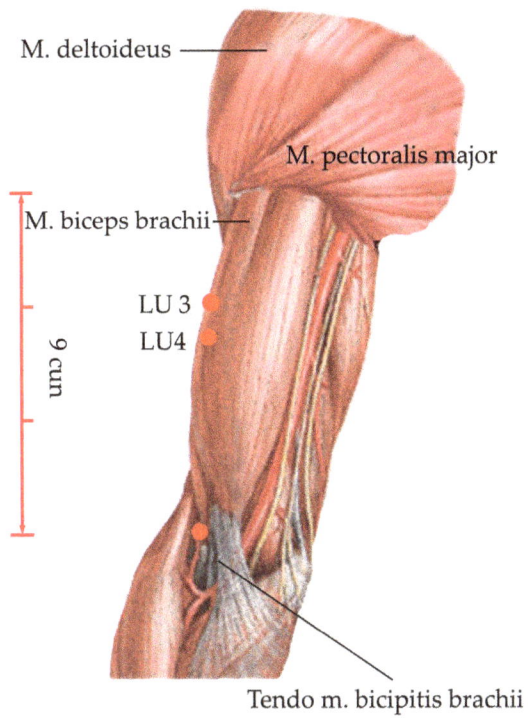

M. deltoideus

M. pectoralis major

M. biceps brachii

LU 3
LU4

9 cun

Tendo m. bicipitis brachii

LU 5 – Chǐ Zé

[Features]	He-sea point of the Lung Channel of Hand *Taiyin*.
[Locating]	The point is located on the cubital crease when the elbow is slightly bent with the palm facing upward, on the radial side of the tendon of biceps brachii.
[Regional Anatomy]	The needle passes through the subcutaneous tissues and deep fascia, penetrates the m. brachioradialis.
[Acupuncture and Moxibustion]	① Insert the needle perpendicularly 0.5~1.0 cun deep and stimulate until there is a sore and numbing sensation in the local area with an electric sensation radiating to the forearm and palm. ② Prick with a three-edged needle to bleed. This point can be moxibusted.
[Indications]	Cough, asthma, hemoptysis, sore throat, chest distention, spasmodic pain of the elbow and arm.

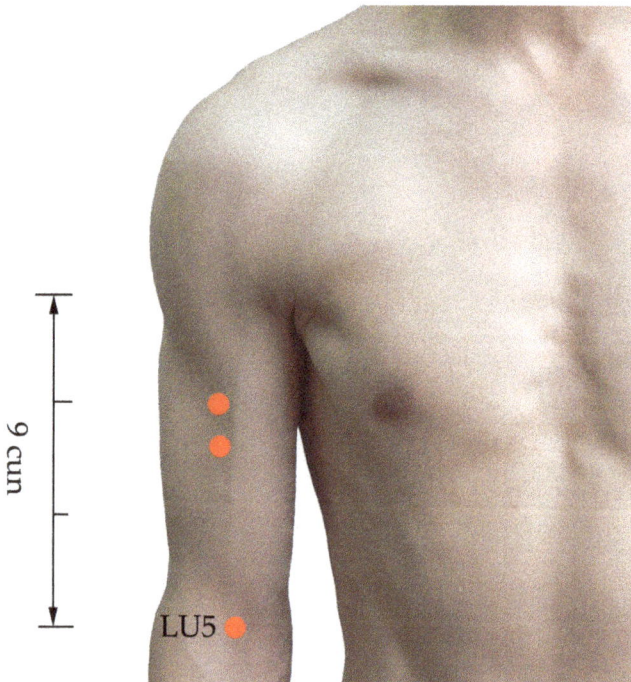

9 cun

LU5

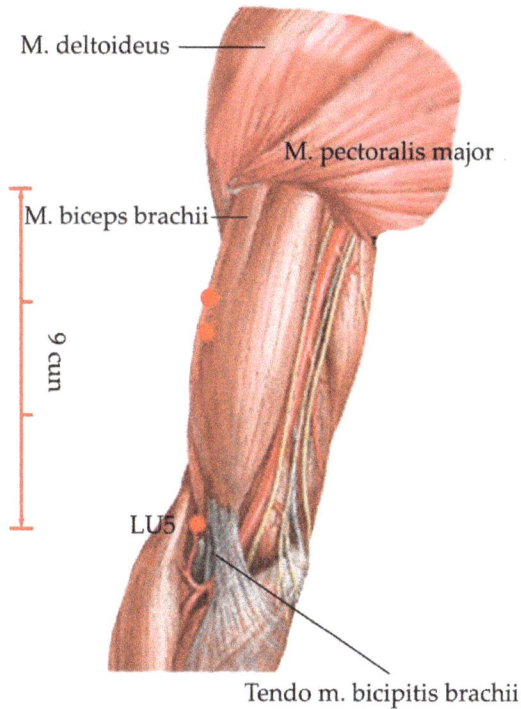

M. deltoideus

M. pectoralis major

M. biceps brachii

9 cun

LU5

Tendo m. bicipitis brachii

LU 6 – Kǒng Zuì

[Features]	Xi-cleft point of the Lung Channel of Hand *Taiyin*.
[Locating]	On the line connecting LU 9 (Tài Yuān) and LU 5 (Chǐ Zé), 7 cun above the transverse crease of the wrist on the palmar aspect of the forearm.
[Regional Anatomy]	The needle passes through the subcutaneous tissues and m. brachioradialis, m. flexor carpi radialis and penetrates the m. flexor digitorum superficialis and m. flexor pollicis longus.
[Acupuncture and Moxibustion]	Insert the needle perpendicularly 0.5~0.8 cun deep and stimulate until there is a sore, numbing and heavy sensation in the local area radiating to the forearm. This point can be moxibusted.
[Indications]	Hemoptysis, epistaxis.

LU 7 – Liè Quē

[Features]	Luo-connecting point of the Lung Channel of Hand Taiyin; one of the eight confluent points associated with the Ren Vessel.
[Locating]	The point is located by crossing the webs of the thumbs and placing the index finger on the styloid process of the radius of the other hand. The point located under the tip of the index finger in the depression of the styloid process.
[Regional Anatomy]	The needle passes through the subcutaneous tissues and vagina tendinum musculorum abductoris longi et extensoris brevis pollicis and penetrates m. pronator quadratus.
[Acupuncture and Moxibustion]	Insert the needle obliquely upward 0.2~0.3 cun deep and stimulate until there is a sore, heavy and numbing sensation in the local area. This point can be moxibusted.
[Indications]	Headache, neck stiffness and sore throat.

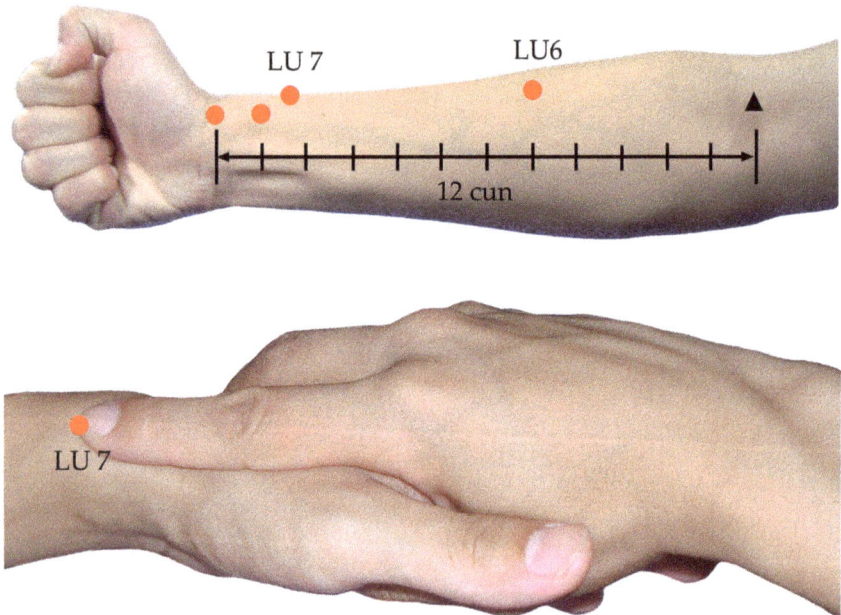

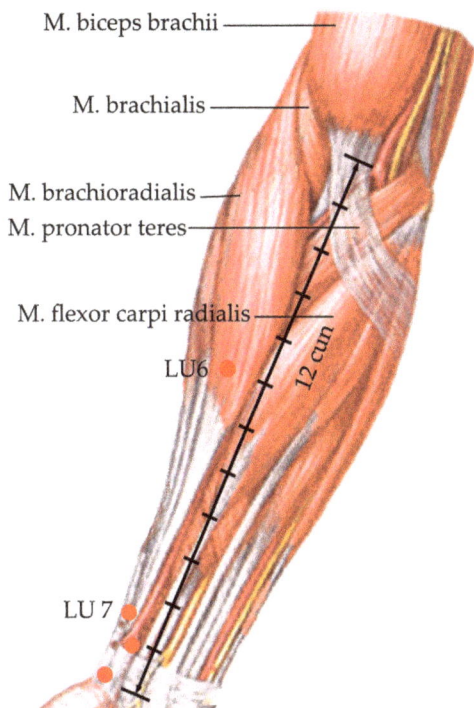

M. biceps brachii

M. brachialis

M. brachioradialis
M. pronator teres

M. flexor carpi radialis

LU6

12 cun

LU 7

LU 8 – Jīng Qú

[Features]	Jing-river point of the Lung Channel of Hand Taiyin.
[Locating]	On the radial side of the palmar surface of the forearm, 1 cun proximal to the transverse crease of the wrist, in the depression between the styloid process of the radius and the radial artery.
[Regional Anatomy]	The needle passes through the subcutaneous tissues, runs through the medial border of the superficial branch of the n. radialis, penetrates through subcutaneous fascia, the radial side of a. radialis and v. radialis, and enters the m. pronator quadratus.
[Acupuncture and Moxibustion]	Insert the needle perpendicularly 0.1~0.3 cun deep and stimulate until there is a sore and numbing sensation in the local area.This point can be moxibusted.
[Indications]	Pharyngitis, pain of the chest and back.

LU 9 – Tài Yuān

[Features]	Shu-stream point and yuan-source point of the Lung Channel of Hand *Taiyin*; influential point of the vessels.
[Locating]	On the radial end of the wrist crease, where the radial pulse is palpable.
[Regional Anatomy]	The needle passes through the subcutaneous tissues and reaches m. flexor carpi radialis.
[Acupuncture and Moxibustion]	Insert the needle perpendicularly 0.2~0.3 cun deep and stimulate until there is a numbing and distending sensation in the local area. This point can be moxi-busted.
[Indications]	Cough, asthma, pain in the wrist and pulseless disease.

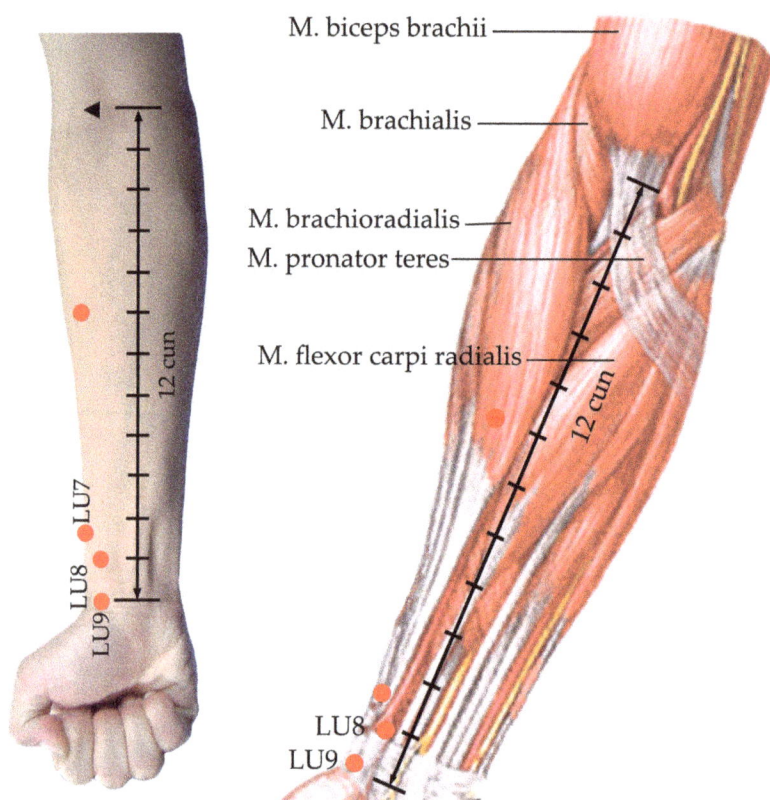

M. biceps brachii

M. brachialis

M. brachioradialis
M. pronator teres

M. flexor carpi radialis

12 cun

LU7
LU8
LU9

12 cun

LU8
LU9

LU 10 – Yú Jì

[Features]	Ying-spring point of the Lung Channel of Hand *Taiyin*.
[Locating]	The point is located when the hand is in a loose fist with the palm facing upwards, at the juncture of the red and white skin in the middle of the first metacarpal bone.
[Regional Anatomy]	The needle passes through the subcutaneous tissues and m. abductor pollicis brevis, and penetrates m. opponens pollicis and m. flexor pollicis brevis.
[Acupuncture and Moxibustion]	① Insert the needle perpendicularly 0.3~0.5 cun deep and stimulate until there is a distending sensation in the local area, which radiates to the thumb. ② Prick with a three-edged needle to bleed. This point can be moxibusted.
[Indications]	Hemoptysis, loss of voice, sore throat, dry throat and asthma.

LU 11 – Shào Shāng

[Features]	Jing-well point of the Lung Channel of Hand *Taiyin*.
[Locating]	The point is located when the hand is in a loose fist with the thumb pointing upward, on the line crossing the radial border and the base of the nail of the thumb. 0.1 cun lateral to the corner of the nail.
[Regional Anatomy]	The needle passes through the subcutaneous tissues and penetrates the base of fingernail.
[Acupuncture and Moxibustion]	① Insert the needle subcutaneously 0.1~0.2 cun deep and stimulate until there is a distending sensation in the local area. ② Prick with three-edged needle and press tightly to expel 5-13 drops of blood. This point can be moxibusted.
[Indications]	Pharyngitis, epistaxis, coma, heatstroke and vomit.

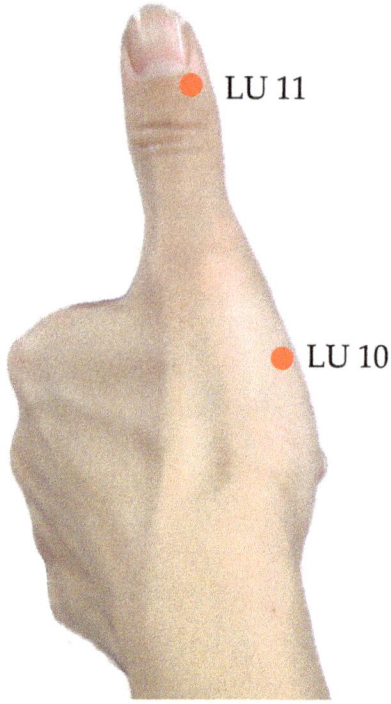

LU 11

LU 10

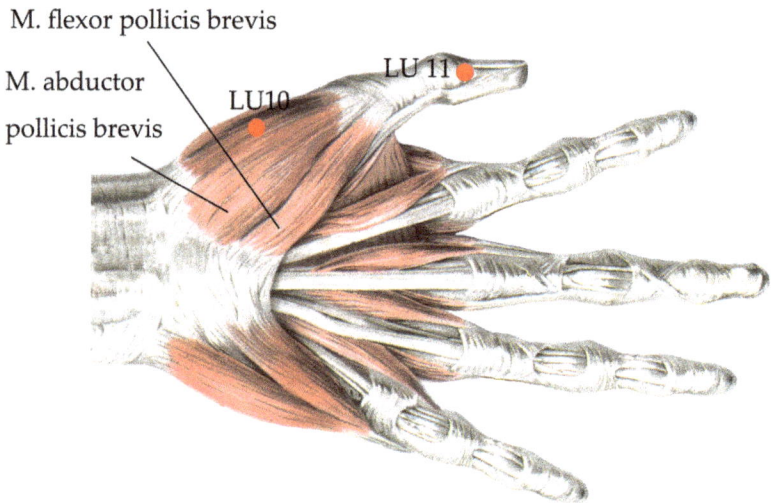

M. flexor pollicis brevis

M. abductor
pollicis brevis

LU10

LU 11

CHAPTER 3

Large Intestine Channel of Hand Yanming; LI

There are twenty points on the Large Intestine Channel of Hand *Yangming* and forty points in total on both sides. There are two points located on the face, three points located on the shoulder and the neck, and fifteen points distributed on the radial side of the dorsum of the upper limb. The first point is LI 1 (Shāng Yáng) and the last is LI 20 (Yíng Xiāng). The main indications of this channel are diseases of the eyes, ears, mouth, teeth, nose, throat, etc., as well as diseases of the abdomen, stomach and intestines and disorders along the course of the channel.

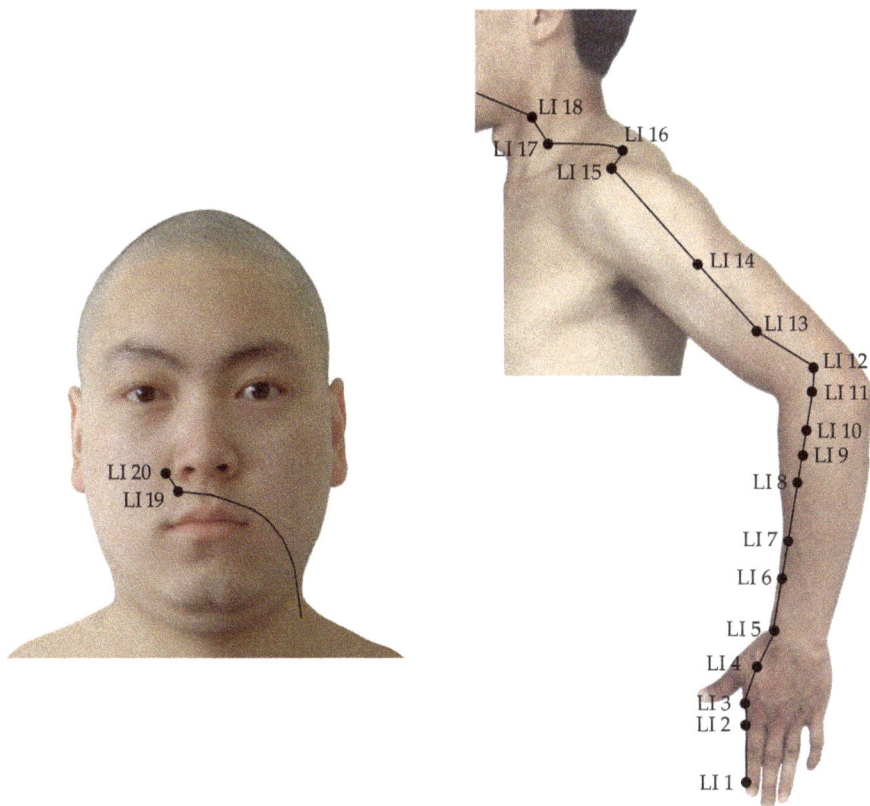

LI 1 – Shāng Yáng

[Features]	Jing-well point of the Large Intestine Channel of Hand *Yangming*.
[Locating]	The point is located when the hand is in a loose fist and the index points forward, at the line crossing the radial border and the base of the nail of the index finger. 0.1 cun medial to the corner of the nail.
[Regional Anatomy]	The needle passes through the skin and penetrates the subcutaneous tissues.
[Acupuncture and Moxibustion]	① Insert the needle perpendicularly 0.1~0.2 cun deep and stimulate until there is a distending sensation in the local area. ② Prick with a three-edged needle to bleed. This point can be moxibusted.
[Indications]	Pharyngitis, fainting, fever and febrile diseases with anhidrosis.

LI 2 – Èr Jiān

[Features]	Ying-spring point of the Large Intestine Channel of Hand *Yangming*.
[Locating]	On the radial side of the index finger, in the depression distal to the metacarpal phalangeal joint, at the junction of the red and white skin when the hand is in a loose fist.
[Regional Anatomy]	The needle passes through the subcutaneous tissues and penetrates the dorsal digital aponeurosis and periost of the index finger.
[Acupuncture and Moxibustion]	Insert the needle perpendicularly 0.2~0.4 cun deep and stimulate until there is a distending sensation in the local area. This point can be moxibusted.
[Indications]	Pharyngitis and toothache.

LI 3 – Sān Jiān

[Features]	Shu-stream point of the Large Intestine Channel of Hand *Yangming*.
[Locating]	On the radial side of the index finger, in the depression proximal to the head of the second metacarpal bone when the hand is in a loose fist.
[Regional Anatomy]	The needle passes through subcutaneous fascia, dorsal fascia of hand, m. interosse dorsales (1st), and runs between m. lumbricales (1st) and 2nd metacarpal bone, and arrives at the space between dorsal side of the tendon of the index finger and 2nd metacarpal bone.
[Acupuncture and Moxibustion]	Insert the needle perpendicularly 0.3~0.5 cun deep and stimulate until there is a numbing and distending sensation in the local area radiating to the dorsum of hand. This point can be moxibusted.
[Indications]	Sore throat and fever.

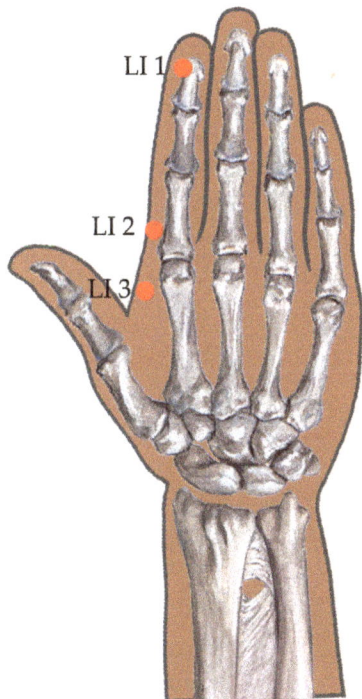

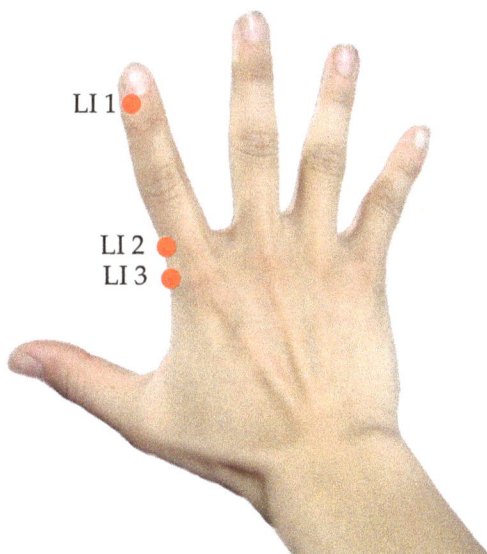

LI 4 – Hé Gǔ

[Features]	Yuan-source point of the Large Intestine Channel of Hand *Yangming*.
[Locating]	On the dorsum of the hand, between the first and second metacarpal bones, on the radial side of the middle of the second metacarpal bone. The point is located in the web between the index finger and the thumb when the thumb and index are stretched apart, at the middle point of the first metacarpal bone.
[Regional Anatomy]	The needle passes through the subcutaneous tissues, enters the m. interosse dorsales (1ˢᵗ), and penetrates the m. adductor pollicis from the medial side of the dorsal venous network and deep palmar artery.
[Acupuncture and Moxibustion]	① Insert the needle perpendicularly 0.5~1.0 cun deep and stimulate until there is a sore and numbing sensation in the local area radiating to the elbow, shoulder and face. ② Insert the needle at LI 4 (Hé Gǔ) until it reaches the points PC 8 (Láo Gōng) or SI 3 (Hòu Xī) and stimulate until there is a sore and numbing sensation radiating to the palm and the tip of the finger. This point can be moxibusted.
[Indications]	Fever, adiaphoresis, headache, nasal obstruction, toothache, mouth ulcers, facial nerve palsy, abdominal pain and dysmenorrhea.
[Note]	It is an important acupuncture point to relieve pain, control sweating and remove phlegm.

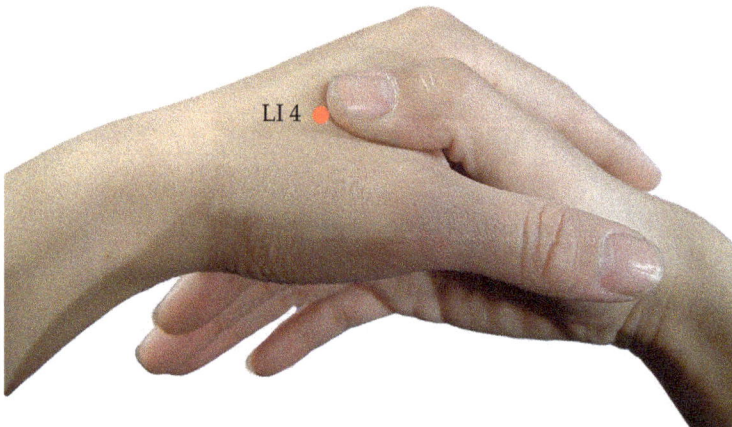

LI 4

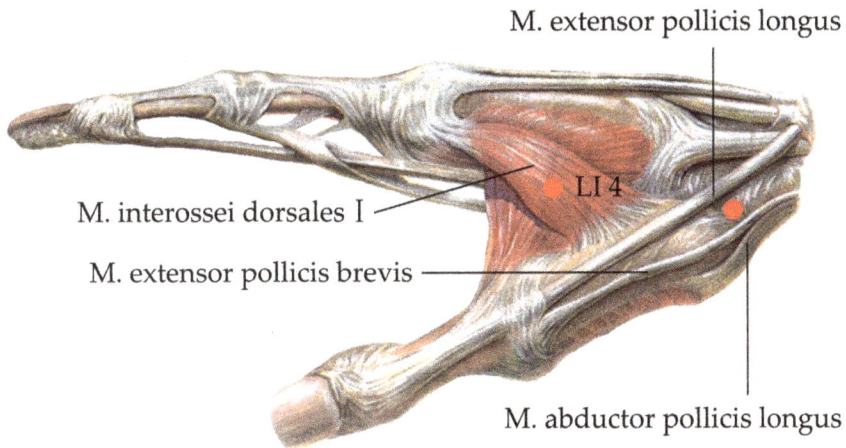

M. extensor pollicis longus

M. interossei dorsales I

M. extensor pollicis brevis

LI 4

M. abductor pollicis longus

LI 5 – Yáng Xī

[Features]	Jing-river point of the Large Intestine Channel of Hand *Yangming*.
[Locating]	The point is located in the depression between the tendons of m. extensor pollicis longus and brevis on the dorsal side of the wrist when the thumb is pointing upward.
[Regional Anatomy]	The needle passes through this ligament, runs between the tendons of m. extensor pollicis longus and m. extensor pollicis brevis, and arrives at the dorsal side of the tendon of m. extensor carpi radialis longus.
[Acupuncture and Moxibustion]	Insert the needle perpendicularly 0.5~0.8 cun deep and stimulate until there is a sore and numbing sensation in the local area. This point can be moxibusted.
[Indications]	Headache, deafness, sore throat, and pain in the wrist.

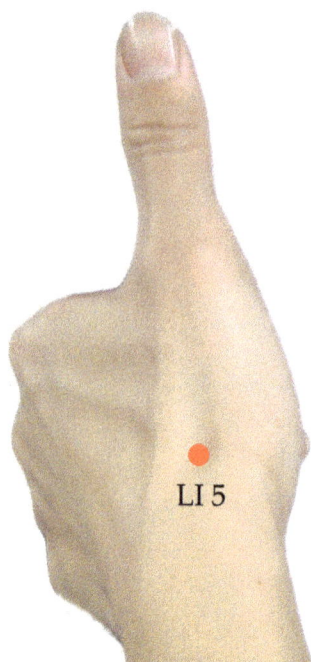

LI 5

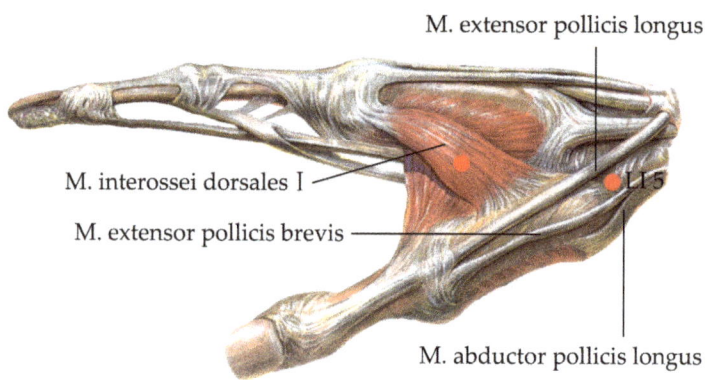

M. extensor pollicis longus

M. interossei dorsales I

M. extensor pollicis brevis

LI 5

M. abductor pollicis longus

LI 6 – Piān Lì

[Features]	Luo-connecting point of the Large Intestine Channel of Hand *Yangming*.
[Locating]	The point is located on the radial side of the forearm when the elbow is flexed and the thumb is pointing upward, 3 cun proximal to the wrist crease on the line connecting LI 5 (Yáng Xī) and LI 11 (Qǔ Chí).
[Regional Anatomy]	The needle penetrates through tendo m. extensoris pollicis brevis and tendo m. extensor carpi radialis longus and reaches the tendo m. extensor pollicis longus.
[Acupuncture and Moxibustion]	① Insert the needle perpendicularly 0.3~0.5 cun deep and stimulate until there is a sore and numbing sensation in the local area. ② Insert the needle obliquely towards the elbow 0.5~0.8 cun deep and stimulate until there is a sore and numbing sensation in the local area radiating to the forearm and the elbow. This point can be moxibusted.
[Indications]	Fever, deafness, nosebleed, and abdominal pain.

LI 7 – Wēn Liū

[Features]	Xi-cleft point of the Large Intestine Channel of Hand *Yangming*.
[Locating]	The point is located on the radial side of the arm when the elbow is flexed, 5 cun proximal to the wrist crease, on the line connecting LI 5 (Yáng Xī) and LI 11 (Qǔ Chí).
[Regional Anatomy]	The needle passes through the subcutaneous tissues from the posterior side of the v. cephalica, penetrates through antebrachial fascia, enters the tendo m. extensor carpi radialis longus and the tendo m. extensor carpi radialis brevis, and reaches the periost of the radius.
[Acupuncture and Moxibustion]	Insert the needle perpendicularly 0.5~1.0 cun deep and stimulate until there is a sore and numbing sensation in the local area radiating to the hand. This point can be moxibusted.
[Indications]	Headache, toothache and swelling of the pharynx.

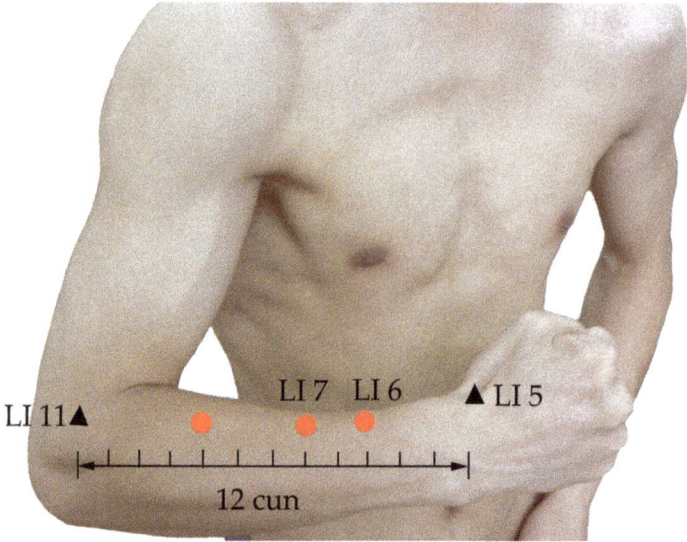

LI 11▲ LI 7 LI 6 ▲ LI 5

12 cun

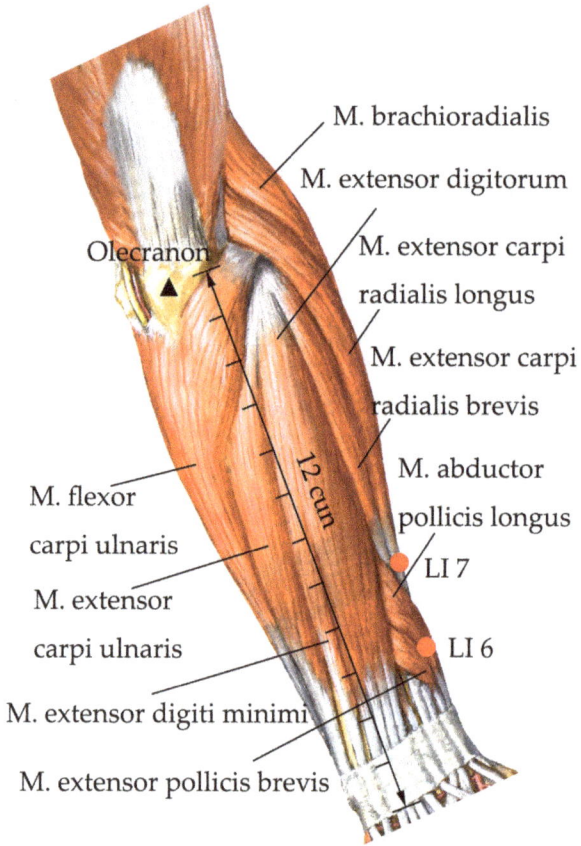

M. brachioradialis

M. extensor digitorum

M. extensor carpi radialis longus

Olecranon

M. extensor carpi radialis brevis

M. abductor pollicis longus

M. flexor carpi ulnaris

12 cun

LI 7

M. extensor carpi ulnaris

LI 6

M. extensor digiti minimi

M. extensor pollicis brevis

LI 8 – Xià Lián

[Locating]	The point is located when the elbow is flexed on the radial side of the forearm, 4 cun distal to the cubital crease on the line connecting LI 5 (Yáng Xī) and LI 11 (Qǔ Chí).
[Regional Anatomy]	The needle passes through the subcutaneous tissues at the front of the n. cutaneus antebrachii lateralis, and runs through the dorsal surface of tendo m. extensor carpi radialis longus, and the tendo m. extensor carpi radialis brevis, and enters into the m. supinator.
[Acupuncture and Moxibustion]	Insert the needle perpendicularly 1.0~1.5 cun deep and stimulate until there is a sore and numbing sensation in the local area radiating to the arm and fingers. This point can be moxibusted.
[Indications]	Abdominal pain, abdominal distention, swelling and pain of the hand and arm, paralysis of the upper limb and weakness and disability of the hand, elbow and shoulder.

LI 9 – Shàng Lián

[Locating]	The point is located when the elbow is flexed on the radial side of the forearm, 3 cun distal to the cubital crease on the line connecting LI 5 (Yáng Xī) and LI 11 (Qǔ Chí).
[Regional Anatomy]	The needle passes through the subcutaneous tissues and penetrates through the antebrachial fascia, m. extensor carpi radialis brevis and m. supinator, and arrives at the m. abductor pollicis longus.
[Acupuncture and Moxibustion]	Insert the needle perpendicularly 1.0~1.5 cun deep and stimulate until there is a sore and numbing sensation in the local area radiating to the hand. This point can be moxibusted.
[Indications]	Abdominal pain and distention, vomiting, swelling and pain of the hand, arm, shoulder and elbow and paralysis of the upper limb.

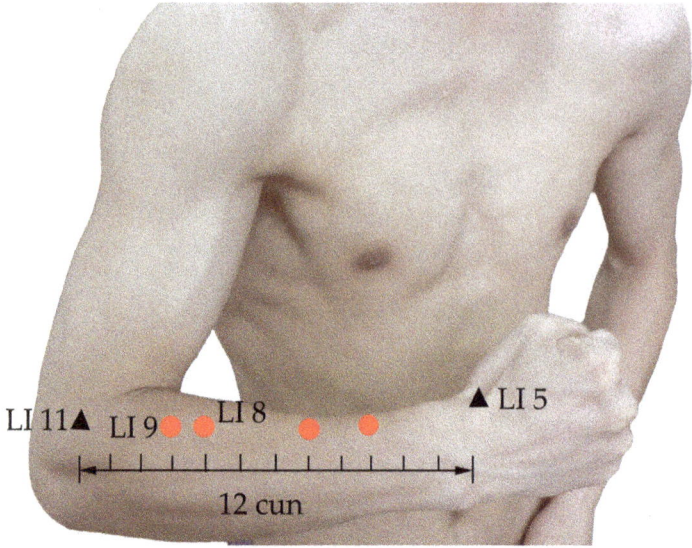

LI 11▲ LI 9 LI 8 ▲LI 5

12 cun

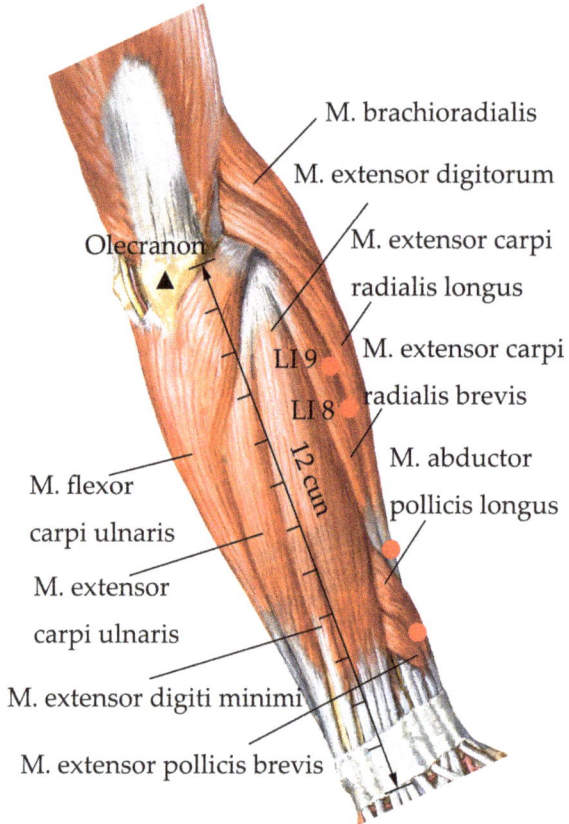

M. brachioradialis

M. extensor digitorum

Olecranon

M. extensor carpi
radialis longus

LI 9

M. extensor carpi

LI 8

radialis brevis

M. flexor

12 cun

M. abductor

carpi ulnaris

pollicis longus

M. extensor

carpi ulnaris

M. extensor digiti minimi

M. extensor pollicis brevis

LI 10 – Shǒu Sān Lǐ

[Locating]	The point is located when the elbow is flexed, 2 cun distal to the transverse cubital crease on the line connecting LI 5 (Yáng Xī) and LI 11 (Qǔ Chí).
[Regional Anatomy]	The needle passes through the subcutaneous tissues and antebrachial fascia, penetrates through the m. extensor carpi radialis longus and m. extensor carpi radialis brevis, and reaches the m. supinator.
[Acupuncture and Moxibustion]	Insert the needle perpendicularly 1~2 cun deep and stimulate until there is a sore, heavy and numbing sensation in the local area radiating to the dorsum of hand. This point can be moxibusted.
[Indications]	Abdominal pain and distention, vomiting, swelling and pain of the hand, arm, shoulder and elbow and paralysis of the upper limb.

LI 11 – Qǔ Chí

[Features]	He-sea point of the Large Intestine Channel of Hand *Yangming* .
[Locating]	In the depression of the radial side of the transverse cubital crease when elbow flexed.
[Regional Anatomy]	The needle passes through the subcutaneous tissues, enters the m. extensor carpi radialis longus and m. extensor carpi radialis brevis, reaches the m. brachioradialis, penetrates through the truncus n. radialis and reaches the m. brachialis.
[Acupuncture and Moxibustion]	Insert the needle perpendicularly 1.0~1.5 cun deep and stimulate until there is a sore and numbing sensation in the local area radiating to the shoulder or the fingers. This point can be moxibusted.
[Locating]	Swelling and pain of throat, fever, abdominal pain, vomiting, swelling of the arm redness, paralysis of the upper limb, pain and paralysis of the elbow and shoulder.

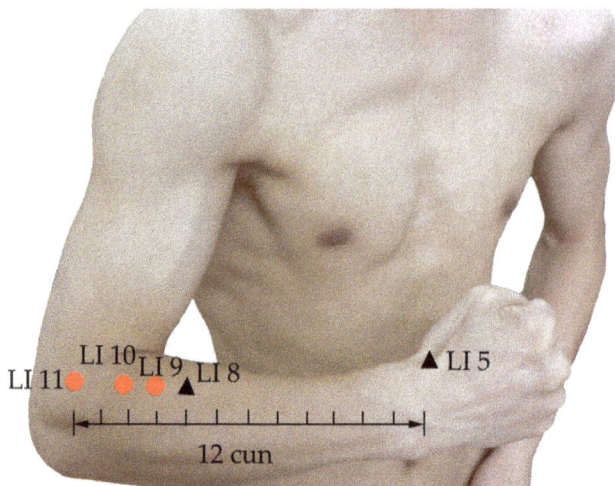

LI 11 LI 10 LI 9 LI 8

LI 5

12 cun

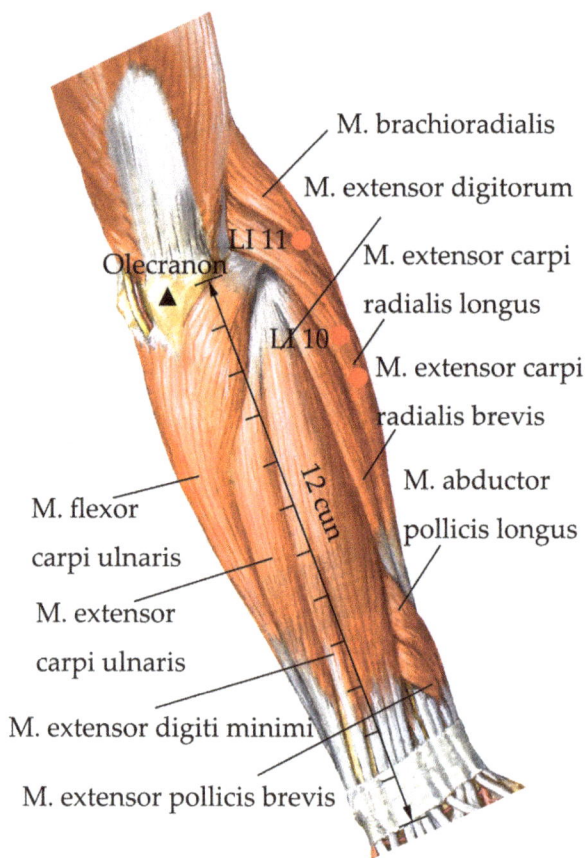

M. brachioradialis

M. extensor digitorum

LI 11

Olecranon

M. extensor carpi
radialis longus

LI 10

M. extensor carpi
radialis brevis

M. flexor
carpi ulnaris

12 cun

M. abductor
pollicis longus

M. extensor
carpi ulnaris

M. extensor digiti minimi

M. extensor pollicis brevis

LI 12 – Zhǒu Liáo

[Locating]	The point is located on the arm, proximal to the lateral epicondyle of the humerus, 1 cun supero-lateral to LI 11 (Qǔ Chí), on the medial side of the humerus triceps.
[Regional Anatomy]	The needle passes through the subcutaneous tissues and penetrates the m. brachioradialis and m. triceps brachii.
[Acupuncture and Moxibustion]	Insert the needle perpendicularly or obliquely 0.5~0.8 cun deep and stimulate until there is a sore and numbing sensation in the local area which radiates to the forearm or elbow. This point can be moxibusted.
[Locating]	Pain of the shoulder, elbow and arm and numbness and inflexibility of the upper limb.

LI 13 – Shǒu Wǔ Lǐ

[Locating]	The point is located when the elbow is flexed, 3 cun proximal to LI 11 (Qǔ Chí) on the line connecting LI 11 (Qǔ Chí) and LI 15 (Jiān Yú).
[Regional Anatomy]	The needle passes through the subcutaneous tissues and penetrates the m. brachialis.
[Acupuncture and Moxibustion]	Insert the needle perpendicularly 0.5~1 cun deep and stimulate until there is a sore and numbing sensation in the local area radiating to the shoulder or elbow. This point can be moxibusted.
[Locating]	Swelling and pain of the arm and paralysis of the upper limb.

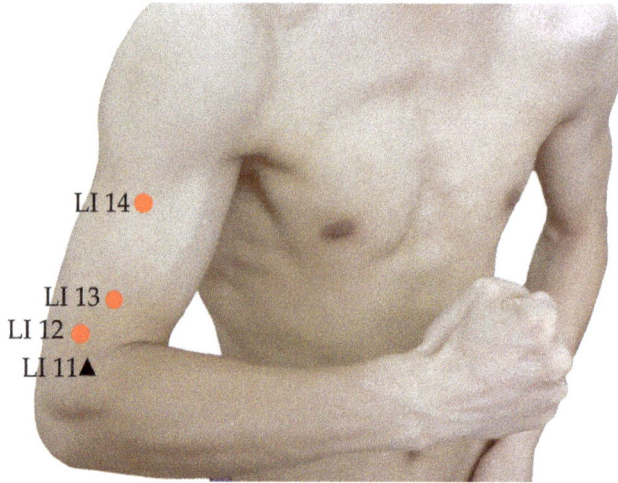

LI 14

LI 13
LI 12
LI 11▲

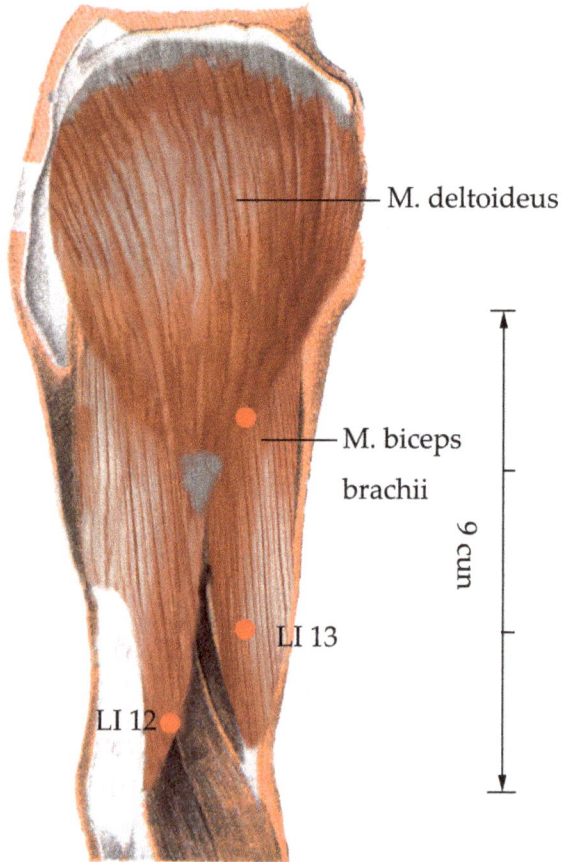

M. deltoideus

M. biceps
brachii

9 cun

LI 13

LI 12

LI 14 – Bì Nào

[Locating]	The point is located on the lateral aspect of the upper arm when the elbow is flexed and the arm is adducted, 7 cun proximal to LI 11 (Qǔ Chí) on the line connecting LI 11 (Qǔ Chí) and LI 15 (Jiān Yú), in the depression formed by the distal insertion of the m.deltoideus and m. brachialis.
[Regional Anatomy]	The needle passes through the skin and subcutaneous tissue and penetrates the midpoint of the m. deltoideus.
[Acupuncture and Moxibustion]	Insert the needle perpendicularly 0.5~1 cun deep and stimulate until there is a sore and numbing sensation in the local area radiating to the forearm; insert the needle obliquely upward 1~2 cun deep and stimulate until there is a sore or numbing sensation radiating to the tricorner muscle and the shoulder.
	This point can be moxibusted.
[Indications]	Pain and redness of the eyes, blurred vision, shoulder and arm pain, paralysis of upper limb, and rigidity of the neck.

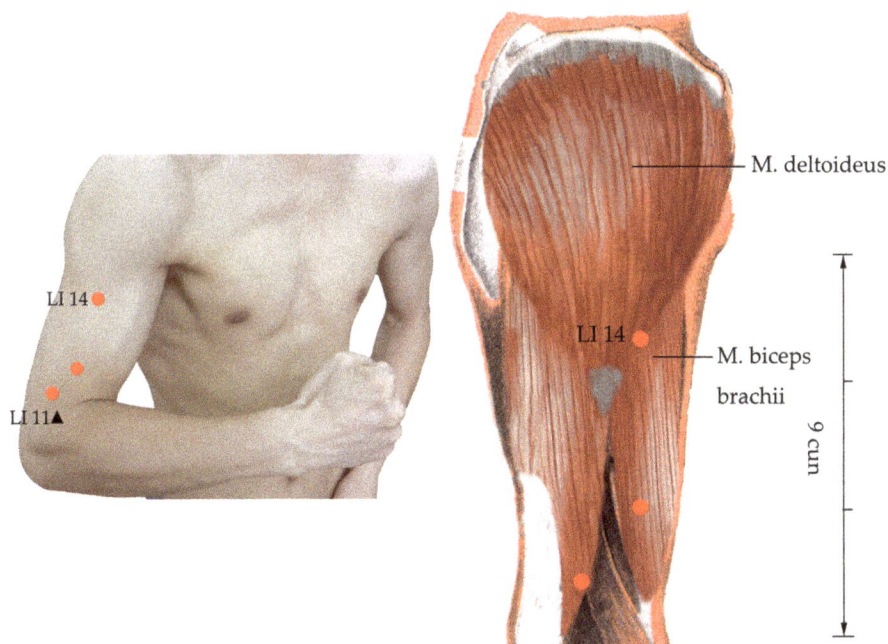

LI 14

LI 11

M. deltoideus

LI 14

M. biceps brachii

9 cun

LI 15 – Jiān Yú

[Locating]	In the anterior and inferior aspect of the acromion, in the depression between the acromion and the greater tubercle of the humerus.
[Regional Anatomy]	The needle passes through the subcutaneous tissues and deeply towards HT 1 (Jí Quán) and reaches the plexus brachialis.
[Acupuncture and Moxibustion]	Insert the needle perpendicularly 1~1.5 cun deep and stimulate until there is a sore and distending sensation around the shoulder. This point can be moxibusted.
[Indications]	Pain of the shoulder and arm, spasm of the arm and hand and hemiplegia.

LI 16 – Jù Gǔ

[Locating]	The point is located in the sitting position when the arm is adducted, on the posterior border of the acromioclavicular joint at the depression between the clavicle and the scapular spine.
[Regional Anatomy]	The needle penetrates the skin, subcutaneous tissue and the m. trapezius, and reaches the m. supraspinatus.
[Acupuncture and Moxibustion]	Insert the needle perpendicularly 0.4~0.6 cun deep and stimulate until there is a sore and distending sensation around the shoulder joint radiating to the clavicle or scapular bone. This point can be moxibusted.
[Indications]	Pain of the arm and the shoulder, spasm of the hand and arm and hemiplegia.

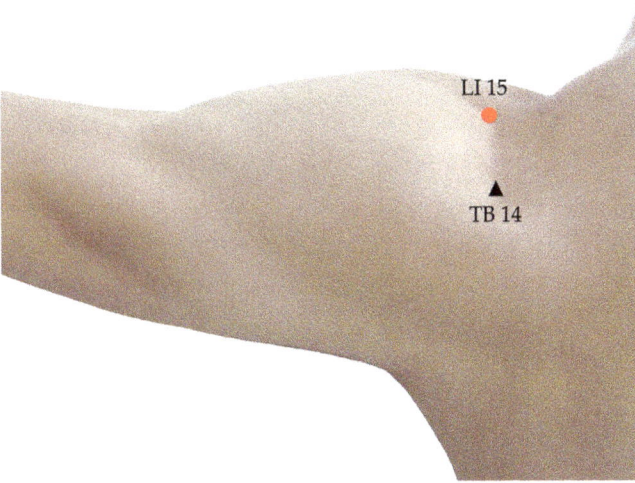

LI 15

TB 14

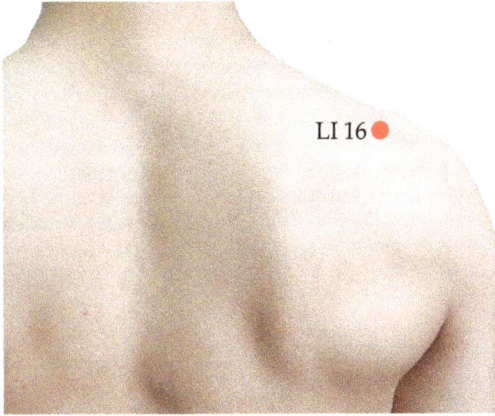

LI 16

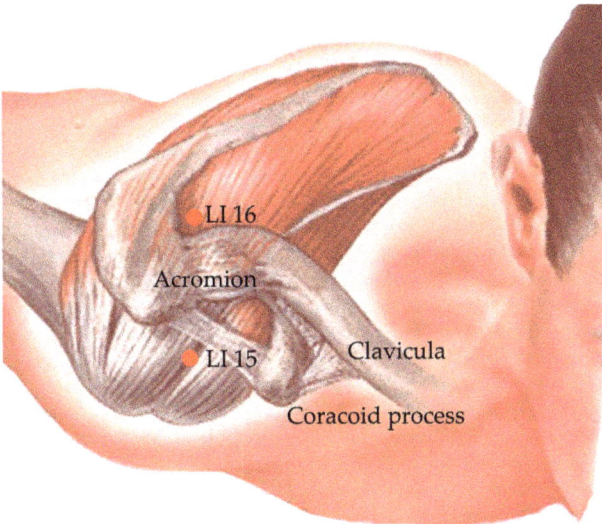

LI 16

Acromion

LI 15

Clavicula

Coracoid process

LI 17 – Tiān Dǐng

[Locating]	The point is located in the sitting position while looking forward, on the posterior aspect of m. sternocleidomastoideus, 3 cun lateral to the laryngeal prominence and 1 cun inferior to LI 18 (Fú Tū).
[Regional Anatomy]	The needle passes through the skin, subcutaneous tissue, the posterior border of m. sternocleidomastoideus, and reaches the root of the plexus brachialis.
[Acupuncture and Moxibustion]	Insert the needle perpendicularly 0.3~0.5 cun deep and stimulate until there is a sore and numbing sensation in the local area radiating to the throat. This point can be moxibusted.
[Indications]	Cough, asthma, sore throat and sudden loss of voice.

LI 18 – Fú Tū

[Locating]	The point is located in the sitting position, 3 cun lateral to RN 23 (Lián Quán), between the anterior and posterior border of the m. sternocleidomastoideus.
[Regional Anatomy]	The needle passes through the skin, subcutaneous tissue, and the posterior border of m. sternocleidomastoideus. It then reaches the medial side of enters the vagina carotica.
[Acupuncture and Moxibustion]	Insert the needle perpendicularly 0.5~0.8 cun and stimulate until there is a sore and numbing sensation in the local area radiating to the throat. This point can be moxibusted.
[Indications]	Cough, asthma, sore throat, phlegm sensation in the throat and sudden loss of voice.

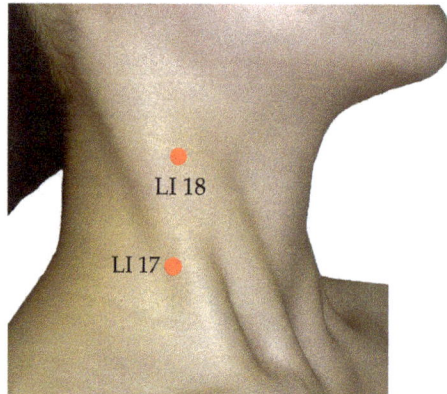

LI 18

LI 17

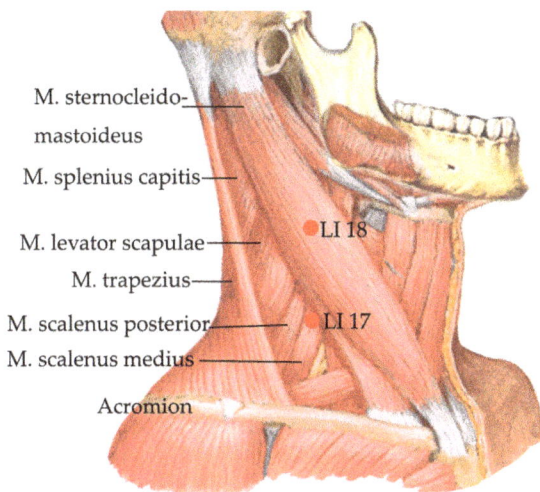

M. sternocleido-mastoideus

M. splenius capitis

M. levator scapulae

M. trapezius

M. scalenus posterior

M. scalenus medius

LI 18

LI 17

Acromion

LI 19 – Kŏu Hé Liáo

[Locating]	The point is located in the sitting or supine position, 0.5 cun lateral to the exterior part of the nostril, at the level with DU 26 (Shuĭ Gōu).
[Regional Anatomy]	The needle passes through the subcutaneous tissues and penetrates into the m. orbicularis oris.
[Acupuncture and Moxibustion]	Insert the needle perpendicularly 0.3~0.5 cun deep and stimulate until there is a local sore or distending sensation. Moxibustion is prohibited.
[Indications]	Nasal obstruction, epistaxis and dry mouth.

LI 20 – Yíng Xiāng

[Locating]	The point is located in the sitting or supine position, at the middle point of the lateral side of the nostril in the nasolabial groove.
[Regional Anatomy]	The needle passes through the skin, subcutaneous fascia and reaches the m. levator labii superioris.
[Acupuncture and Moxibustion]	Insert the needle horizontally towards Bí Tōng EX-HN8 0.5~1.0 cun deep and stimulate until there is a sore and numbing sensation in local area and radiating to the nasal area. This point is not suitable for moxibustion.
[Indications]	Nasal obstruction, hyposmia, epistaxis and rhinorrhea.

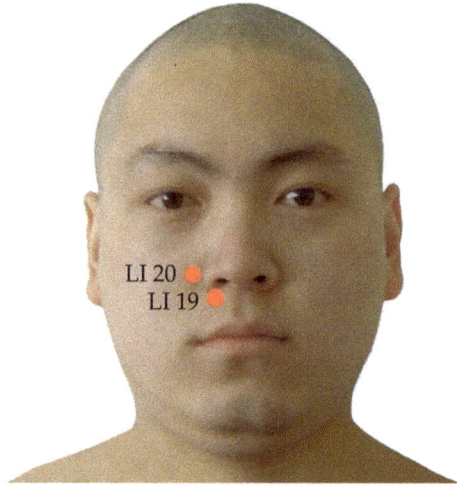

LI 20
LI 19

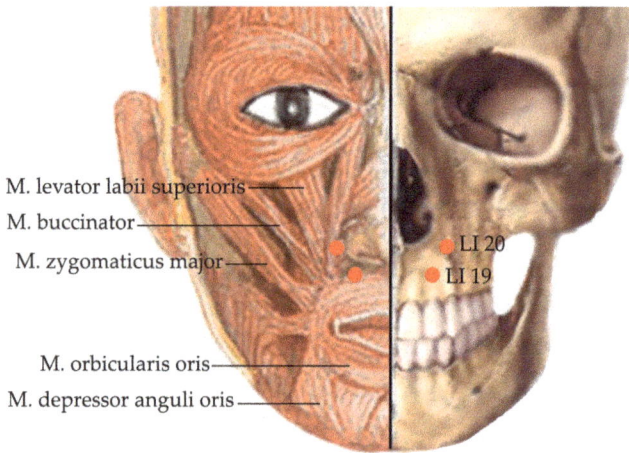

M. levator labii superioris
M. buccinator
M. zygomaticus major

LI 20
LI 19

M. orbicularis oris
M. depressor anguli oris

CHAPTER 4

Stomach Channel of Foot Yangming; ST

There are forty-five points on the Stomach Channel of the Foot *Yangming* and ninety in total including both sides. There are four points on the neck and the shoulder, fifteen points are distributed on the lateral anterior side of the lower limb, twenty-six points are distributed on the abdomen, chest and the head. The first point is ST 1 (Chéng Qì) and the last is ST 45 (Lì Duì). The indications of this channel are the diseases of the eyes, ears, mouth, teeth, nose, throat, stomach, intestines, abdomen, etc. as well as the syndromes along the course of the channel.

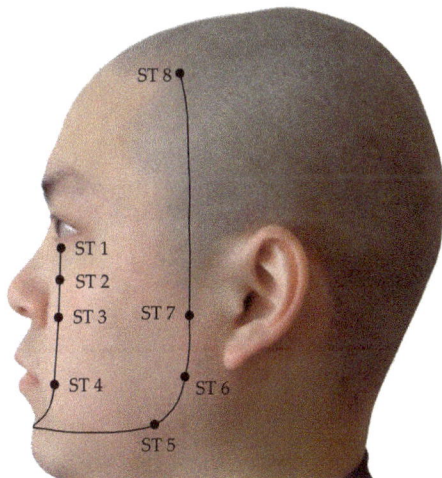

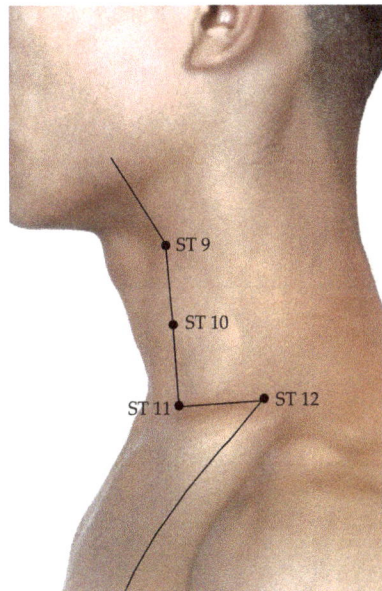

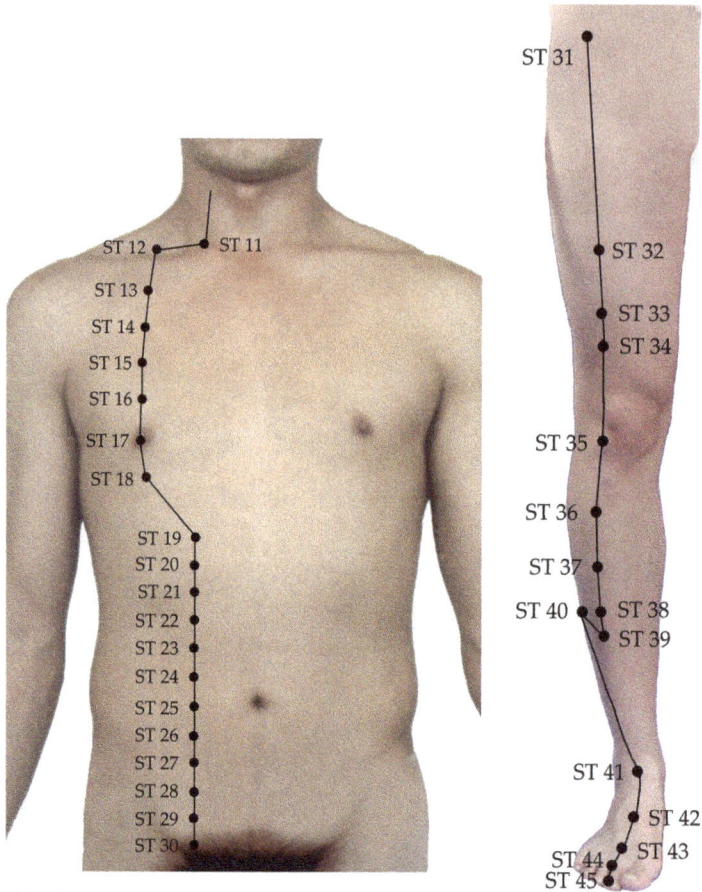

ST 31
ST 12 • • ST 11
ST 13
ST 14
ST 15
ST 16
ST 17
ST 18
ST 19
ST 20
ST 21
ST 22
ST 23
ST 24
ST 25
ST 26
ST 27
ST 28
ST 29
ST 30
ST 32
ST 33
ST 34
ST 35
ST 36
ST 37
ST 40 • • ST 38
ST 39
ST 41
ST 42
ST 44 • ST 43
ST 45

ST 1 – Chéng Qì

[Locating]	On the face, directly inferior to the pupil while looking forward, between the eyeball and the infraorbital margin.
[Regional Anatomy]	The needle passes through the subcutaneous tissues and m. tarsalis inferior and enters the m. oblique inferior and m. rectus inferior.
[Acupuncture and Moxibustion]	Push the eyeball upwards and hold with the left thumb. Insert the needle, slowly, perpendicularly 0.5~0.8 cun deep along the infraorbital ridge. Avoid manipulating the needle with large amplitude. Moxibustion is prohibited.
[Indications]	Acute or chronic conjunctivitis,, inflammation of the eyelid, cornea inflammation, optic nerve inflammation, optic nerve atrophy and infraorbital neuralgia.

ST 2 – Sì Bái

[Locating]	On the face, inferior to the pupil in the depression of the infraorbital foramen.
[Regional Anatomy]	The needle passes through the subcutaneous tissues and penetrates the posterior structure of the infraorbital wall.
[Acupuncture and Moxibustion]	Insert the needle perpendicularly 0.5~0.8 cun deep until there is soreness and a numbness sensation in the local area. This point is not suitable for moxibustion.
[Indications]	Pain, redness and itching of the eyes, lacrimation, facial paralysis, spasm of the facial muscle, myopia and pain of the head and face.

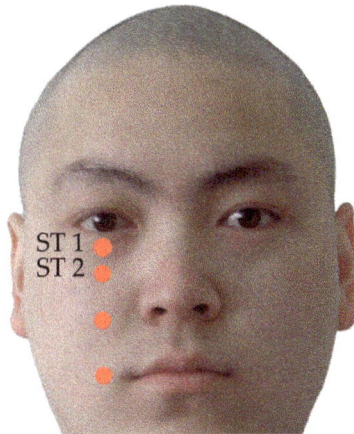

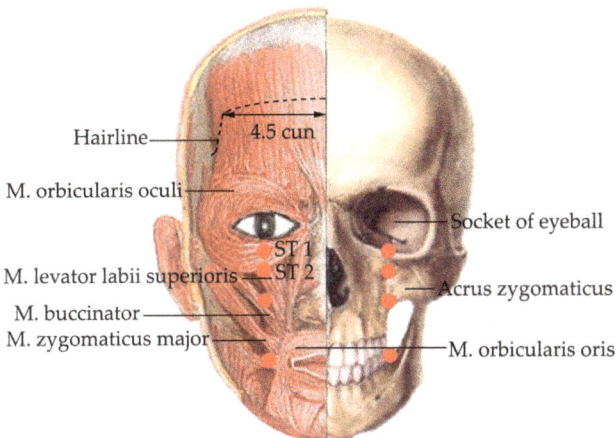

ST 3 – Jù Liáo

[Locating]	On the face, inferior to the pupil at the level with the inferior boarder of the nostril, on the outside of the nasolabial fold.
[Regional Anatomy]	The needle passes through the subcutaneous tissues and penetrates into the m. levator labii superioris and m. levator anguli oris from the lateral side of the facial artery and superficial facial vein.
[Acupuncture and Moxibustion]	Insert the needle perpendicularly 0.3~0.6 cun deep and stimulate until there is a sore and numbing sensation in the local area. This point can be moxibusted.
[Indications]	Facial paralysis, spasm of the facial muscle, myopia, epistaxis and toothache.

ST 4 – Dì Cāng

[Locating]	The point is located in the sitting or supine position while looking forward, the point is directly inferior to the pupil at the level of the corner of the mouth.
[Regional Anatomy]	The needle passes through the subcutaneous tissues, penetrates between m. risorius and m. buccinator and enters the masseter.
[Acupuncture and Moxibustion]	① Insert the needle perpendicularly 0.2 cun deep and stimulate until there is a sore and numbing sensation in the local area radiating to the lateral aspect of the face. ② Insert the needle subcutaneously 1.0~2.5 cun deep towards ST 6 (Jiáchē) and stimulate until there is a sore and numbing sensation in the local area radiating to the lateral aspect of the face to treat facial paralysis. This point can be moxibusted.
[Indications]	Facial paralysis, spasm of the facial muscle, trifacial neuralgia, Cheilitis and drooling.

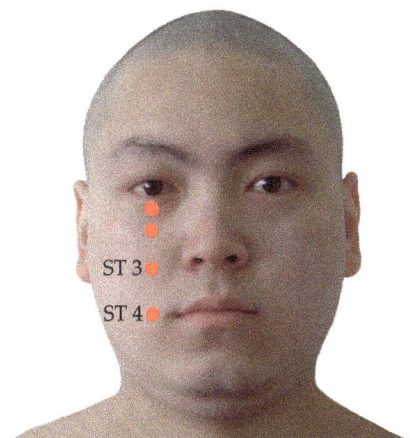

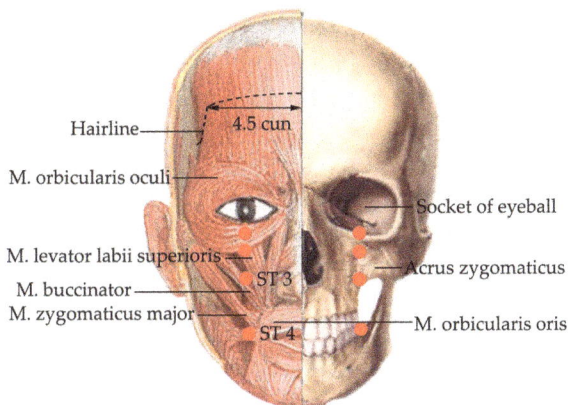

Hairline
4.5 cun
M. orbicularis oculi
Socket of eyeball
M. levator labii superioris
Acrus zygomaticus
M. buccinator
ST3
M. zygomaticus major
ST4
M. orbicularis oris

ST 5 – Dà Yíng

[Locating]	On the lateral side of the face, 1.3 cun anterior and inferior to the corner of the jaw, on the anterior part of the masseter muscle where the pulse of the facial artery can be felt.
[Regional Anatomy]	The needle passes through the subcutaneous tissues, penetrates m. depressor anguli oris, and reaches the anterior border of masseter.
[Acupuncture and Moxibustion]	Insert the needle perpendicularly 0.2~0.5 cun deep and stimulate until there is a sore and numbing sensation in the local area radiating to the lateral aspect of the face. This point can be moxibusted.
[Indications]	Facial paralysis, spasm of the facial muscle and myopia.

ST 6 – Jiá Chē

[Locating]	On the cheek, in the depression one finger-breadth anterior and superior to the corner of the mandible, on the prominence of the muscle when the teeth are clenched.
[Regional Anatomy]	The needle passes through the subcutaneous tissues, penetrates the deep fascia of masseter and enters the masseter.
[Acupuncture and Moxibustion]	Insert the needle perpendicularly 0.5~0.8 cun deep and stimulate until there is a sore and numbing sensation in the local area radiating to the cheek. This point can be moxibusted.
[Indications]	Deviation of the eye, lockjaw, swelling of the cheek, toothache, loss of voice and neck stiffness.

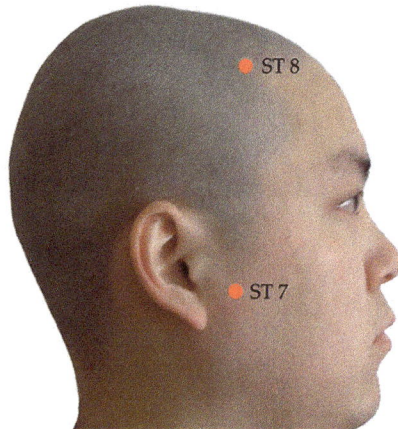

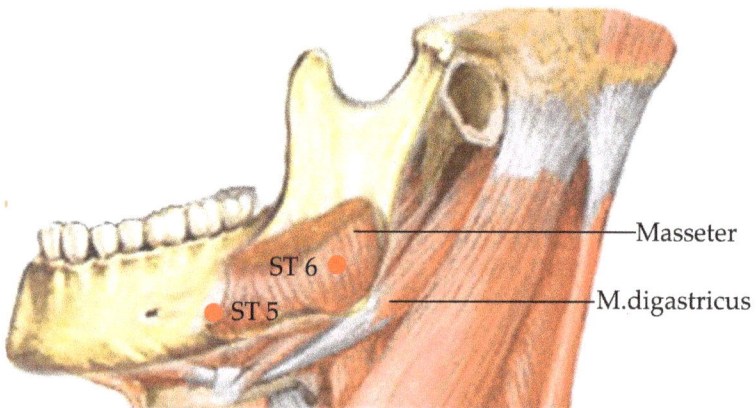

ST 7 – Xià Guān

[Locating]	The point is located in the sitting or recumbent position, on the inferior border of the zygomatic arch, anterior to the condyloid process of the mandible when the mouth is open.
[Regional Anatomy]	The needle passes through the posterior aspect of the parotid, penetrates the tendo m. temporalis, and enters infratemporal fossa.
[Acupuncture and Moxibustion]	Insert the needle perpendicularly 0.3~0.5 cun deep until there is a sore sensation radiating to the auricular region. This point can be moxibusted.
[Indications]	Deviation of the eye and mouth, pain in the cheek, toothache, tremors of the mouth, deafness, tinnitus and dizziness.

ST 8 – Tóu Wéi

[Locating]	On the head, 0.5 cun inside the anterior hairline above the temples and 4.5 cun from the midline.
[Regional Anatomy]	The needle passes through the subcutaneous tissues and enters the m. temporalis.
[Acupuncture and Moxibustion]	Insert the needle subcutaneously towards the back of the head 0.5~1.0 cun deep until there is a sore or distending sensation in the local area. This point can be moxibusted.
[Indications]	Headache, migraine, blurred vision, eye ache, lacrimation and drooping of the eyelid.

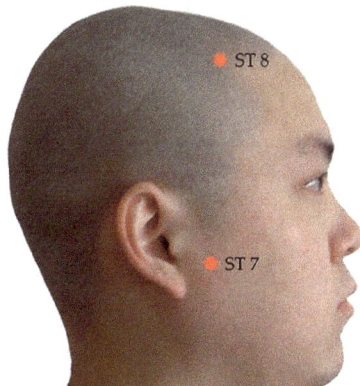

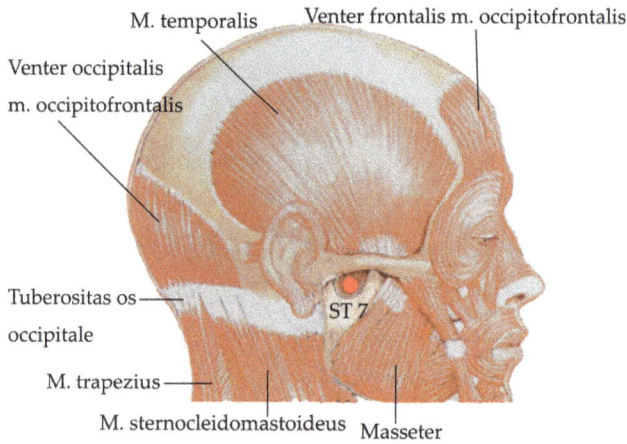

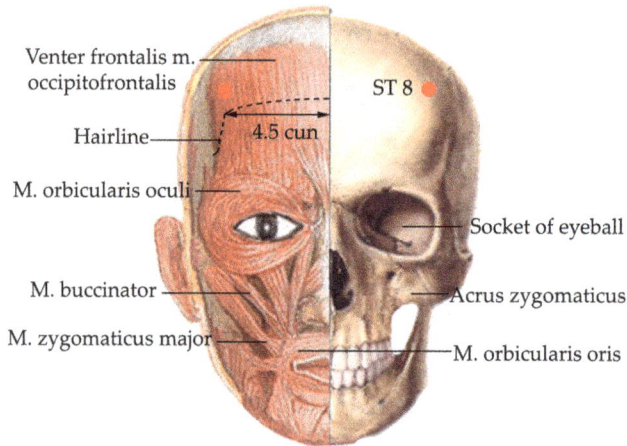

Venter occipitalis
m. occipitofrontalis

M. temporalis

Venter frontalis m. occipitofrontalis

Tuberositas os occipitale

ST 7

M. trapezius

M. sternocleidomastoideus

Masseter

Venter frontalis m. occipitofrontalis

ST 8

Hairline

4.5 cun

M. orbicularis oculi

Socket of eyeball

M. buccinator

Acrus zygomaticus

M. zygomaticus major

M. orbicularis oris

ST 9 – Rén Yíng

[Locating]	On the neck, at the level of the Adam's apple, on the anterior aspect of the sternocleidomastoid muscle.
[Regional Anatomy]	The needle passes through the anterior border of m. sternocleidomastoideus, enters the carotid triangle.
[Acupuncture and Moxibustion]	Insert the needle perpendicularly 0.2~0.4 cun deep and stimulate until there is a sore and numbing sensation in the local area radiating to the shoulder. This point can be moxibusted.
[Indications]	Chest distention, sore throat, hypertension.
[Note]	Avoid puncturing the artery.

ST 10 – Shuǐ Tū

[Locating]	On the neck, on the anterior aspect of the sterno-cleidomastoid muscle, at the midpoint between ST 9 (Rén Yíng) and ST 11 (Qì Shè).
[Regional Anatomy]	The needle passes through the superficial layer of deep fasciae, enters m. sternohyoideus and m. sternothyroideus, and penetrates the thyroid gland.
[Acupuncture and Moxibustion]	Insert the needle perpendicularly 0.3~0.4 cun deep and stimulate until there is a sore and numbing sensation in the local area. This point can be moxibusted.
[Indications]	Cough, sore throat, and asthma.

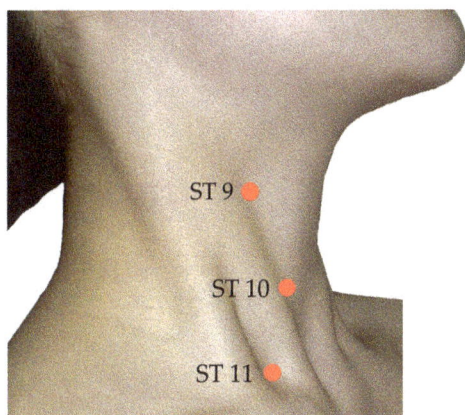

ST 9

ST 10

ST 11

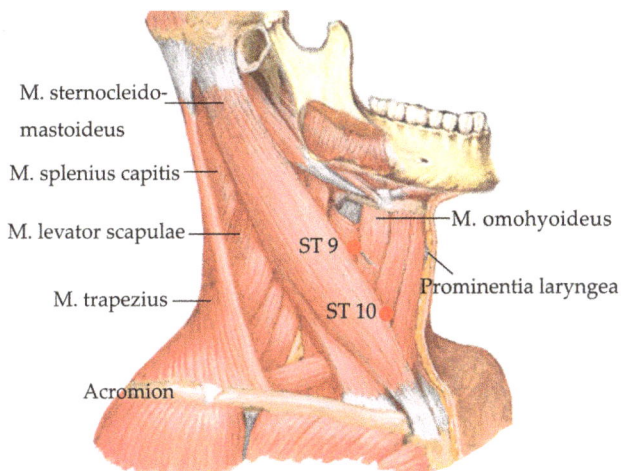

M. sternocleido-mastoideus

M. splenius capitis

M. levator scapulae

M. trapezius

Acromion

M. omohyoideus

ST 9

Prominentia laryngea

ST 10

ST 11 – Qì Shè

[Locating]	On the superior aspect of the internal end of clavicle of the neck, between the sternal end and clavicle end of the m. sternocleidomastoideus.
[Regional Anatomy]	The needle penetrates the space between the sternal and clavicular ends of m. sternocleidomastoideus.
[Acupuncture and Moxibustion]	Insert the point perpendicularly 0.3~0.5 cun deep and stimulate until there is a sore and numbing sensation in the local area. This point can be moxibusted.
[Indications]	Cough and sore throat.

ST 12 – Quē Pén

[Locating]	The point is located in the sitting position while looking upwards, in the centre of the supraclavicular fossae, 4 cun lateral to the anterior midline.
[Regional Anatomy]	The needle passes through the subcutaneous tissues and penetrates the anterior tracheal fascia.
[Acupuncture and Moxibustion]	Insert the needle perpendicularly 0.3~0.5 cun deep and stimulate until there is a sore and numbing sensation in the local area radiating to the upper arm. This point can be moxibusted.
[Indications]	Cough, sore throat and shoulder pain.

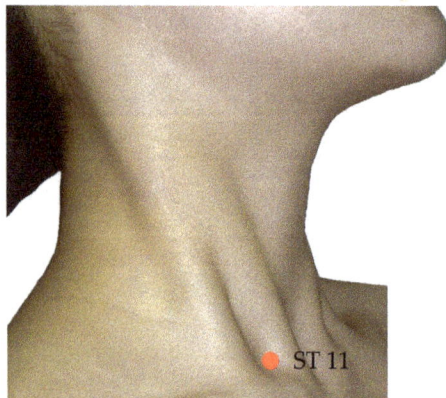

ST 11

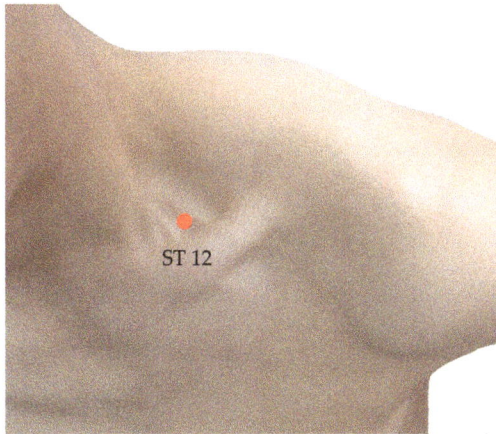

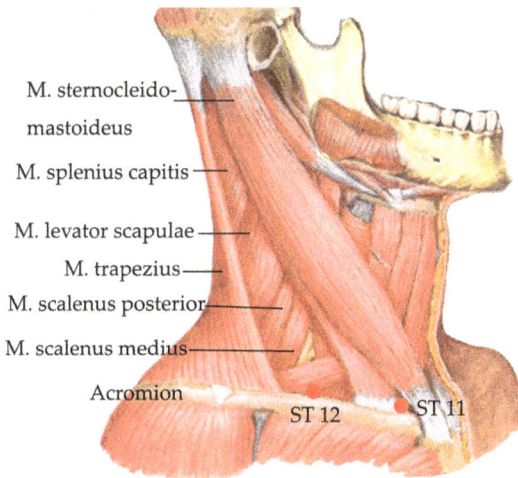

ST 12

M. sternocleido-
mastoideus

M. splenius capitis

M. levator scapulae

M. trapezius

M. scalenus posterior

M. scalenus medius

Acromion

ST 12   ST 11

ST 13 – Qì Hù

[Locating]	On the inferior boarder of middle point of clavicle of the chest, 4 cun lateral to the anterior midline.
[Regional Anatomy]	The needle passes through the subcutaneous tissues and penetrates the clavicular end of m. pectoralis major and m. subclavius.
[Acupuncture and Moxibustion]	Insert the needle obliquely or subcutaneously 0.5~0.8 cun deep and stimulate until there is a sore and numbing sensation in the local area but avoid lifting and pulling the needle. This point can be moxibusted.
[Indications]	Cough, sore throat and asthma.
[Note]	Avoid deep insertion to prevent pneumothorax.

ST 14 – Kù Fáng

[Locating]	The point is located in the supine position, in the first intercostal space, directly above the mamilla.
[Regional Anatomy]	The needle passes through the subcutaneous tissues and enters the m. intercostales externi and m. intercostales interni within in the 1st intercostal space.
[Acupuncture and Moxibustion]	Insert the needle obliquely 0.5~0.8 cun deep and stimulate until there is a sore and numbing sensation in the local area. This point can be moxibusted.
[Indications]	Chest congestion, cough and asthma.

ST 15 – Wū Yì

[Locating]	The point is located in the supine position, on the chest, in the second intercostal space, directly above the mamilla.
[Regional Anatomy]	The needle passes through the subcutaneous tissues and penetrates the m. intercostales externi and m. intercostales interni.
[Acupuncture and Moxibustion]	Insert the needle obliquely 0.5~0.8 cun deep and stimulate until there is a sore and numbing sensation in the local area. This point can be moxibusted.
[Indications]	Mastitis, cough, and asthma.

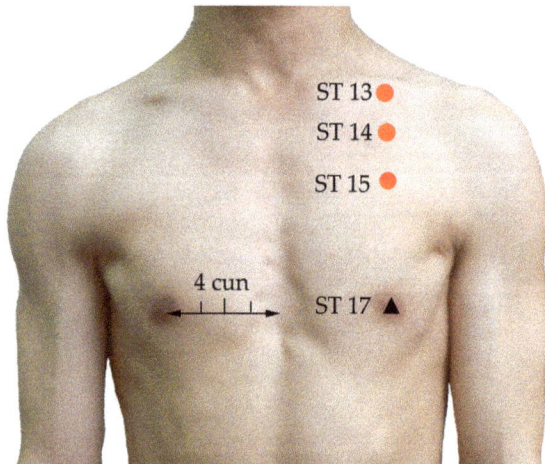

ST 13
ST 14
ST 15

4 cun

ST 17

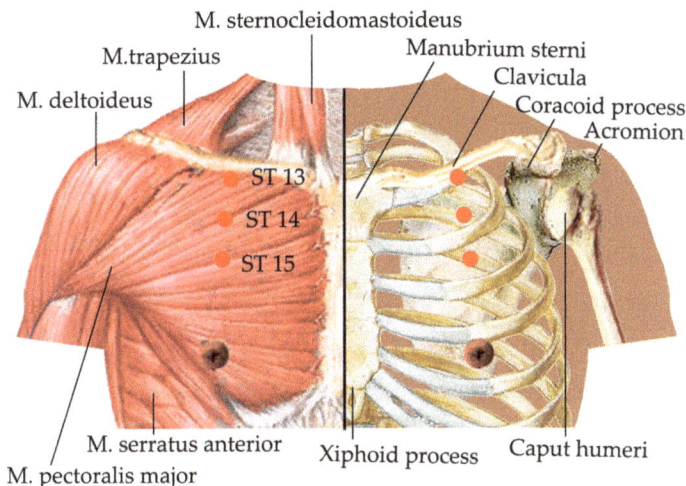

M. sternocleidomastoideus
M.trapezius
M. deltoideus
Manubrium sterni
Clavicula
Coracoid process
Acromion

ST 13
ST 14
ST 15

M. serratus anterior
M. pectoralis major
Xiphoid process
Caput humeri

ST 16 – Yīng Chuāng

[Locating]	The point is located in the supine position, on the chest in the third intercostal space, one costal space above the mamilla.
[Regional Anatomy]	The needle passes through the subcutaneous tissues and penetrates m. pectoralis major, and enters m. pectoralis minor.
[Acupuncture and Moxibustion]	Insert the needle obliquely 0.5~0.8 cun deep and stimulate until there is a sore and numbing sensation in the local area. This point can be moxibusted.
[Indications]	Cough and asthma .

ST 17 – Rǔ Zhōng

[Locating]	The point is located in the supine position, on the chest, in the fourth intercostal space.
[Regional Anatomy]	Muscular: M. pectoralis major. Gland: Mammary gland. Innervations: Supraclavicular nerve, the anterior cutaneous branches of the 3rd, 4th and 5th intercostal nerves.
[Acupuncture and Moxibustion]	Acupuncture is prohibited. Moxibustion is prohibited.
[Note]	This point is mostly used as a landmark for the location of other points.

ST 18 – Rǔ Gēn

[Locating]	The point is located in the supine position, on the chest, in the fifth intercostal space, 4 cun from the midline, inferior to the mamilla.
[Regional Anatomy]	The needle passes through the subcutaneous tissues and penetrates m. pectoralis major and m. obliquus externus abdominis.
[Acupuncture and Moxibustion]	Insert the needle obliquely outward or upward 0.5~0.8 cun deep and stimulate until there is a sore and numbing sensation in the local area radiating to the breast.
	This point can be moxibusted.
[Indications]	Chest pain, chest distention, cough and cardiac spasm.

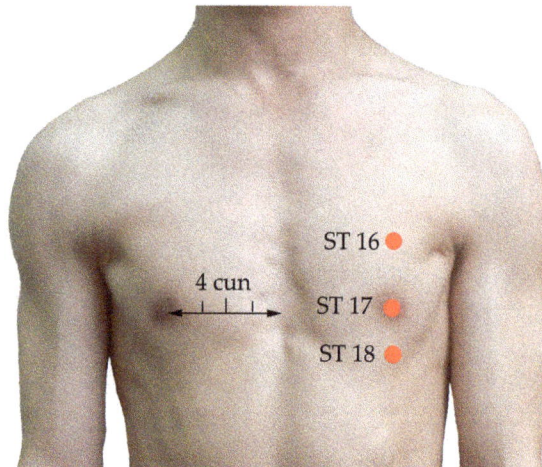

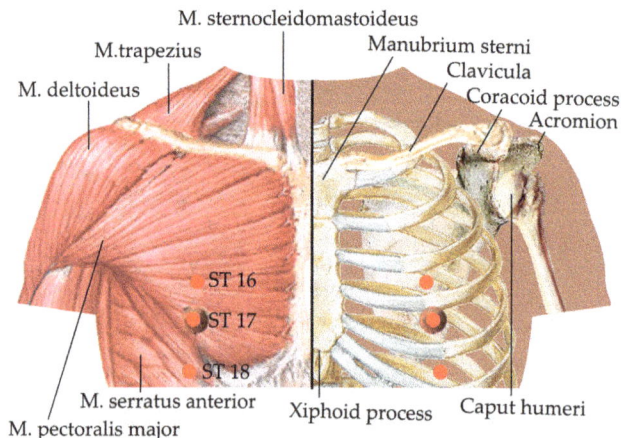

4 cun

ST 16
ST 17
ST 18

M. sternocleidomastoideus
M.trapezius
Manubrium sterni
M. deltoideus
Clavicula
Coracoid process
Acromion

ST 16
ST 17
ST 18

M. serratus anterior
M. pectoralis major
Xiphoid process
Caput humeri

ST 19 – Bù Róng

[Locating]	On the upper abdomen, 6 cun superior to the umbilicus and 2 cun lateral to the anterior midline.
[Regional Anatomy]	The needle passes through the subcutaneous tissues and enters m. rectus abdominis or endothoracic fascia.
[Acupuncture and Moxibustion]	Insert the needle perpendicularly 0.5~0.8 cun deep and stimulate until there is a sore and numbing sensation in the local area. This point can be moxibusted.
[Indications]	Abdominal distention, stomach ache, vomiting, anorexia and hematemesis.
[Note]	Avoid deep insertion to prevent puncturing the liver and stomach.

ST 20 – Chéng Mǎn

[Locating]	On the upper abdomen, 5 cun superior to the umbilicus, 2 cun lateral to the anterior midline.
[Regional Anatomy]	The needle passes through the subcutaneous tissues, penetrates the anterior layer of sheath of m. rectus abdominis, and enters m. rectus abdominis.
[Acupuncture and Moxibustion]	Insert the needle perpendicularly 0.5~0.8 cun deep and stimulate until there is a heavy and distending sensation in the upper abdomen. This point can be moxibusted.
[Indications]	Stomach ache, vomiting.
[Note]	Avoid deep insertion to prevent puncturing the liver and stomach.

ST 21 – Liáng Mén

[Locating]	On the upper abdomen, 4 cun superior to umbilicus, 2 cun lateral to the anterior midline.
[Regional Anatomy]	The needle passes through the subcutaneous tissues and penetrates the posterior layer of sheath of m. rectus abdominis and m. rectus abdominis.
[Acupuncture and Moxibustion]	Insert the needle perpendicularly 0.5~1.0 cun deep and stimulate until there is a sore and numbing sensation in the local area. This point can be moxibusted.
[Indications]	Stomach ache, vomiting.

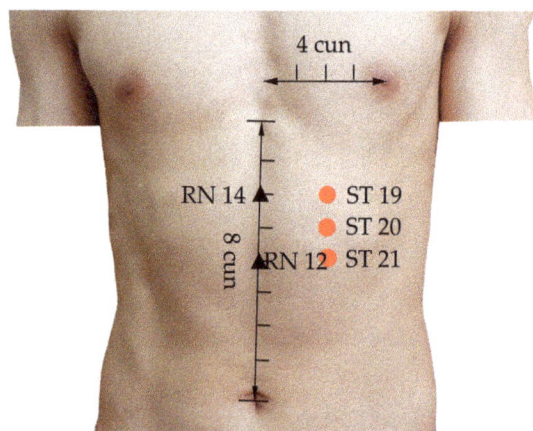

4 cun

RN 14   ● ST 19
         ● ST 20
8 cun RN 12 ● ST 21

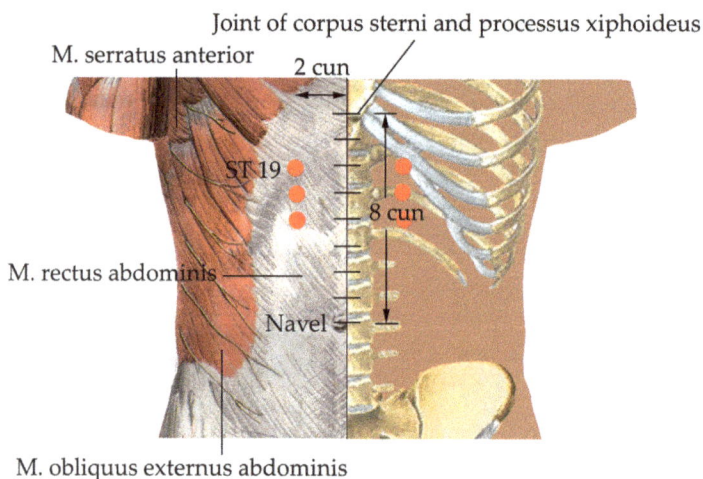

Joint of corpus sterni and processus xiphoideus

M. serratus anterior   2 cun

ST 19

8 cun

M. rectus abdominis

Navel

M. obliquus externus abdominis

ST 22 – Guān Mén

[Locating]	On the upper abdomen, 3 cun superior to the umbilicus, 2 cun lateral to the anterior midline.
[Regional Anatomy]	The needle passes through the subcutaneous tissues and penetrates the posterior layer of sheath of m. rectus abdominis and m. rectus abdominis.
[Acupuncture and Moxibustion]	Insert the needle perpendicularly 1.0~1.5 cun deep and stimulate until there is a heavy and distending sensation in the local area. This point can be moxibusted.
[Indications]	Stomach ache, vomiting, abdominal distention, borborygums, anorexia and hematemesis.

ST 23 – Tài Yĭ

[Locating]	On the upper abdomen, 2 cun superior to the umbilicus, 2 cun lateral to the anterior midline.
[Regional Anatomy]	The needle passes through the subcutaneous tissues and penetrates the posterior layer of sheath of m. rectus abdominis and m. rectus abdominis.
[Acupuncture and Moxibustion]	Insert the needle perpendicularly 1.0~1.5 cun deep and stimulate until there is a sore, heavy and numbing sensation in the local area. This point can be moxibusted.
[Indications]	Stomach ache, vomiting, abdominal distention, borborygums, anorexia and hematemesis.

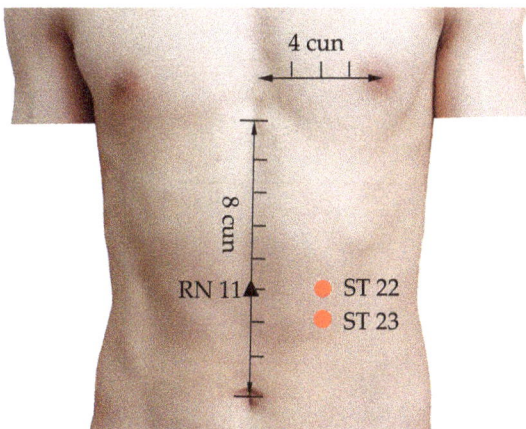

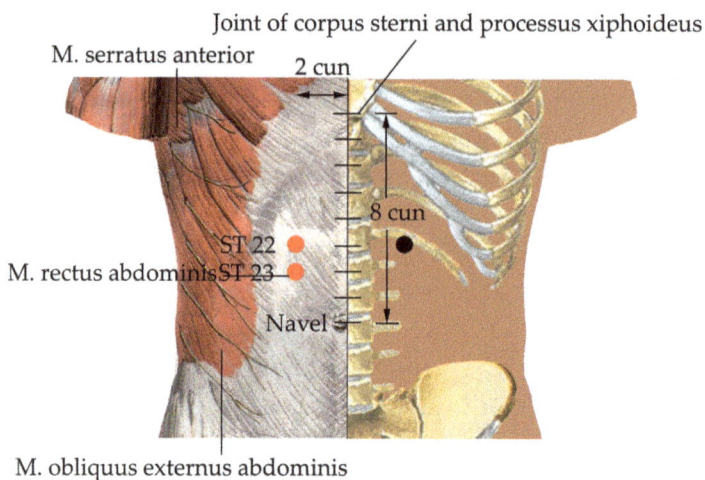

Joint of corpus sterni and processus xiphoideus

M. serratus anterior

2 cun

8 cun

ST 22

M. rectus abdominis ST 23

Navel

M. obliquus externus abdominis

ST 24 – Huá Ròu Mén

[Locating]	On the upper abdomen, 1 cun superior to the umbilicus, 2 cun lateral to the anterior midline.
[Regional Anatomy]	The needle passes through the subcutaneous tissues and penetrates the posterior layer of sheath of m. rectus abdominis and m. rectus abdominis.
[Acupuncture and Moxibustion]	Insert the needle perpendicularly 1.0~1.5 cun deep and stimulate until there is a sore and numbing sensation in the local area radiating downward. This point can be moxibusted.
[Indications]	Stomach ache, vomiting, abdominal distention, borborygmus, anorexia, hydroperitonia and hematemesis.

ST 25 – Tiān Shū

[Features]	Front-mu point of the Large Intestine Channel of the Hand *Yangming*.
[Locating]	The point is located in the supine position, on the abdomen, 2 cun lateral to the umbilicus.
[Regional Anatomy]	The needle passes through the subcutaneous tissues and penetrates the posterior layer of sheath of m. rectus abdominis and m. rectus abdominis.

[Acupuncture and Moxibustion]	Insert the needle perpendicularly 1.0~1.5 cun deep and stimulate until there is a sore and numbing sensation in the local area. This point can be moxibusted.
[Indications]	Vomiting, hematemesis, abdominal distention, borborygums, pain around the umbilicus, dysentery, constipation and hernia.

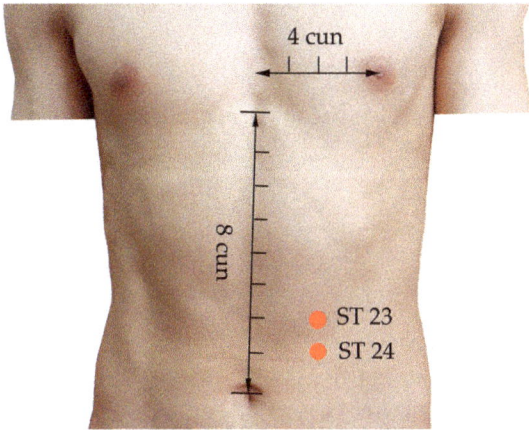

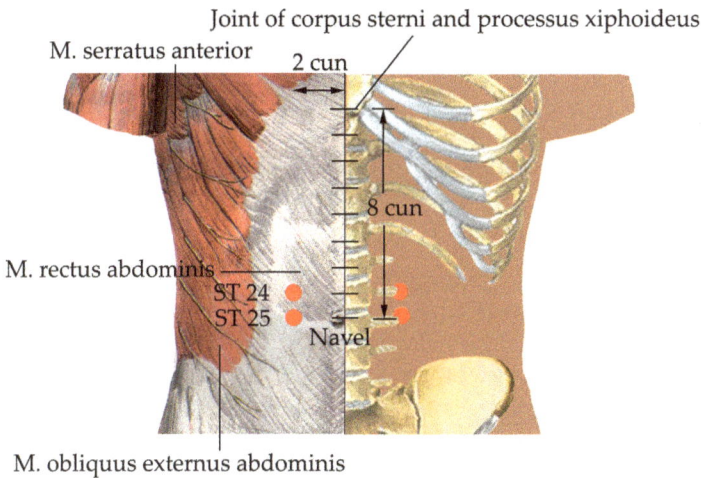

4 cun

8 cun

ST 23
ST 24

Joint of corpus sterni and processus xiphoideus

M. serratus anterior   2 cun

8 cun

M. rectus abdominis

ST 24
ST 25

Navel

M. obliquus externus abdominis

ST 26 – Wài Líng

[Locating]	On the lower abdomen, 1 cun inferior to the umbilicus, 2 cun lateral to the anterior midline.
[Regional Anatomy]	The needle passes through the subcutaneous tissues and penetrates the posterior layer of sheath of m. rectus abdominis and m. rectus abdominis.
[Acupuncture and Moxibustion]	Insert the needle perpendicularly 1.0~1.5 cun deep and stimulate until there is a sore and numbing sensation in the local area. This point can be moxibusted.
[Indications]	Stomach ache, abdominal pain, abdominal distention, hernia and dysmenorrhea.

ST 27 – Dà Jù

[Locating]	On the lower abdomen, 2 cun inferior to the umbilicus, 2 cun lateral to the anterior midline.
[Regional Anatomy]	The needle passes through the subcutaneous tissues and penetrates the posterior layer of sheath of m. rectus abdominis and m. rectus abdominis.
[Acupuncture and Moxibustion]	Insert the needle perpendicularly 1.0~1.5 cun deep and stimulate until there is a sore and numbing sensation in the local area. This point can be moxibusted.
[Indications]	Constipation, abdominal pain, spermatorrhea, premature ejaculation, impotence, hernia and difficult urination.

ST 28 – Shuǐ Dào

[Locating]	On the lower abdomen, 3 cun inferior to the umbilicus, 2 cun lateral to the anterior midline.
[Regional Anatomy]	The needle passes through the subcutaneous tissues and penetrates the posterior layer of sheath of m. rectus abdominis and m. rectus abdominis.
[Acupuncture and Moxibustion]	Insert the needle perpendicularly 1.0~1.5 cun deep and stimulate until there is a sore and numbing sensation in the local area. This point can be moxibusted.
[Indications]	Constipation, abdominal pain, distention, dysmenorrhea, hernia and difficult urination.

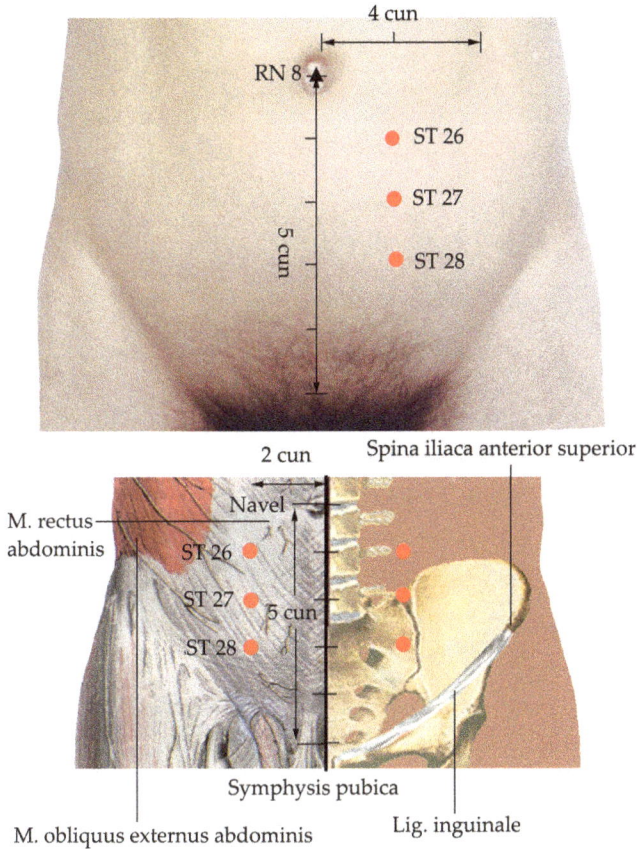

4 cun

RN 8

ST 26

ST 27

ST 28

5 cun

2 cun   Spina iliaca anterior superior

M. rectus abdominis   Navel

ST 26

ST 27   5 cun

ST 28

Symphysis pubica

M. obliquus externus abdominis   Lig. inguinale

ST 29 – Guī Lái

[Locating]	On the lower abdomen, 4 cun inferior to the umbilicus, 2 cun lateral from the anterior midline.
[Regional Anatomy]	The needle passes through the subcutaneous tissues and penetrates the posterior layer of sheath of m. rectus abdominis, m. rectus abdominis and peritoneum.
[Acupuncture and Moxibustion]	Insert the needle perpendicularly 1.0~1.5 cun deep and stimulate until there is a sore heavy sensation in the lower abdomen. This point can be moxibusted.
[Indications]	Abdominal pain, Irregular menstruation, dysmenorrhea, pelvic inflammation, leucorrhea and menoschesis.

ST 30 – Qì Chōng

[Locating]	On the lower abdomen, 5 cun inferior to the umbilicus, slightly above the groin, 2 cun lateral to the anterior midline.
[Regional Anatomy]	The needle passes through the subcutaneous tissues and penetrates the posterior layer of sheath of m. rectus abdominis, m. rectus abdominis and peritoneum.
[Acupuncture and Moxibustion]	Insert the needle perpendicularly 0.5~1.0 cun deep and stimulate until there is a heavy and distending sensation in the local area. This point can be moxibusted.
[Indications]	Impotence, hernia, infertility, swelling and pain of the vulva, pain of the external genitalia, irregular menstruation and abdominal pain.

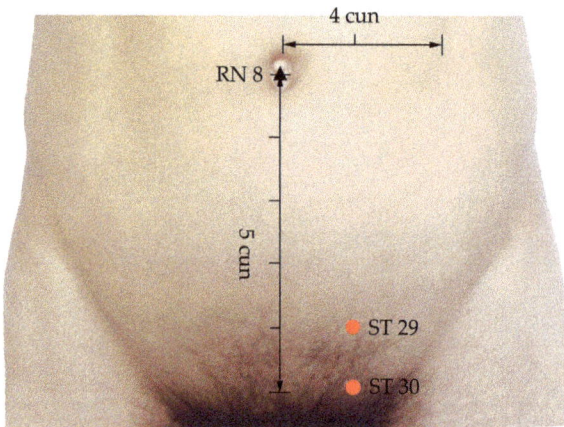

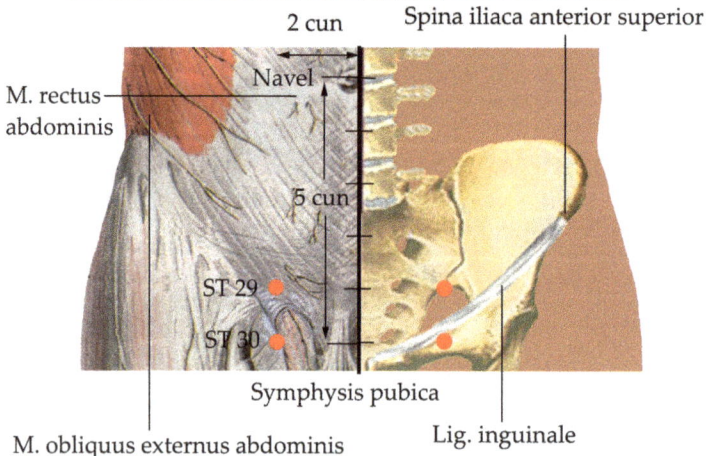

4 cun

RN 8

5 cun

ST 29

ST 30

2 cun   Spina iliaca anterior superior

M. rectus abdominis

Navel

5 cun

ST 29

ST 30

Symphysis pubica

M. obliquus externus abdominis   Lig. inguinale

ST 31 – Bì Guān

[Locating]	On the anterior aspect of the thigh, on the line connecting the anterior superior iliac spine and lateral end of the patella when the leg is flexed, in the notch lateral to the m. sartorius.
[Regional Anatomy]	The needle passes through the subcutaneous tissues and m. tensor fasciae latae, penetrates m. rectus femoris and m. vastus lateralis.
[Acupuncture and Moxibustion]	Insert the needle perpendicularly 1.5~2.0 cun deep and stimulate until there is a sore and numbing sensation in the local area radiating to the lateral side of the thigh. This point can be moxibusted.
[Indications]	Pain of the knee and waist and numbness and weakness of the lower extremities.

ST 32 – Fú Tù

[Locating]	On the anterior aspect of the thigh, on the line connecting the anterior superior iliac spine and lateral end of the patella, 6 cun proximal to the superior border of patella.
[Regional Anatomy]	The needle passes through the subcutaneous tissues and penetrates the m. rectus femoris and m. vastus intermedius.
[Acupuncture and Moxibustion]	Insert the needle perpendicularly 1.5~2.5 cun deep and stimulate until there is a sore and numbing sensation in the local area radiating to the knee. This point can be moxibusted.
[Indications]	Numbness and pain of the waist, leg and knee.

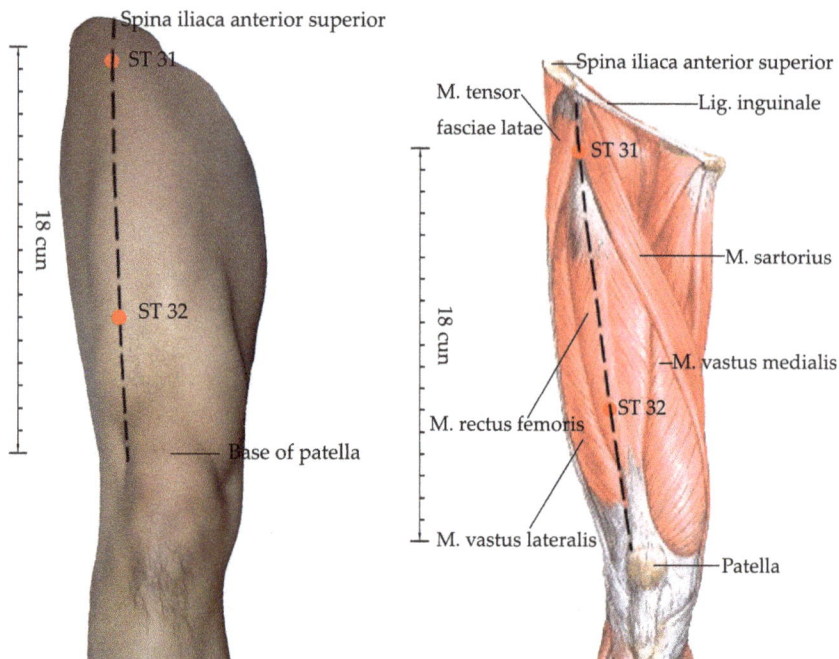

Labels: Spina iliaca anterior superior, ST 31, 18 cun, ST 32, Base of patella. M. tensor fasciae latae, Spina iliaca anterior superior, Lig. inguinale, ST 31, M. sartorius, 18 cun, M. vastus medialis, M. rectus femoris, ST 32, M. vastus lateralis, Patella.

ST 33 – Yīn Shì

[Locating]	On the anterior aspect of the thigh, on the line connecting the anterior superior iliac spine and the lateral end of the patella, 3 cun proximal to the patella.
[Regional Anatomy]	The needle passes through the subcutaneous tissues and penetrates the m. vastus lateralis.
[Acupuncture and Moxibustion]	Insert the needle perpendicularly 1.0~1.5 cun deep and stimulate until there is a sore and numbing sensation in the local area radiating to the knee. This point can be moxibusted.
[Indications]	Coldness, pain and paralysis of the leg and knee.

ST 34 – Liáng Qiū

[Features]	Xi-cleft point of the Stomach Channel of the Foot *Yangming*.
[Locating]	On the anterior aspect of the thigh, on the line connecting the anterior superior iliac spine and lateral end of the patella, 2 cun proximal to the patella when the knee is bent.

[Regional Anatomy]	The needle passes through the subcutaneous tissues and penetrates the m. vastus lateralis.
[Acupuncture and Moxibustion]	Insert the needle perpendicularly 1.0~1.5 cun deep until there is a sore and numbing sensation in the local area radiating to the knee. This point can be moxibusted.
[Indications]	Stomach ache, borborygums diarrhea and knee pain.

ST 35 – Dú Bí

[Locating]	The point is located in the sitting position when the knee is bent, in the depression inferior and lateral to the ligament of the patella.
[Regional Anatomy]	The needle passes through the subcutaneous tissues and penetrates the capsule of knee joint from the lateral side of patellar ligament.
[Acupuncture and Moxibustion]	Insert the needle obliquely 0.8~1.2 cun deep and stimulate until there is a sore and heavy sensation spreading in the knee. This point can be moxibusted.
[Indications]	Coldness, pain and paralysis of the leg and knee.

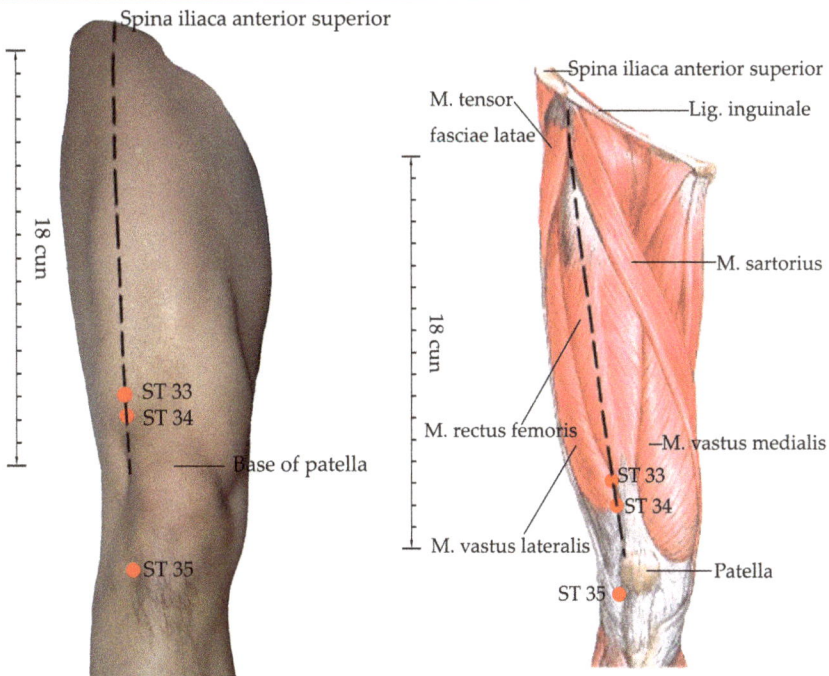

ST 36 – Zú Sān Lǐ

[Features]	He-sea and lower he-sea point of the Stomach Channel of the Foot *Yangming*.
[Locating]	On the anterior aspect of the lower leg, 3 cun distal to ST 35 (Dú Bí), one finger width lateral from the anterior ridge of the tibia.
[Regional Anatomy]	The needle passes through the subcutaneous tissues and penetrates m. tibialis anterior and m. extensor hallucis longus.
[Acupuncture and Moxibustion]	Insert the needle perpendicularly 0.5~1.5 cun deep and stimulate until there is a sensation radiating to the ankle and dorsum of the foot and toes. This point can be moxibusted.
[Indications]	Stomach ache, vomiting, abdominal distention, borborygums, indigestion, diarrhea, constipation, dysentery and palpitation.

ST 37 – Shàng Jù Xū

[Features]	Lower he-sea point of the Large Intestine Channel of the Hand *Yangming*.
[Locating]	The point is located in the sitting position when the knee is bent or in the supine position, 6 cun distal to ST 35 (Dú Bí), one finger width lateral to the anterior ridge of the tibia.
[Regional Anatomy]	The needle passes through the subcutaneous tissues and penetrates m. tibialis anterior and m. extensor hallucis longus.
[Acupuncture and Moxibustion]	Insert the needle perpendicularly 0.5~1.5 cun deep and stimulate until there is a sore and numbing sensation in the local area radiating upwards or domnwards. This point can be moxibusted.
[Indications]	Dyspepsia, dysentery, diarrhea, constipation, abdominal distention and borborygums.

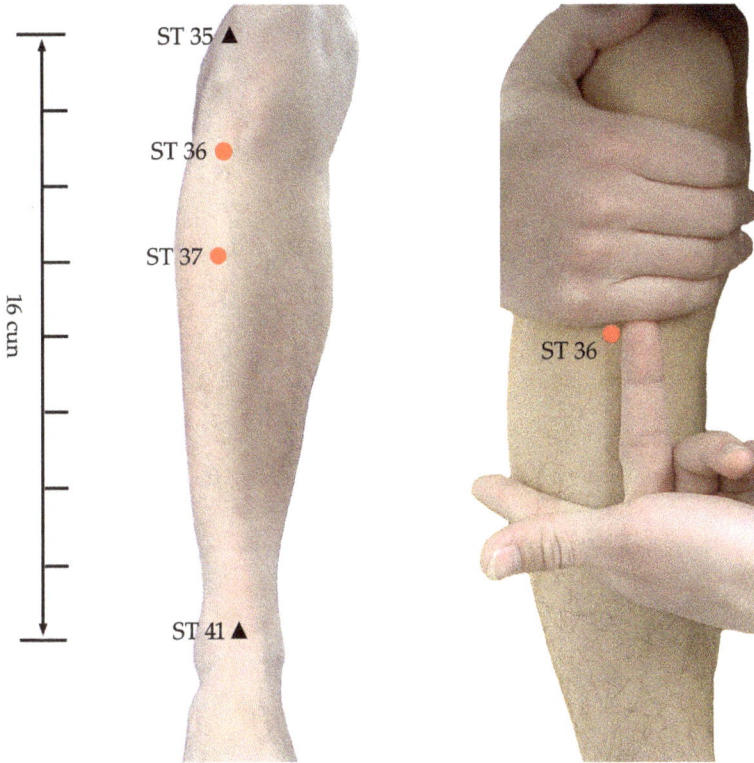

16 cun

ST 35 ▲

ST 36 ●

ST 37 ●

ST 41 ▲

ST 36 ●

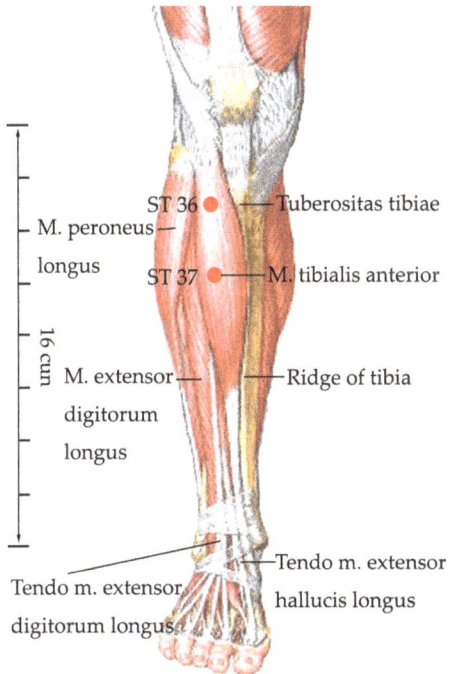

ST 36 ● — Tuberositas tibiae

M. peroneus longus

ST 37 ● — M. tibialis anterior

16 cun

M. extensor digitorum longus — Ridge of tibia

Tendo m. extensor digitorum longus — Tendo m. extensor hallucis longus

ST 38 – Tiáo Kǒu

[Locating]	On anterior and lateral side of the leg, 8 cun distal to ST 35 (Dú Bí), one finger width lateral to the anterior ridge of the tibia.
[Regional Anatomy]	The needle passes through the subcutaneous tissues and penetrates m. tibialis anterior and m. extensor hallucis longus.
[Acupuncture and Moxibustion]	Insert the needle perpendicularly 0.5~1.0 cun deep and stimulate until there is a sore, heavy and numbing sensation in the local area radiating to the leg and dorsum of the foot. This point can be moxibusted.
[Indications]	Pain of the shoulder and back.

ST 39 – Xià Jù Xū

[Features]	Lower he-sea point of the Small Intestine Channel of the Hand *Taiyang*.
[Locating]	On anterior and lateral side of the leg, 9 cun distal to ST 35 (Dú Bí), one finger lateral to the anterior ridge of the tibia.
[Regional Anatomy]	The needle passes through the subcutaneous tissues and penetrates m. tibialis anterior and m. extensor hallucis longus.
[Acupuncture and Moxibustion]	Insert the needle perpendicularly 0.5~1.0 cun deep and stimulate until there is a sore and numbing sensation in the local area which radiates to the dorsum of the foot. This point can be moxibusted.
[Indications]	Low appetite, borborygums, abdominal pain and dysentery.

ST 40 – Fēng Lóng

[Features]	Luo-connecting point of the Stomach Channel of the Foot *Yangming*.
[Locating]	On the anterior and lateral aspect of the leg, 8 cun superior to the tip of the lateral malleolus, two finger width lateral from the anterior ridge of the tibia.

[Regional Anatomy]	The needle passes through the subcutaneous tissues and penetrates the lateral side of m. extensor digitorum longus, m. peroneus longus and m. peroneus brevis.
[Acupuncture and Moxibustion]	Insert the needle perpendicularly 0.5~1.0 cun deep and stimulate until there is a sensation radiating to the foot.
	This point can be moxibusted.
[Indications]	Hiccough, vomiting, stomach ache, constipation and difficult urination.

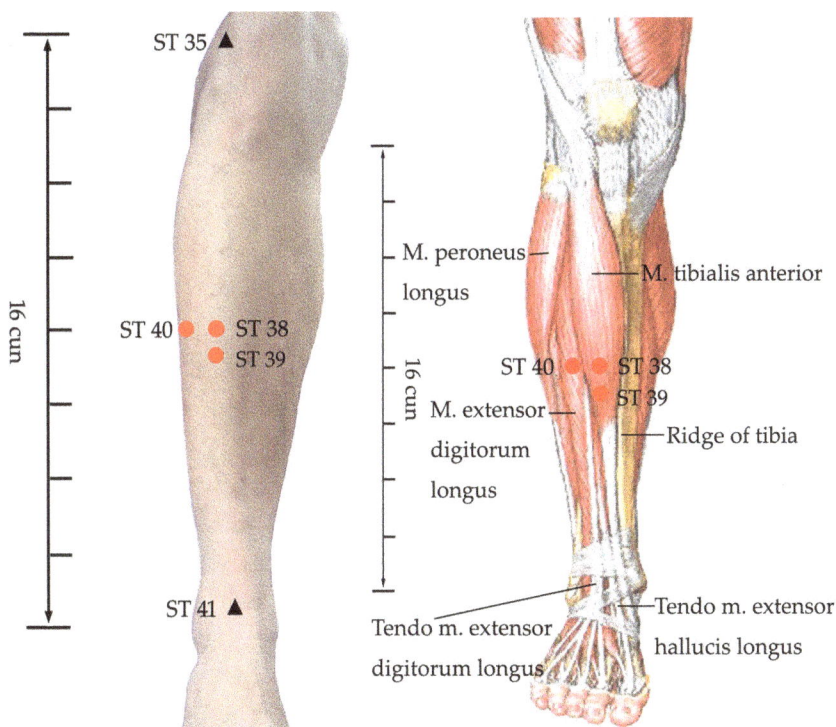

16 cun

ST 35 ▲

ST 40 ● ● ST 38
ST 39

ST 41 ▲

M. peroneus longus
M. tibialis anterior

16 cun

ST 40 ● ● ST 38
ST 39
M. extensor digitorum longus
Ridge of tibia

Tendo m. extensor digitorum longus
Tendo m. extensor hallucis longus

ST 41 – Jiě Xī

[Features]	Jing-river point of the Stomach Channel of the Foot *Yangming*.
[Locating]	In the horizontal stria of the dorsum of foot, between the extensor pollicis longus muscle tendon and the extensor digitorum longus.
[Regional Anatomy]	The needle passes through the subcutaneous tissues and penetrates the tibiofibular syndesmosis.

[Acupuncture and Moxibustion]	Insert the needle perpendicularly 0.3~0.5 cun deep and stimulate until there is a sore and numbing sensation in the local area radiating to the ankle.
	This point can be moxibusted.
[Indications]	Headache, abdominal distention, constipation, pain, weakness and numbness of the leg and ankle.

ST 42 – Chōng Yáng

[Features]	Yuan-source point of the Stomach Channel of the Foot *Yangming*.
[Locating]	On the dorsum of the foot, between the extensor pollicis longus muscle tendon and extensor digitorum longus where the pulse of the dorsal artery can be felt.
[Regional Anatomy]	The needle passes through the subcutaneous tissues and penetrates the periost of the second cuneiform bone.
[Acupuncture and Moxibustion]	Insert the needle perpendicularly 0.2~0.3 cun deep.
	This point can be moxibusted.
[Indications]	Paralysis of the foot.
[Note]	Avoid puncturing the artery.

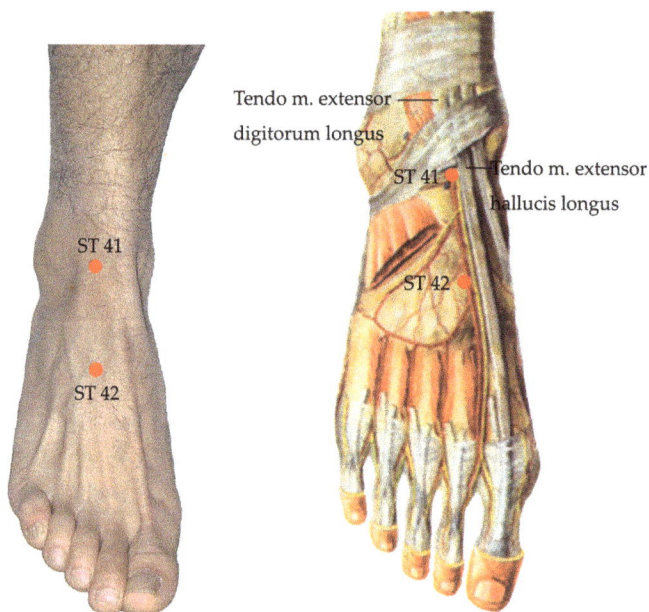

Tendo m. extensor digitorum longus

Tendo m. extensor hallucis longus

ST 41

ST 42

ST 41

ST 42

ST 43 – Xiàn Gǔ

[Features]	Shu-stream points of the Stomach Channel of the Foot *Yangming*.
[Locating]	The point is located in the sitting position with the foot resting on the ground or in the supine position, proximal to the second and third metatarsophalangeal joint, in depression distal to the junction of the second and third metatarsal bones.
[Regional Anatomy]	The needle passes through the subcutaneous tissues and penetrates m. extensor digitorum brevis.
[Acupuncture and Moxibustion]	Insert the needle perpendicularly 0.2~0.3 cun deep and stimulate until there is a sore and numbing sensation in the local area. This point can be moxibusted.
[Indications]	Borborygums and abdominal pain.

ST 44 – Nèi Tíng

[Features]	Ying-spring point of the Stomach Channel of the Foot *Yangming*.
[Locating]	The point is located in the sitting position when the foot is resting on the ground or in the supine position, in distal to the second metatarsophalangeal joint, in the web between the second and third toes.
[Regional Anatomy]	The needle passes through the subcutaneous tissues, penetrates the dorsal deep fascia, and enters interosseous muscles.
[Acupuncture and Moxibustion]	Insert the needle perpendicularly or obliquely 0.2~0.3 cun deep and stimulate until there is a sore and numbing sensation in the local area. This point can be moxibusted.
[Indications]	Abdominal pain and distention, diarrhea, dysentery, toothache, sore throat and epistaxis, irritability, insomnia with many dreams and psychosis.

ST 45 – Lì Duì

[Features]	Jing-well point of the Stomach Channel of the Foot *Yangming*.
[Locating]	On the lateral side of the second toe, 0.1 cun lateral to the corner of the nail.
[Regional Anatomy]	The needle passes through the subcutaneous tissues and penetrates m. extensor digitorum longus and lateral bundle of tendo m. extensor Digitorum of digiti pedis Ⅱ.
[Acupuncture and Moxibustion]	① Insert the needle 0.1~0.2 cun deep and stimulate until there is sore and distending sensation in the local area. ② Prick with three-edged needle to bleed.
[Indications]	Insomnia with many dreams.

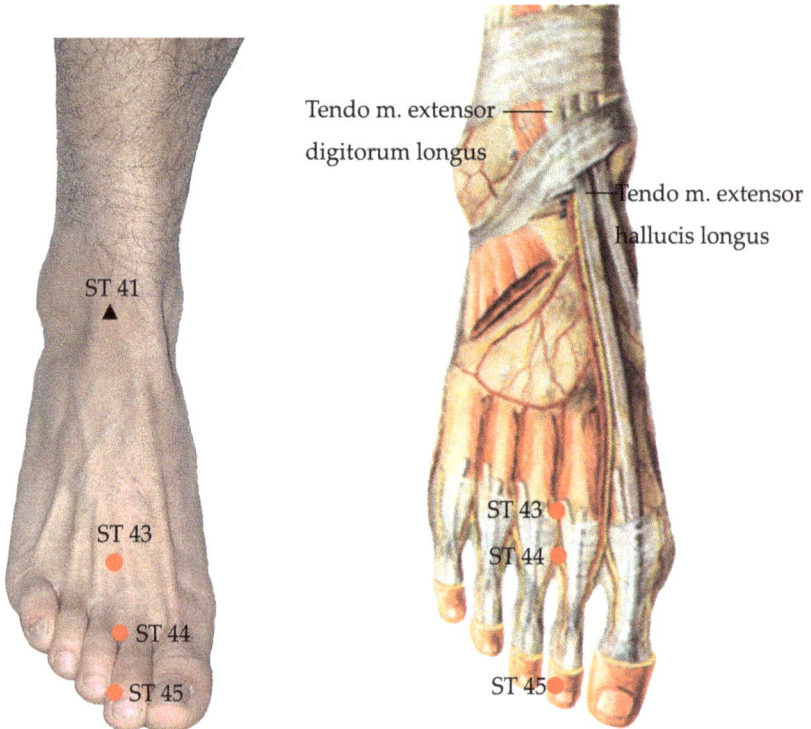

Tendo m. extensor
digitorum longus

Tendo m. extensor
hallucis longus

ST 41

ST 43

ST 44

ST 45

ST 43

ST 44

ST 45

CHAPTER 5

Spleen Channel of Foot Taiyin; SP

There are twenty-one points on the Spleen Channel of the Foot *Taiyin*, and forty-two points in total on both sides. There are eleven points on medial side of the lower limb and ten points on the abdomen and the lateral part of the chest. The first point is SP 1 (Yǐn Bái) and the last is SP 21 (Dà Bāo). The indications are the diseases of the stomach and intestines and the syndromes along the course of the channel.

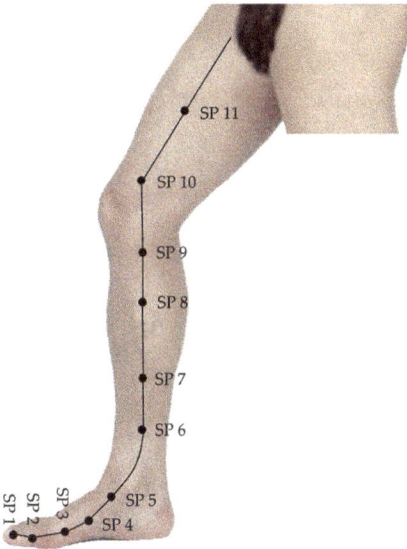

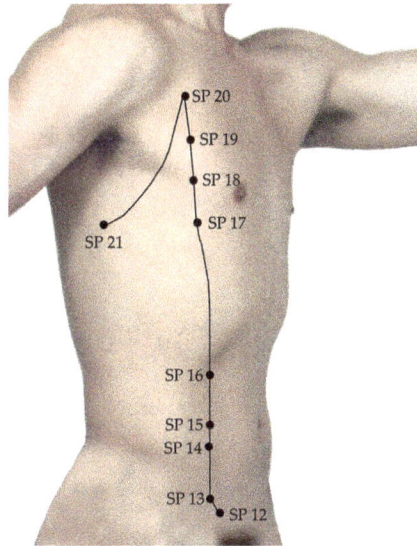

SP 1 – Yĭn Bái

[Features]	Jing-well point of the Spleen Channel of the Foot *Taiyin*.
[Locating]	On the medial side of the the big toe, 0.1 cun lateral to the corner of the nail.
[Regional Anatomy]	The needle passes through the skin and subcutaneous tissue, penetrates the space between the centrifugal phalanx and ends on the medial side of the big toe.
[Acupuncture and Moxibustion]	① Insert the needle 0.1~0.2 cun deep until there is a sore a distending sensation in the local area. ② Prick with the three-edged needle to bleed.This point can be moxibusted.
[Indications]	Irregular menstruation and metrorrhagia, vomiting, abdominal distention, insomnia with many dreams.

SP 2 – Dà Dū

[Features]	Ying-spring point of the Spleen Channel of the Foot *Taiyin*.
[Locating]	On the medial side of foot, in the depression at the junction of the red and white skin anterior and inferior to the proximal metatarsodigital joint of the big toe.
[Regional Anatomy]	The needle passes through the skin and subcutaneous tissue, enters the digital fibrous sheath, penetrates tendo m. flexor hallucis longus and reaches the superior and inferior border of the sheath.
[Acupuncture and Moxibustion]	Insert the needle perpendicularly 0.3~0.5 cun deep and sitmulate until there is a sore and numbing sensation in the local area. This point can be moxibusted.
[Indications]	Abdominal distention and pain and stomach ache.

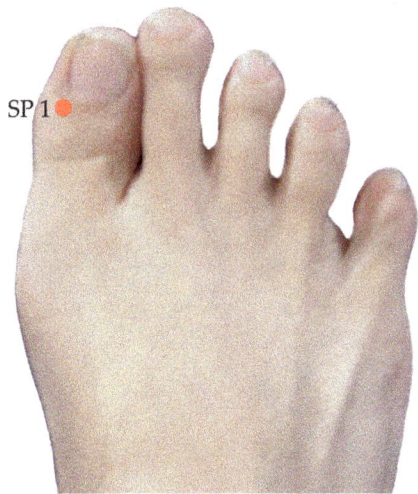

SP 1

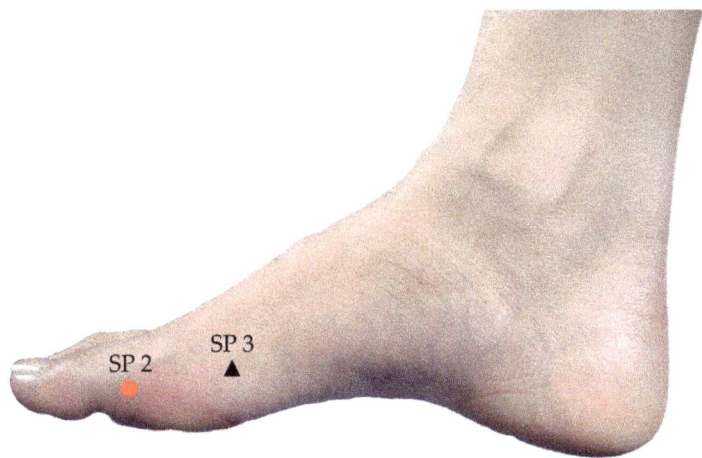

SP 2   SP 3

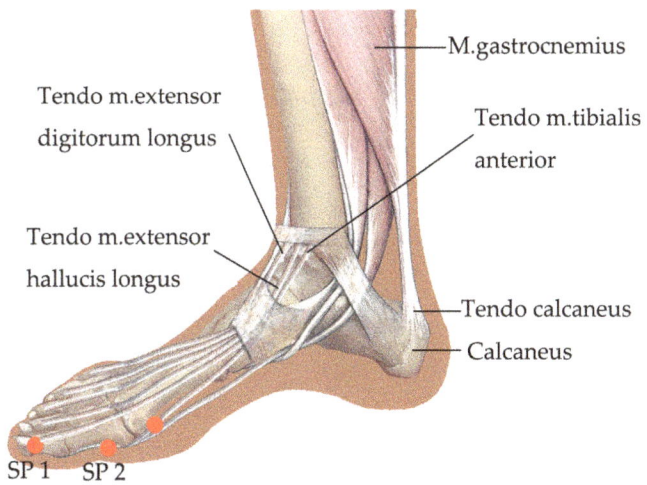

M.gastrocnemius

Tendo m.extensor
digitorum longus

Tendo m.tibialis
anterior

Tendo m.extensor
hallucis longus

Tendo calcaneus

Calcaneus

SP 1   SP 2

SP 3 – Tài Bái

[Features]	Shu-stream point and yuan-source point of the Spleen Channel of the Foot *Taiyin*.
[Locating]	On the medial side of foot, in the depression at the junction of red and white skin, posterior and inferior to the proximal metatarsodigital joint of the big toe.
[Regional Anatomy]	The needle passes through the skin and subcutaneous tissue, enters the digital fibrous sheath, penetrates tendo m. abductor hallucis and tendo m. flexor hallucis brevis.
[Acupuncture and Moxibustion]	Insert the needle perpendicularly 0.3~0.5 cun deep and stimulate until there is a sore and numbing sensation in the local area. This point can be moxibusted.
[Indications]	Stomach ache, abdominal distention and pain and borborygums.

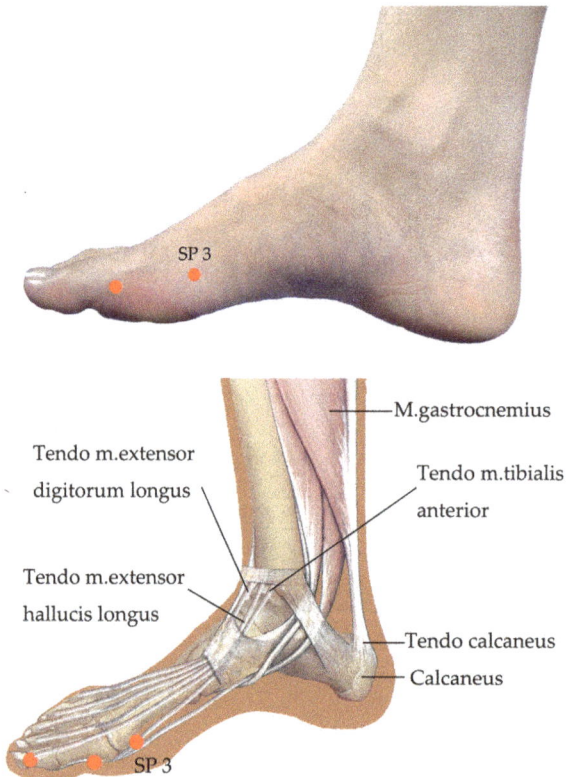

SP 3

M.gastrocnemius

Tendo m.extensor digitorum longus

Tendo m.tibialis anterior

Tendo m.extensor hallucis longus

Tendo calcaneus

Calcaneus

SP 3

SP 4 – Gōng Sūn

[Features]	Luo-connecting point of the Spleen Channel of the Foot *Taiyin*; confluent point of the penetrating vessel.
[Locating]	On the medial side of the foot, in the depression anterior and inferior to the base of the first metatarsal bone, at the junction of the red and white skin, 1 cun proximal to SP 3 (Tài Bái).
[Regional Anatomy]	The needle passes by the metatarsophalangeal fascia and plantar aponeurosis, enters the m. abductor hallucis and m. flexor hallucis brevis.
[Acupuncture and Moxibustion]	Insert the needle perpendicularly towards KI 1 (Yǒng Quán) 0.5~0.8 cun deep and stimulate until there is a sore and numbing sensation in the local area radiating to the sole of the foot. This point can be moxibusted.
[Indications]	Vomiting, hiccough, abdominal pain and stomach ache.

SP 5 – Shāng Qiū

[Features]	Jing-river point of the Spleen Channel of the Foot *Taiyin*.
[Locating]	In the depression anterior and inferior to the medial malleolus, at the midpoint between the tuberosity of the navicular bone and the tip of the medial malleolus.
[Regional Anatomy]	The needle passes through the skin and subcutaneous fasica, penetrates the dorsal fascia and the posteroinferior aspect of the m. tibialis anterior, and reaches the periost of the medial side of talus.
[Acupuncture and Moxibustion]	Insert the needle perpendicularly 0.3~0.5 cun deep and stimulate until there is a sore and numbing sensation in the local area radiating to the ankle. This point can be moxibusted.
[Indications]	Ankle pain.

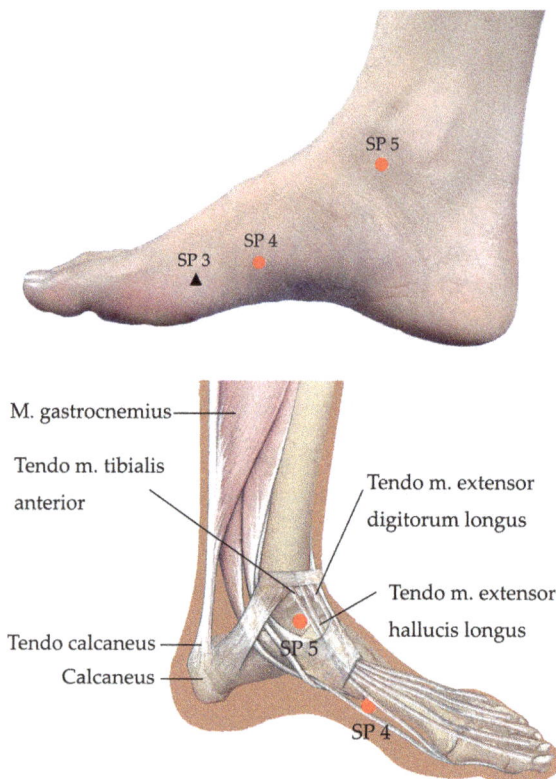

M. gastrocnemius

Tendo m. tibialis anterior

Tendo m. extensor digitorum longus

Tendo m. extensor hallucis longus

Tendo calcaneus

Calcaneus

SP 5

SP 4

SP 6 – Sān Yīn Jiāo

[Locating]	On the medial part of the leg, 3 cun superior to the tip of medial malleolus, posterior to the medial edge of the tibia.
[Regional Anatomy]	The needle passes through the skin and subcutaneous fascia and enters m. flexor digitorum longus and m. flexor hallucis longus medial to m. triceps surae.
[Acupuncture and Moxibustion]	Insert the needle perpendicularly 0.5~1.0 cun deep and stimulate until there is a sore and numbing sensation in the local area with an electric sensation radiating to the sole of the foot. This point can be moxibusted.
[Indications]	Abdominal distention and pain, irregular menstruation, metrorrhagia, bloody and excessive leucorrhea, amenorrhea, infertility, edema, dysuria, nocturnal emission and impotence.
[Note]	Prohibited during pregnancy.

SP 7 – Lòu Gǔ

[Locating]	On the medial aspect of the lower extremities, on the line connecting the medial malleolus to SP 9 (Yīn Líng Quán), 6 cun superior to the medial malleolus, posterior to the medial edge of the tibia.
[Regional Anatomy]	The needle passes through the skin and subcutaneous fascia, penetrates the deep fascia of the lower limb, and enters m. flexor digitorum longus and m. tibialis posterior at the front of m. triceps surae.
[Acupuncture and Moxibustion]	Insert the needle perpendicularly 1.0~1.5 cun deep and stimulate until there is a sore and numbing sensation in the local area radiating to the lateral aspect of the leg. This point can be moxibusted.
[Indications]	Abdominal distention and pain, edema, and dysuria.

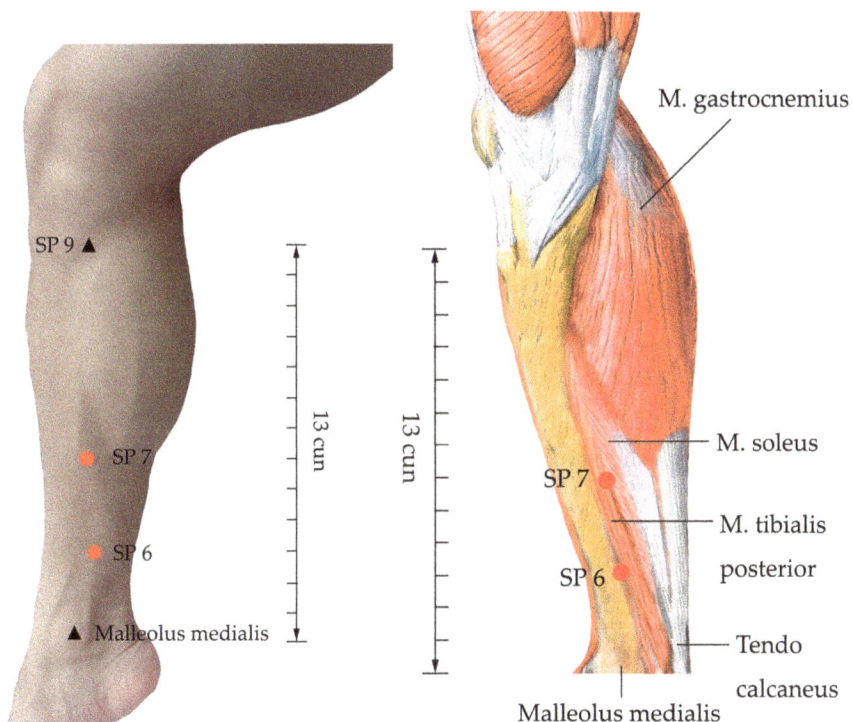

SP 8 – Dì Jī

[Features]	Xi-cleft point of the Spleen Channel of the Foot *Taiyin*.
[Locating]	On the medial aspect of the lower leg, on the line connecting the medial malleolus to SP 9 (Yīn Líng Quán), 3 cun inferior to SP 9 (Yīn Líng Quán).
[Regional Anatomy]	The needle passes through the skin, subcutaneous fascia and m. triceps surae, penetrates the deep fascia of the leg, and enters m. flexor digitorum longus and m. tibialis.
[Acupuncture and Moxibustion]	Insert the needle perpendicularly 1.0~1.5 cun deep and stimulate until there is a sore and numbing sensation in the local area radiating to the calf. This point can be moxibusted.
[Indications]	Abdominal distention and pain, irregular menstruation and dysmenorrhea.

SP 9 – Yīnlíngquán

[Features]	He-sea point of the Spleen Channel of the Foot Taiyin.
[Locating]	On the medial part of the lower leg, in the depression of the lower border of the medial condyle of the tibia.
[Regional Anatomy]	The needle penetrates the deep fascia of the lower limb, reaches the m. sartorius, m. semitendinosus and m. semimembranosus and enters m. popliteus.
[Acupuncture and Moxibustion]	Insert the needle perpendicularly 1.0-1.5 deep and stimulate until there is a sensation in the local area. This point can be moxibusted.
[Indications]	Abdominal pain and distention, edema, incontinence.

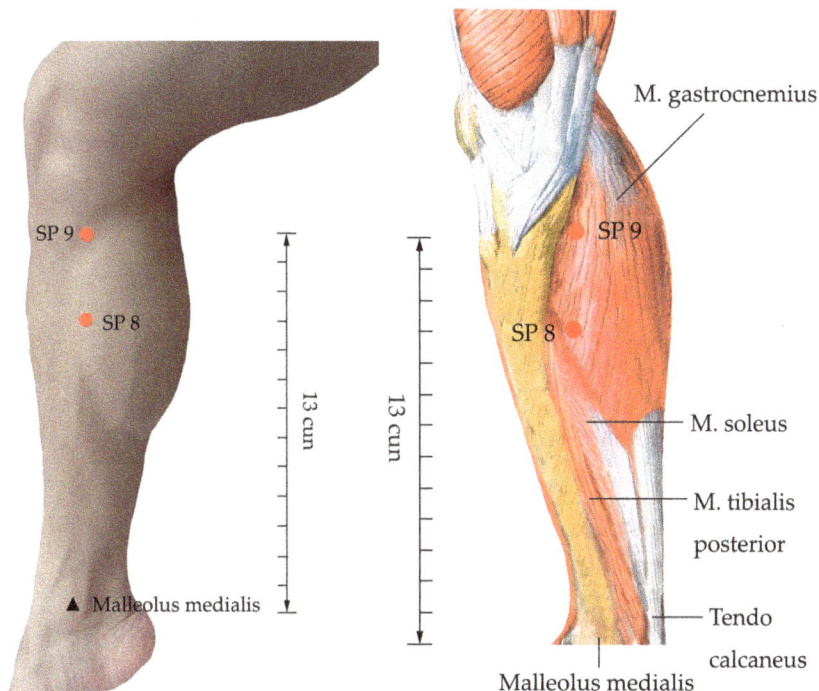

SP 9

M. gastrocnemius

SP 9

SP 8

SP 8

13 cun

13 cun

M. soleus

M. tibialis posterior

▲ Malleolus medialis

Tendo calcaneus

Malleolus medialis

SP 10 – Xuè Hǎi

[Locating]	The point is located in the sitting position with the knee flexed, 2 cun proximal to the medial and superior border of the patella. Also located when the patient is in the sitting position with the knee flexed, the doctor faces the patient and places the center of their palm on the center of the patient's patella with the thumb towards the medial side of the body. The point is located under the tip of the thumb.
[Regional Anatomy]	The needle passes through the skin and subcutaneous fascia, penetrates the ascia lata, and enters m. vastus medialis.
[Acupuncture and Moxibustion]	Insert the needle perpendicularly 1.0~2.0 cun deep and stimulate until there is a sore and numbing sensation in the local area. This point can be moxibusted.
[Indications]	Abdominal distention, irregular menstruation, dysmenorrhea, eczema, urticaria, erysipelas and scabies.

SP 11 – Jī Mén

[Locating]	In the medial aspect of the thigh, on the line connecting SP 10 (Xuè Hǎi) to SP 12 (Chōng Mén), 6 cun proximal to SP 10 (Xuè Hǎi).
[Regional Anatomy]	The needle passes through the skin and subcutaneous fascia, penetrates the fascia lata of the thigh, and enters m. adductor magnus from the medial side of m. sartorius.
[Acupuncture and Moxibustion]	Insert the needle perpendicularly 0.5~1.0 cun deep and stimulate until there is a sore and numbing sensation in the local area radiating up to the medial aspect of the thigh and down to the ankle. This point can be moxibusted.
[Indications]	Dysuria, enuresis, and eczema of the scrotum.

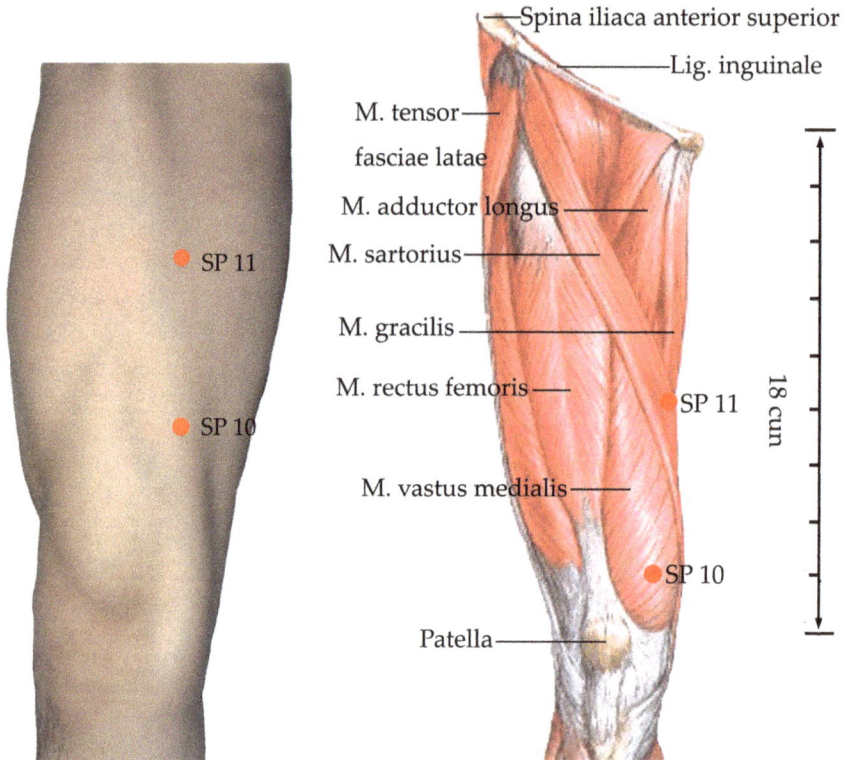

Spina iliaca anterior superior

Lig. inguinale

M. tensor fasciae latae

M. adductor longus

M. sartorius

M. gracilis

M. rectus femoris

M. vastus medialis

SP 11

SP 10

18 cun

Patella

SP 12 – Chōng Mén

[Locating]	The point is located in the supine position, 3.5 cun lateral to RN 2 (Qū Gǔ), lateral to the pulse of the femoral artery.
[Regional Anatomy]	The needle passes through the skin and subcutaneous fascia, penetrates the aponeurosis of m. obliquus externus abdominis, and enters m. obliquus internus abdominis and m. transversus abdominis.
[Acupuncture and Moxibustion]	Insert the needle perpendicularly 0.5~1.0 cun deep and stimulate until there is a sore and distending sensation in the inguinal groove spreading to the external genitalia. This point can be moxibusted.
[Indications]	Abdominal pain and distention.

SP 13 – Fǔ Shè

[Locating]	The point is located in the supine position, 0.7 cun superior lateral to SP 12 (Chōng Mén), 4 cun lateral to the anterior midline.
[Regional Anatomy]	The needle passes through the skin and subcutaneous fascia, penetrates m. obliqus internus abdominis and m. transversus abdominis, and enters fascia transversalis and subperitoneal fascia.
[Acupuncture and Moxibustion]	Insert the needle perpendicularly 0.5~1.0 cun deep and stimulate until there is a sore and numbing sensation in the local area radiating to the external genitalia. This point can be moxibusted.
[Indications]	Abdominal pain, cholera, vomiting, diarrhea, hernia and abdominal distention.

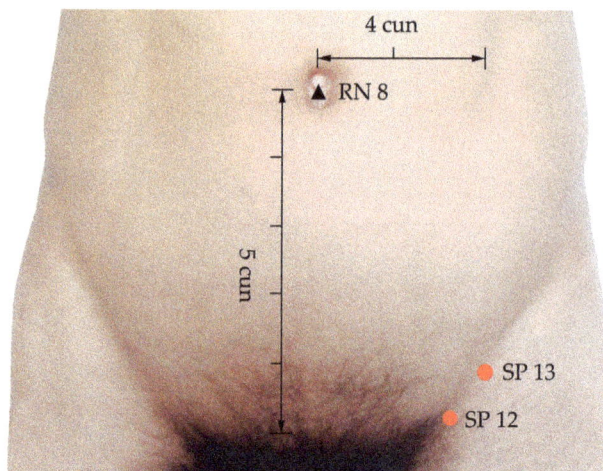

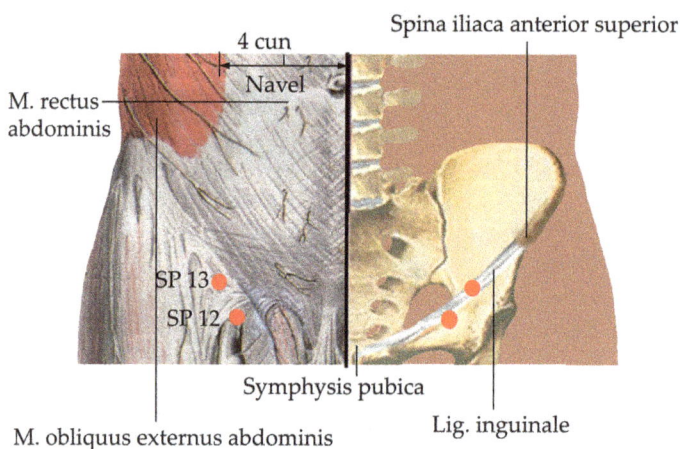

4 cun

RN 8

5 cun

SP 13

SP 12

Spina iliaca anterior superior

4 cun

Navel

M. rectus abdominis

SP 13

SP 12

Symphysis pubica

M. obliquus externus abdominis

Lig. inguinale

SP 14 – Fù Jié

[Locating]	The point is located in the supine position, 1.3 cun inferior to SP 15 (Dà Héng), 4 cun lateral to the anterior midline.
[Regional Anatomy]	The needle passes the skin and subcutis and penetrates the parietal peritoneum.
[Acupuncture and Moxibustion]	Insert the needle perpendicularly 1.0~1.5 cun deep and stimulate until there is a sore, heavy and distending sensation in the loca area. This point can be moxibusted.
[Indications]	Abdominal pain around the umbilicus and diarrhea.

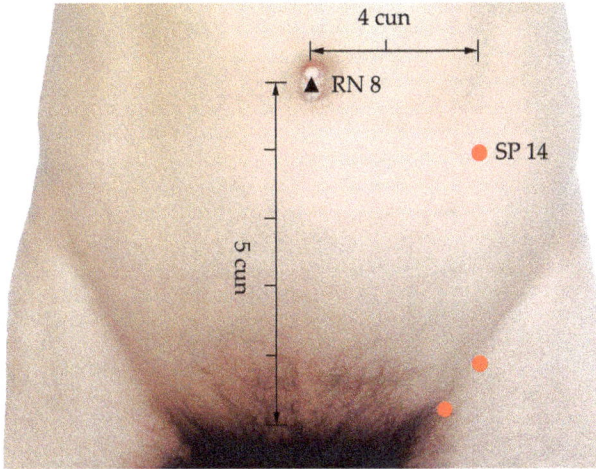

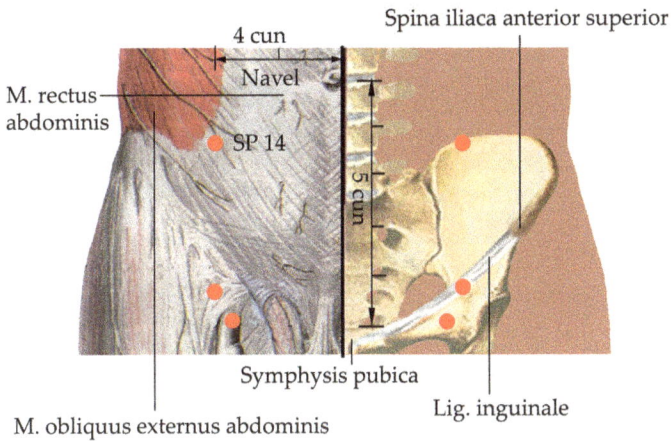

4 cun

▲ RN 8

● SP 14

5 cun

Spina iliaca anterior superior

4 cun

Navel

M. rectus abdominis

SP 14

5 cun

Symphysis pubica

Lig. inguinale

M. obliquus externus abdominis

SP 15 – Dà Héng

[Locating]	The point is located in the supine position, 4 cun lateral to RN 8 (Shén Què).
[Regional Anatomy]	The needle passes the skin and subcutis, and penetrates m. obliquus internus abdomini and m. transversus abdominis.
[Acupuncture and Moxibustion]	Insert the needle perpendicularly 1.0~1.5 cun deep and stimulate until there is a sore and numbing sensation in the local area. This point can be moxibusted.
[Indications]	Abdominal distention and pain, diarrhea and constipation.

SP 16 – Fù Āi

[Locating]	The point is located in the supine position, 3 cun superior to SP 15 (Dà Héng).
[Regional Anatomy]	The needle passes the skin and subcutis, penetrates m. obliquus externus abdominis, m. obliquus internus abdominis and m. transversus abdominis. The ascending colon is under the point on the right side.
[Acupuncture and Moxibustion]	Insert the needle perpendicularly 1.0~1.5 cun deep until there is a sore, heavy and distending sensation in the local area. This point can be moxibusted.
[Indications]	Abdominal pain around the umbilicus, dyspepsia, constipation, dysentery and diarrhea.

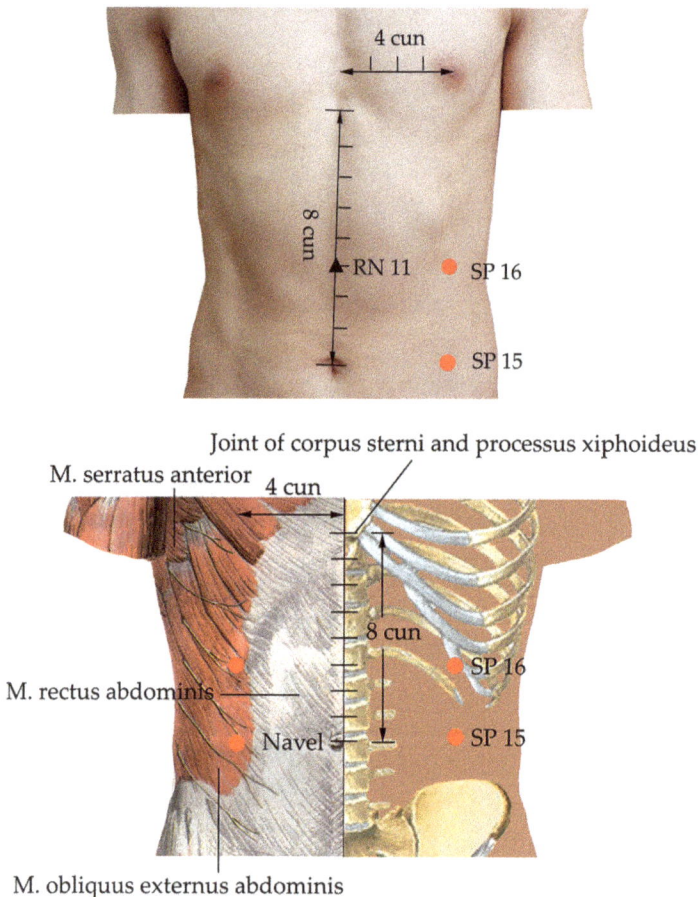

SP 17 – Shí Dòu

[Locating]	On the lateral aspect of the chest, in the fifth intercostal space, 6 cun lateral to the anterior midline.
[Regional Anatomy]	The needle passes through the skin and subcutaneous fascia, penetrates the deep fascia at the surface of m. pectoralis major and the inferior border of m. pectoralis major and enters m. serratus anterior. When puncturing deeply, the needle will penetrate m. intercostales interni and m. intercostales externi.
[Acupuncture and Moxibustion]	Insert the needle obliquely outwards 0.5~0.8 cun deep and stimulate until there is a sore and numbing sensation in the local area. This point can be moxibusted.
[Indications]	Chest and hypochondrium pain.
[Note]	Avoid deep puncture to prevent pneumothorax.

SP 18 – Tiān Xī

[Locating]	On the lateral aspect of the chest, in the fourth intercostal space, 6 cun lateral to the anterior midline.
[Regional Anatomy]	The needle passes through the skin and subcutaneous fascia, penetrates the deep fascia at the surface of m. pectoralis major and the inferior border of m. pectoralis major, enters m. serratus anterior. When puncturing deeply, the needle penetrates m. intercostales interni and m. intercostales externi.
[Acupuncture and Moxibustion]	Insert the needle obliquely or perpendicularly 0.5~0.8 cun and stimulate until there is a sore and numbing sensation in the local area. This point can be moxibusted.
[Indications]	Costal pain, cough, chest and hypochondrium pain.
[Note]	Avoid deep puncture to prevent pneumothorax.

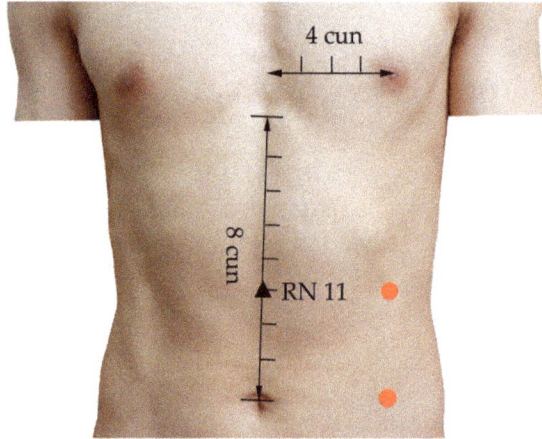

4 cun

8 cun

▲ RN 11

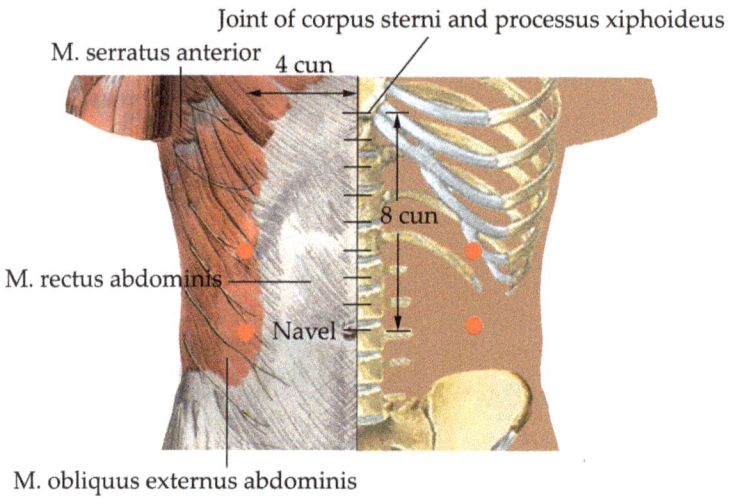

Joint of corpus sterni and processus xiphoideus

M. serratus anterior

4 cun

8 cun

M. rectus abdominis

Navel

M. obliquus externus abdominis

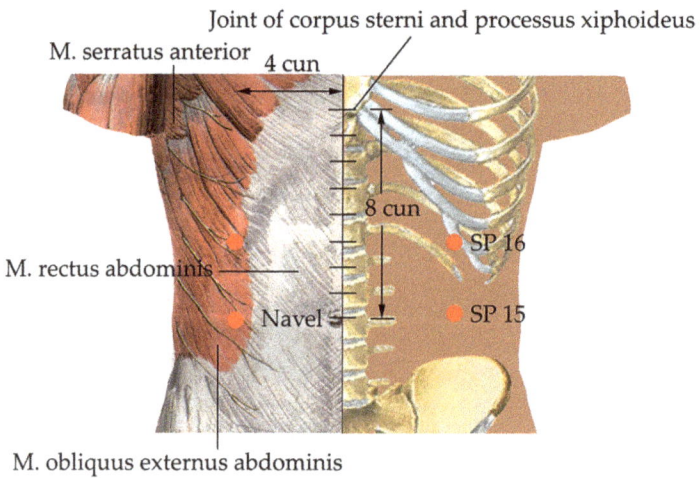

Joint of corpus sterni and processus xiphoideus

M. serratus anterior

4 cun

8 cun

SP 16

M. rectus abdominis

Navel

SP 15

M. obliquus externus abdominis

SP 19 – Xiōng Xiāng

[Locating]	On the lateral aspect of the chest, in the third intercostal space, 6 cun lateral to the anterior midline.
[Regional Anatomy]	The needle passes through the skin and subcutaneous fascia, penetrates the deep fascia at the surface of m. pectoralis major and the inferior border of m. pectoralis major, and enters m. serratus anterior. When puncturing deeply, the needle penetrates m. intercostales interni and m. intercostales externi.
[Acupuncture and Moxibustion]	Insert the needle obliquely outwards 0.5~0.8 cun deep and stimulate until there is a sore and numbing sensation in the local area. This point can be moxibusted.
[Indications]	Chest and hypochondrium pain.
[Note]	Avoid deep puncture to prevent pneumothorax.

SP 20 – Zhōu Róng

[Locating]	At the lateral aspect of chest, in the second intercostal space, 6 cun lateral from the anterior midline.
[Regional Anatomy]	The needle passes through the skin and subcutaneous fascia, penetrates the deep fascia at the surface of m. pectoralis major and enters endothoracic fascia.
[Acupuncture and Moxibustion]	Insert the needle obliquely outwards 0.5~0.8 cun deep and stimulate until there is a sore and numbing sensation in local area. This point can be moxibusted.
[Indications]	Chest distention, costal pain, cough and asthma.
[Note]	Avoid deep puncture to prevent pneumothorax.

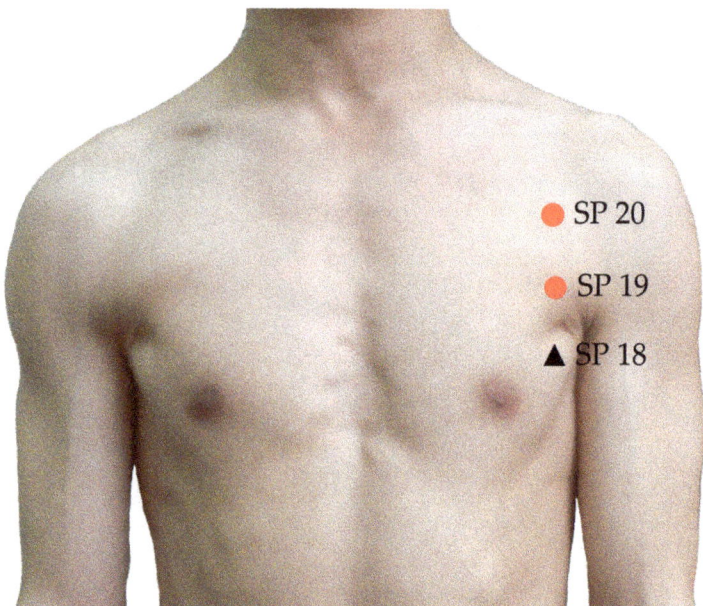

● SP 20

● SP 19

▲ SP 18

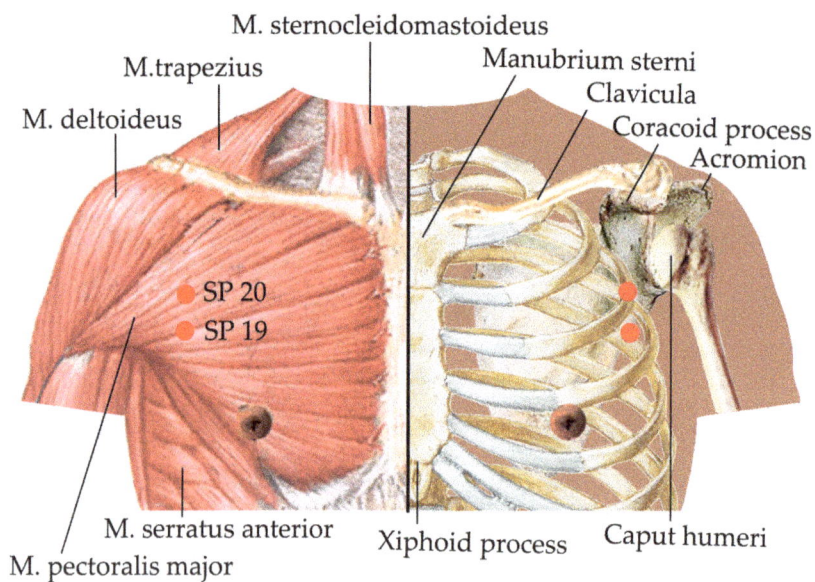

M. sternocleidomastoideus

M.trapezius

Manubrium sterni

Clavicula

M. deltoideus

Coracoid process

Acromion

SP 20

SP 19

M. serratus anterior

Xiphoid process

Caput humeri

M. pectoralis major

SP 21 – Dà Bāo

[Features]	Great luo-connecting point of the Spleen Channel of the Foot *Taiyin*.
[Locating]	On the lateral aspect of the chest, on the mid-axillary line, 6 cun inferior to the center of the axilla, in the sixth intercostal space.
[Regional Anatomy]	The needle passes through the skin and subcutaneous fascia, penetrates the m. serratus anterior and structure of the 6th intercostal space, enters the endothoracic fascia.
[Acupuncture and Moxibustion]	Insert the needle obliquely backwards 0.5~0.8 cun and stimulate until there is a sore and numbing sensation in the local area. This point can be moxibusted.
[Indications]	Costal pain and asthma, bodyaches and weakness of the limbs.

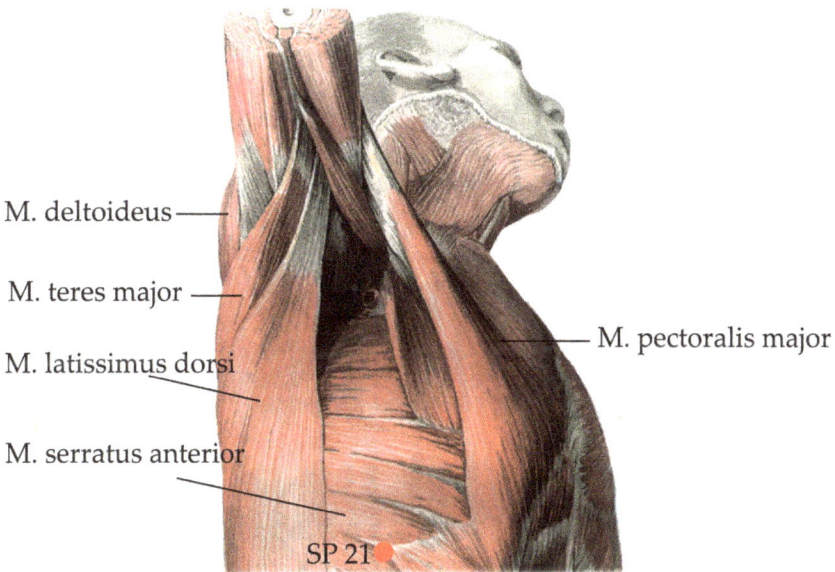

M. deltoideus

M. teres major

M. latissimus dorsi

M. serratus anterior

M. pectoralis major

SP 21

CHAPTER 6

Heart Channel of Hand Shaoyin; HT

There are nine acupuncture points on the Heart Channel of the Hand *Shaoyin* (eighteen in total on both sides). There is one point in the axillary fossa and eight on the ulnar side of the palmar aspect of the upper limb. The first point is HT 1 (Jí Quán) and the last point is HT 9 (Shào Chōng). The indications for this channel are the diseases of the circulatory system and syndromes along the course of the channel.

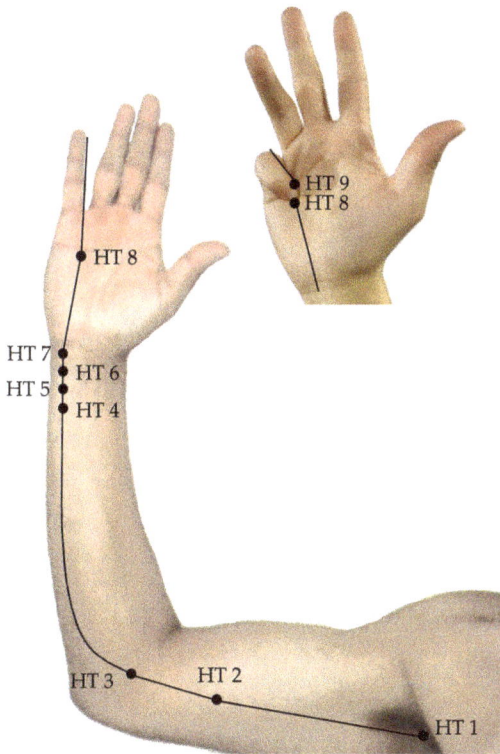

HT 1 – Jí Quán

[Locating]	The point is located when the elbow is flexed and the arm is raised to feel the pulse in the axillary fossa.
[Regional Anatomy]	The needle passes through the skin and subcutaneous fascia and penetrates the m. teres major.
[Acupuncture and Moxibustion]	Insert the needle perpendicularly 0.5~1.0 cun deep and stimulate until there is a sore and distending sensation in the axillary fossa with an electric sensation radiating the forearm causing the arm to twitch 3 times. This point can be moxibusted.
[Indications]	Palpitation, pain and distention of the chest and hypo-chondrium pain.
[Note]	Avoid puncturing the artery.

HT 2 – Qīng Líng

[Locating]	On the medial aspect of the upper limb, on the line connecting HT 1 (Jí Quán) to HT 3 (Shào Hǎi), 3 cun proximal to the transverse elbow crease, in the medial groove of m. biceps brachii.
[Regional Anatomy]	The needle passes through the skin and subcutaneous fascia, and enters the medial intermuscular septum of arm and reaches the humerus.
[Acupuncture and Moxibustion]	Insert the needle perpendicularly 0.5~1.0 cun deep and stimulate until there is a sore and numbing sensation in the local area radiating to the forearm and axilla. This point can be moxibusted.
[Indications]	Shoulder and arm pain.

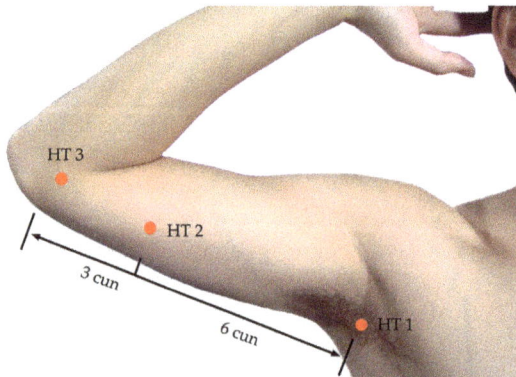

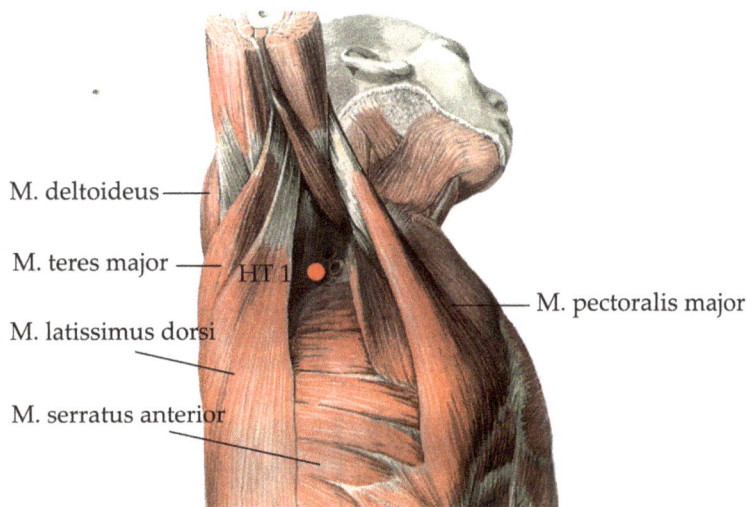

M. deltoideus

M. teres major

M. latissimus dorsi

M. serratus anterior

HT 1

M. pectoralis major

HT 3 – Shào Hǎi

[Features]	He-sea point of the Heart Channel of the Hand *Shao-yin*.
[Locating]	The point is located by flexing the elbow and raising the arm behind the head, in the depression between the medial end of the epicondyle of the humerus and the tranverse elbow crease.
[Regional Anatomy]	The needle passes through the skin and subcutaneous fascia, penetrates the deep fascia of the arm in front of v. basilica, enters m. pronator tere and finally and penetrates n. medianus by running along the medial side of the nerve.
[Acupuncture and Moxibustion]	Insert the needle perpendicularly 0.5~1.0 cun deep and stimulate until there is a sore and numbing sensation in the local area or an electric sensation radiating to the forearm. This point can be moxibusted.
[Indications]	Cardiac pain, spasmodic pain and numbness of the elbow and arm.

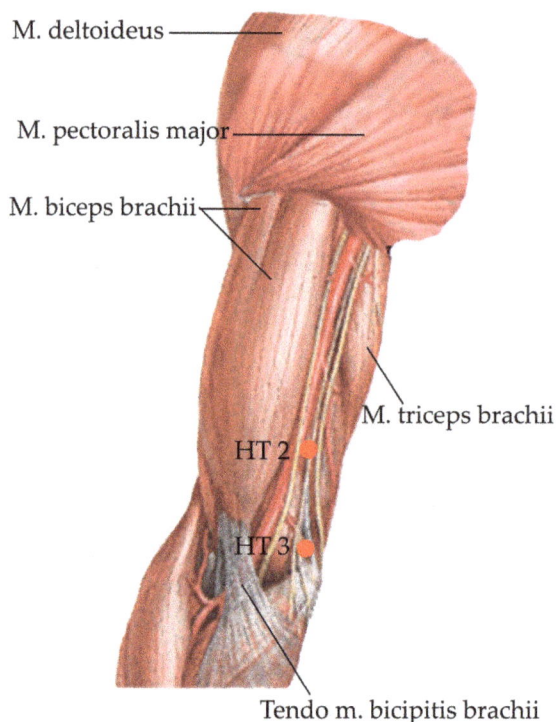

M. deltoideus

M. pectoralis major

M. biceps brachii

M. triceps brachii

HT 2

HT 3

Tendo m. bicipitis brachii

HT 4 – Líng Dào

[Features]	Jing-river point of the Heart Channel of the Hand *Shaoyin*.
[Locating]	The point is located on the radial side of the tendon m. flexor carpi ulnaris, 1.5 cun proximal to the transverse wrist crease when the palm is facing upwards.
[Regional Anatomy]	The needle passes through the skin and subcutaneous tissue, penetrates the deep fascia of the arm and the space between the tendo m. flexor carpi ulnaris and m. flexor digitorum superficialis and enters m. pronator quadratus.
[Acupuncture and Moxibustion]	Insert the needle perpendicularly 0.3~0.5 cun deep and stimulate until there is a sore and numbing sensation in the local area radiating to the elbow and fingers. This point can be moxibusted.
[Indications]	Heart palpitation, terror and cardiac pain.

HT 5 – Tōng Lǐ

[Features]	Luo-connecting point of the Heart Channel of the Hand *Shaoyin*.
[Locating]	The point is located on the radial aspect of the tendon m. flexor carpi ulnaris, 1 cun proximal to the transverse wrist crease when the palm is facing upwards.
[Regional Anatomy]	The needle passes the skin and subcutaneous fascia, penetrates the deep fascia of arm; enters m. flexor digitorum profundus at the radial side of the ulnar artery, vein and nerve and reaches m. pronator quadratus.
[Acupuncture and Moxibustion]	Insert the needle perpendicularly 0.3~0.5 cun deep and stimulate until there is a sore and numbing sensation in the local area. This point can be moxibusted.
[Indications]	Cardiac pain and shock.

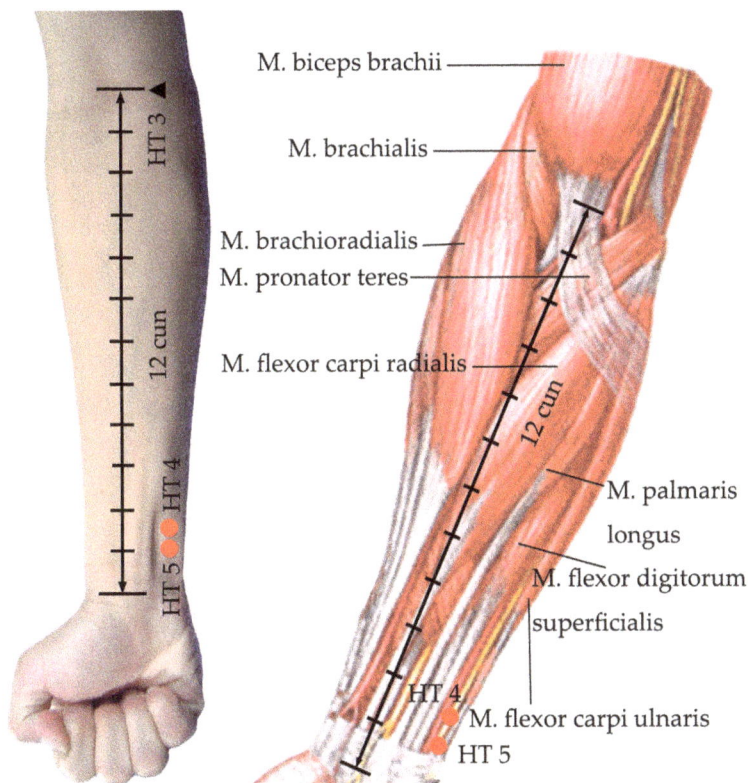

HT 6 – Yīn Xì

[Features]	Xi-cleft point of the Heart Channel of the Hand *Shaoyin*.
[Locating]	The point is located on the radial side of the tendon m. flexor carpi ulnaris, 0.5 cun proximal to the transverse wrist crease when the palm is facing upwards.
[Regional Anatomy]	The needle passes the skin and subcutaneous fascia, penetrates the deep fascia of the arm, and reaches the region between n. ulnaris and the ulnar artery and vein from the radial border of m. flexor carpi ulnaris.
[Acupuncture and Moxibustion]	Insert the needle perpendicularly 0.3~0.5 cun deep and stimulate until there is a sore and numbing sensation in the local area. This point can be moxibusted.
[Indications]	Cardiac pain, night sweat, and loss of voice.

HT 7 – Shén Mén

[Features]	Shu-stream and yuan-source point of the Heart Channel of the Hand *Shaoyin*.
[Locating]	The point is located on the radial side of the tendon m. flexor carpi ulnaris, on the transverse wrist crease when the palm is facing upwards.
[Regional Anatomy]	The needle passes through the skin and subcutis, penetrates the deep fascia of the arm from the radial border of m. flexor carpi ulnaris, reaches the head of the ulna from the medial side of n. ulnaris and the ulnar artery and vein.
[Acupuncture and Moxibustion]	Insert the needle perpendicularly 0.3~0.5 cun deep and stimulates until there is a sore and numbing sensation in the local area with an electricity sensation radiating to the fingers. This point can be moxibusted.
[Indications]	Irritability, amnesia, insomnia, loss of consciousness and epilepsy, cardiac pain and palpitation.

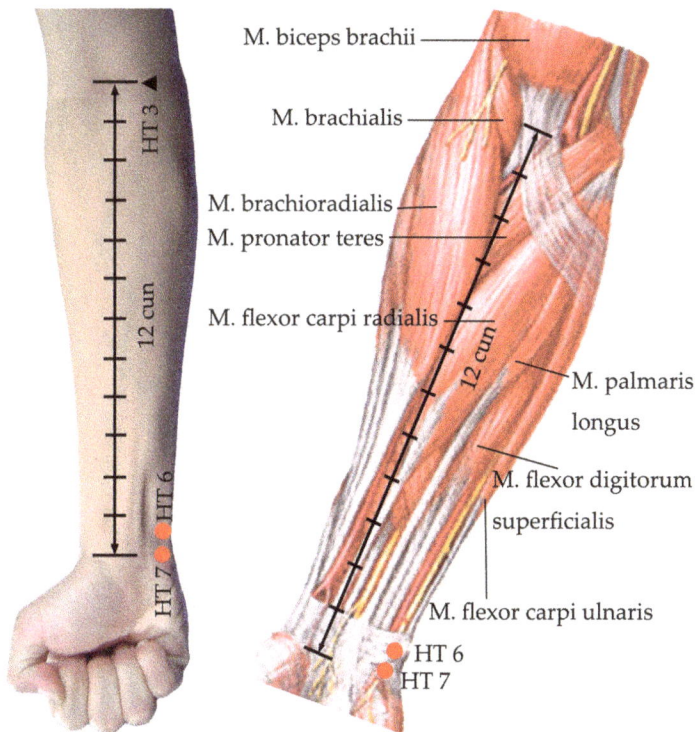

M. biceps brachii

M. brachialis

M. brachioradialis

M. pronator teres

M. flexor carpi radialis

HT 3

12 cun

12 cun

HT 6

HT 7

M. palmaris longus

M. flexor digitorum superficialis

M. flexor carpi ulnaris

HT 6
HT 7

HT 8 – Shào Fǔ

[Features]	Ying-spring point of the Heart Channel of the Hand *Shaoyin*.
[Locating]	In the palm, between the 4th and 5th metacarpal bone. The point is located under the tip of the little finger when the hand makes a loose fist.
[Regional Anatomy]	The needle passes through the skin and subcutaneous fascia, penetrates the palmar aponeurosis, runs between the tendons of m. flexor digitorum superficialis and m. flexor digitorum profundus, enters m. lumbricales IV from the ulnar side of n. digitales palmares proprii and a. digitales palmares communes, and finally reaches m. interossei IV.
[Acupuncture and Moxibustion]	Insert the needle perpendicularly 0.2~0.3 cun deep and stimulate until the needling sensation radiates to the elbow or the little finger.
	This point can be moxibusted.
[Indications]	Heart palpitation and chest pain.

HT 9 – Shào Chōng

[Features]	Jing-well point of the Heart Channel of the Hand *Shaoyin*.
[Locating]	On the radial side of the distal aspect of the little finger, 0.1 cun lateral to the radial corner of the nail.
[Regional Anatomy]	The needle passes through the skin and subcutaneous fascia and arrives at the root of finger nail
[Acupuncture and Moxibustion]	① Insert the needle 0.1~0.2 cun deep and stimulate until there is a sore and distending sensation in the local area. ② Prick with a three-edged needle to bleed. This point can be moxibusted.
[Indications]	Fever, epilepsy, stroke, and loss of consciousnes.

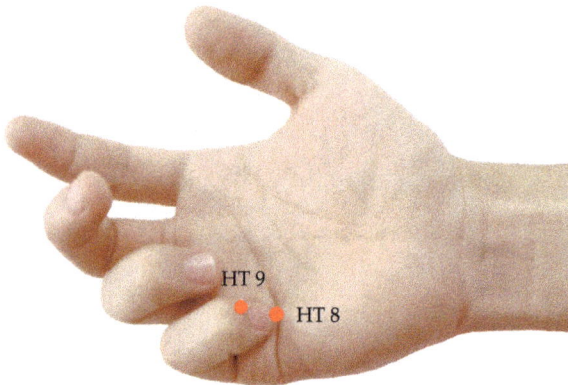

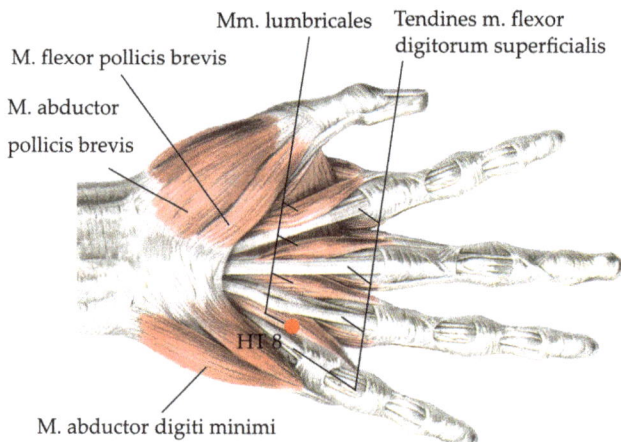

HT 9
HT 8

Mm. lumbricales   Tendines m. flexor
                    digitorum superficialis

M. flexor pollicis brevis

M. abductor
pollicis brevis

HT 8

M. abductor digiti minimi

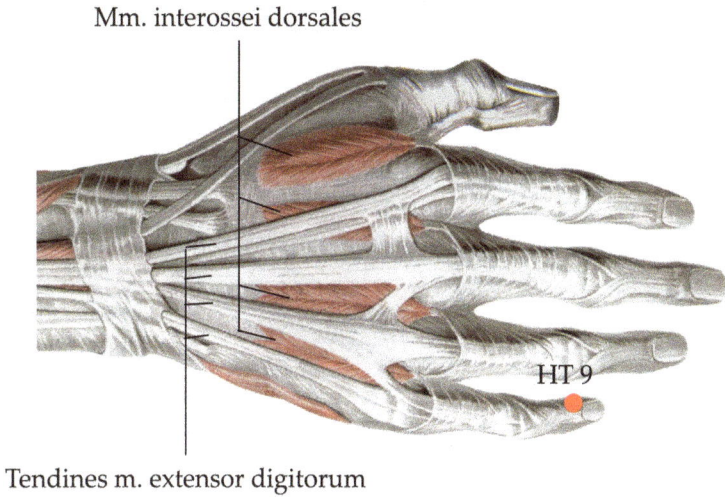

Mm. interossei dorsales

HT 9

Tendines m. extensor digitorum

CHAPTER 7

Small Intestine Channel of Hand Taiyang; SI

There are nineteen points on the Small Intestine Channel of the Hand *Taiyang* (thirty-eight points in total on both sides). There are four points on the head and neck, seven points on the back and shoulder, eight points on the posterior side of the lateral aspect of the upper limb. The first point is SI 1 (Shào Zé) and the last one is SI 19 (Tīng Gōng). The indications of this channel are the diseases of the small intestine, chest, throat, neck, face and the syndromes along the course of the channel.

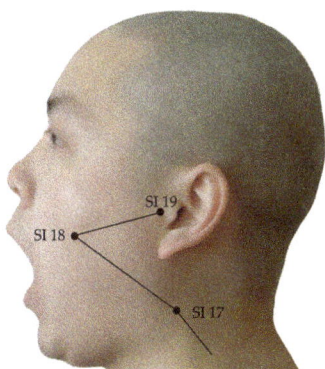

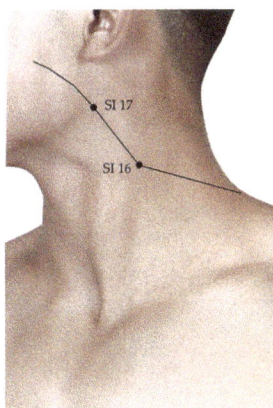

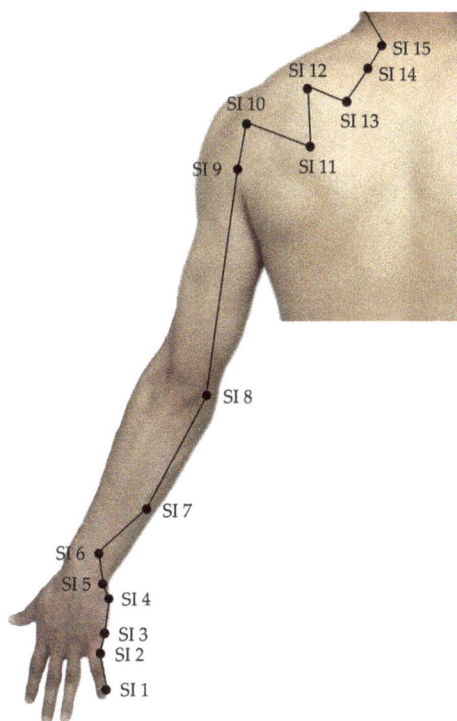

SI 1 – Shào Zé

[Features]	Jing-well point of the Small Intestine Channel of the Hand *Taiyang*.
[Locating]	On the ulnar side of the distal phalanx of the little finger, 0.1 cun lateral to the corner of the nail.
[Regional Anatomy]	The needle passes through the skin and subcutaneous fascia and arrives at the base of the finger nail.
[Acupuncture and Moxibustion]	① Insert the needle 0.1~0.2 cun deep and stimulate until there is a distending and painful sensation in the local area. ② Prick with a three-edged needle to bleed. This point can be moxibusted.
[Indications]	Stroke and loss of conciseness, febrile disease.

SI 2 – Qián Gǔ

[Features]	Ying-spring point of the Small Intestine Channel of the Hand *Taiyang*.
[Locating]	On the ulnar side of the hand, distal to the fifth metacarpophalangeal joint, at the end of the transverse crease, at the the junction of the red and white skin.
[Regional Anatomy]	The needle passes through the skin and subcutaneous tissue and reaches the proximal border of the phalanx of the little finger.
[Acupuncture and Moxibustion]	Insert the needle perpendicularly 0.2~0.3 cun deep and stimulate until there is a sore and distending sensation in the local area. This point can be moxibusted.
[Indications]	Febrile, malaria, pain and rigidity of the head and neck, neck stiffness and arm pain.

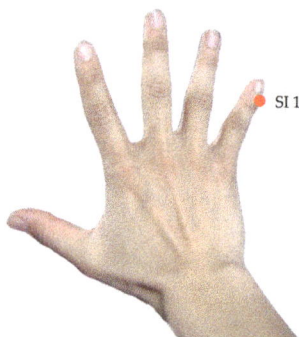

SI 1

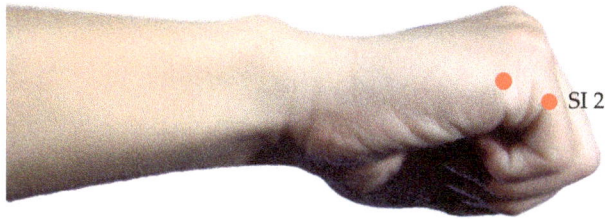

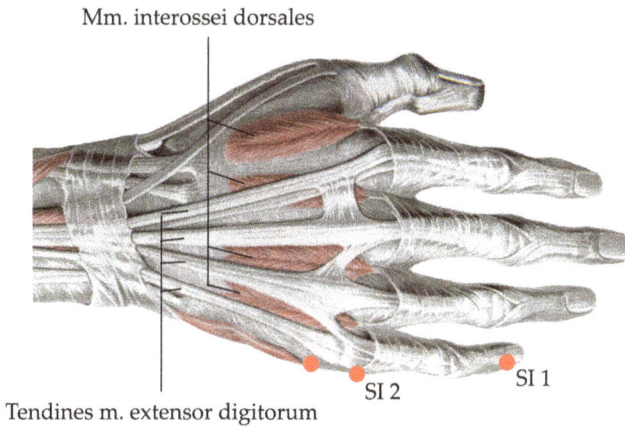

Mm. interossei dorsales

SI 2

SI 2   SI 1

Tendines m. extensor digitorum

SI 3 – Hòu Xī

[Features]	Shu-stream points of the Small Intestine Channel of the Hand *Taiyang*; Confluent points of the Du vessel.
[Locating]	On the ulnar side of the hand, proximal to the fifth metacarpophalangeal joint, at the end of the transverse crease, at the the junction of the red and white skin side.
[Regional Anatomy]	The needle passes through the skin and subcutaneous tissue, enters m. abductor digiti minimi, and reaches the region between m. flexor digiti minimi brevis manus and the 5th metacarpal bone.
[Acupuncture and Moxibustion]	Insert the needle perpendicularly 0.5~0.8 cun deep and stimulate until there is a sore and numbing sensation in the local area spreading in the palm. This point can be moxibusted.
[Indications]	Pain and rigidity of the head and neck, tinnitus, deafness, manic psychosis, epilepsy and stroke.

SI 4 – Wàn Gǔ

[Features]	Yuan-source point of the Small Intestine Channel of the Hand *Taiyang*.
[Locating]	On the ulnar side of the palm, at the junction of the red and white skin, in the depression between the base of the fifth metacarpal bone and the hamate bone.
[Regional Anatomy]	The needle passes through the skin and subcutaneous tissue, penetrates the abductor digiti minimi, and reaches the lig. pisometacarpeum.
[Acupuncture and Moxibustion]	Insert the needle perpendicularly 0.3~0.5 cun deep and stimulate until there is a sore and numbing sensation in the local area spreading in the palm. This point can be moxibusted.
[Indications]	Headache, tinnitus, febrile, jaundice, anhidrosis and malaria.

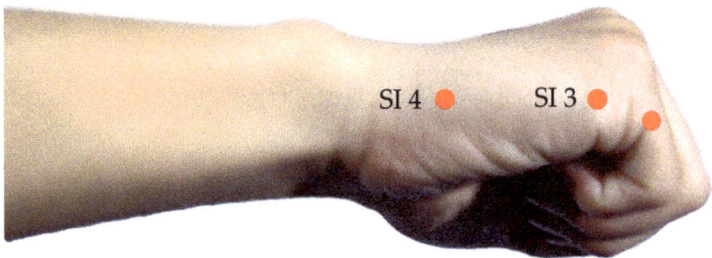

SI 4   SI 3

Mm. interossei dorsales

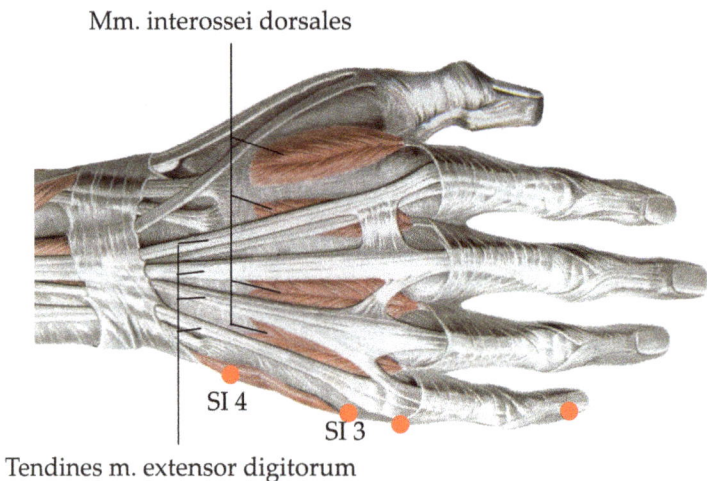

SI 4
SI 3

Tendines m. extensor digitorum

SI 5 – Yáng Gǔ

[Features]	Jing-river point of the Small Intestine Channel of the Hand *Taiyang*.
[Locating]	On the ulnar side of the wrist, in the depression between the styloid process of the ulna and the triangular bone.
[Regional Anatomy]	The needle passes through the skin and subcutaneous tissue, penetrates ligament pisometacarpeum and reaches the periost of the unciform bone.
[Acupuncture and Moxibustion]	Insert the needle perpendicularly 0.3~0.5 cun deep and stimulate until there is a sore and numbing sensation in the local area radiating in the wrist. This point can be moxibusted.
[Indications]	Headache, tinnitus, deafness, and eye pain.

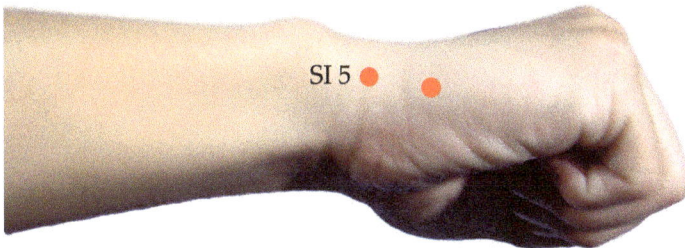

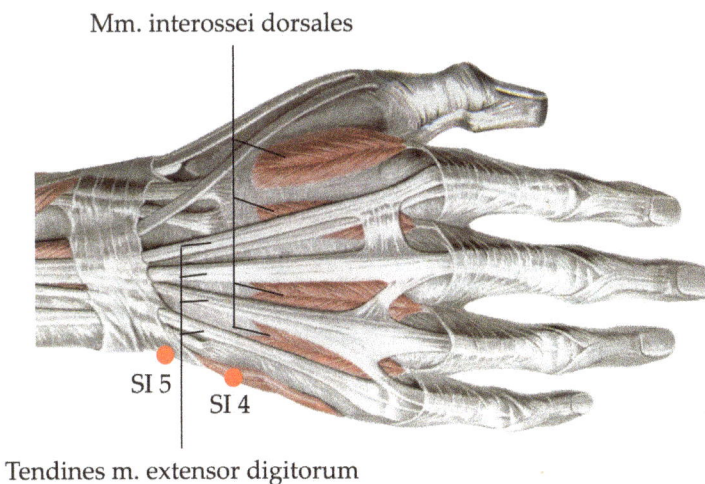

Mm. interossei dorsales

SI 5

SI 4

Tendines m. extensor digitorum

SI 6 – Yăng Lăo

[Features]	Xi-cleft point of the Small Intestine Channel of the Hand *Taiyang*.
[Locating]	On the ulnar rear of forearm, in the depression on the radial side of the styloid process of the ulna.
[Regional Anatomy]	The needle passes through the skin, subcutaneous tissue and the space between the tendons of m. extensor digiti minimi and m. extensor digitorum; penetrates the posterior interosseous artery, vein and nerves and reaches the interosseous membrane of radius and ulna.
[Acupuncture and Moxibustion]	Insert the needle obliquely upwards 0.5~0.8 cun deep and stimulate until there is a sore and numbing sensation in the wrist radiating to the shoulder and elbow. This point can be moxibusted.
[Indications]	Hemiplegia, and acute lumbago.

SI 7 – Zhī Zhèng

[Features]	Luo-connecting point of the Small Intestine Channel of the Hand *Taiyang*.
[Locating]	The point is located on the anterior border of the ulna, 5 cun proximal to the posterior transverse wrist crease when the elbow is flexed and the palm faces down.
[Regional Anatomy]	The needle passes through the skin and subcutis, penetrates m. flexor carpi ulnaris, and reaches m. flexor digitorum profundus.
[Acupuncture and Moxibustion]	Insert the needle perpendicularly or obliquely 0.5~1.0 cun deep and stimulate until there is a distending and heavy sensation radiating to the hand. This point can be moxibusted.
[Indications]	Pain of the elbow and finger and neck stiffness.

SI 8 – Xiǎo Hǎi

[Features]	He-sea point of the Small Intestine Channel of the Hand *Taiyang*.
[Locating]	On the medial aspect of the elbow, in the depression between the olecranon of the ulna and the medial epicondyle of the humerus.
[Regional Anatomy]	The needle passes through the skin and subcutis and reaches the groove of the ulnar nerve.
[Acupuncture and Moxibustion]	Insert the needle perpendicularly 0.2 ~ 0.3 cun deep and stimulate until there is a sore and numbing sensation in the local area or until there is an electric shock sensation down the ulnar aspect of the forearm and hand. This point can be moxibusted.
[Indications]	Headache, deafness, blurred vision, and gum swelling.

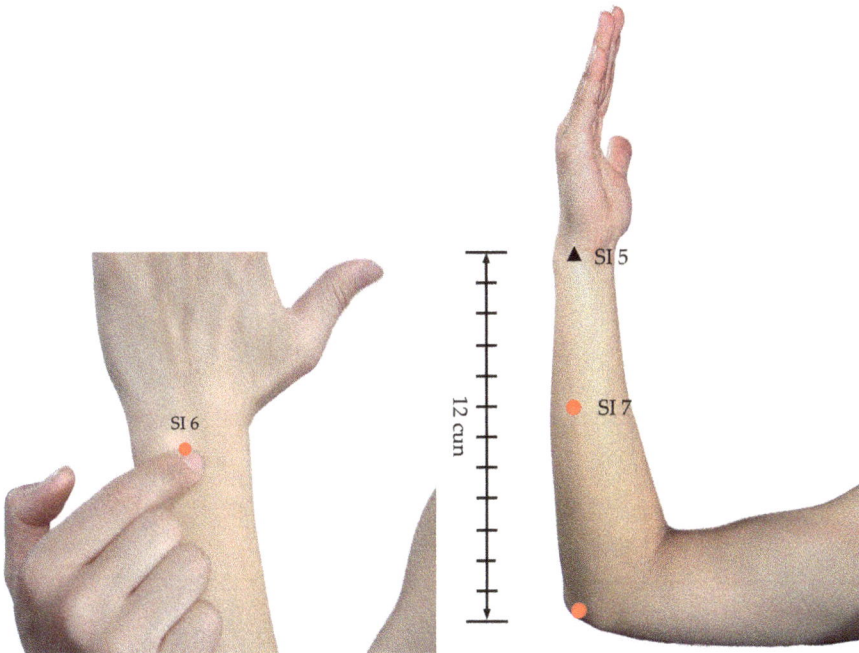

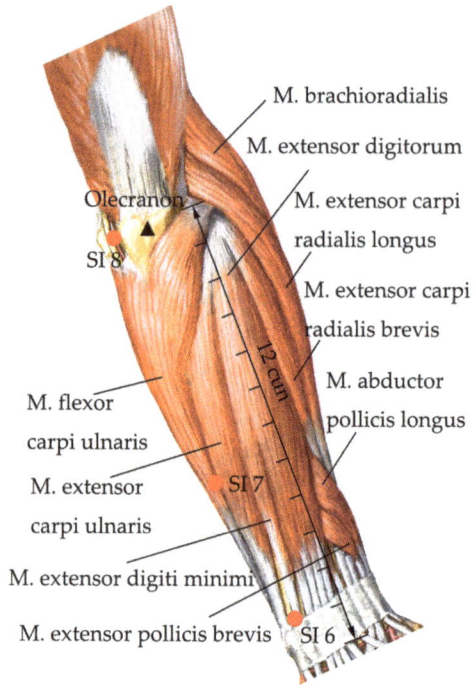

M. brachioradialis

M. extensor digitorum

M. extensor carpi radialis longus

M. extensor carpi radialis brevis

M. abductor pollicis longus

Olecranon

SI 8

12 cun

M. flexor carpi ulnaris

M. extensor carpi ulnaris

M. extensor digiti minimi

M. extensor pollicis brevis

SI 7

SI 6

SI 9 – Jiān Zhēn

[Locating]	The point is located on the posterior and inferior aspect of the shoulder, 1 cun superior to the posterior axilary fold when arm is adducted.
[Regional Anatomy]	The needle passes through the skin and subcutis tissue, penetrates the posterior portion of m. deltoideus; enters caput longum m. tricipitis brachii and m. teres major and m. latissimus dorsi and reaches the axillary cavity.
[Acupuncture and Moxibustion]	Insert the needle perpendicularly 0.5 ~ 1.0 cun deep and stimulate until there is a sore and ditending sensation spreading in the shoulder joint or radiating down to the finger tips. This point can be moxibusted.
[Indications]	Pain of the shoulder and arm.

SI 10 – Nào Shū

[Locating]	On the posterior aspect of the shoulder, directly above the posterior end of the axilla fold, in the depression inferior to the scapular spine.
[Regional Anatomy]	The needle passes through the skin and subcutis and enters m. deltoideus and m. supraspinatus.
[Acupuncture and Moxibustion]	Insert the needle perpendicularly 0.5~1.0 cun deep and stimulate until there is a sore and numbing sensation in the local area radiating to the shoulder. This point can be moxibusted.
[Indications]	Pain and weakness of the shoulder and arm and swelling of the shoulder.

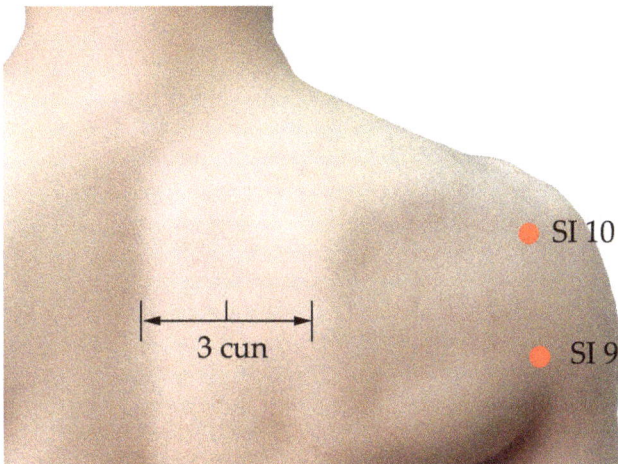

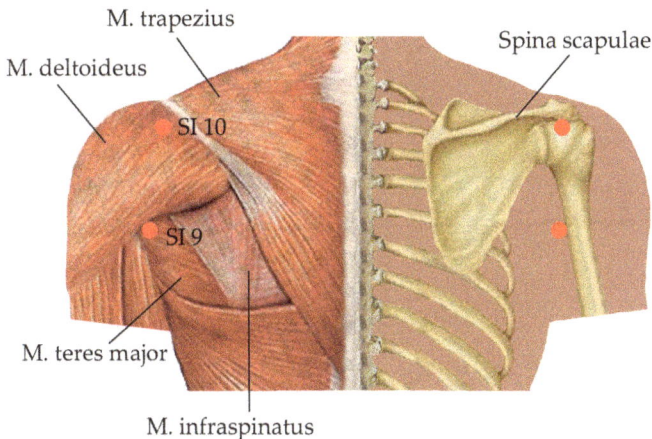

SI 10

SI 9

3 cun

M. trapezius

M. deltoideus

Spina scapulae

SI 10

SI 9

M. teres major

M. infraspinatus

SI 11 – Tiān Zōng

[Locating]	On the scapula, in the depression one third of the distance from the center of the inferior border of the scapular spine to the inferior angle of the scapula, at the level with the fourth thoratic vertebra.
[Regional Anatomy]	The needle passes through the skin and subcutis, penetrates m. trapezius and reaches m. infraspinatus.
[Acupuncture and Moxibustion]	Insert the needle perpendicularly 0.5~1.0 cun deep and stimulate until there is a sore and numbing sensation in the local area radiating to the scapula and down to the fingers. This point can be moxibusted.
[Indications]	Pain in shoulder, arm, elbow, asthma, and carbuncle.

SI 12 – Bǐng Fēng

[Locating]	The point is located in the sitting or prone position, in the center of the supraspinous fossa, 1 cun superior to the spinous border forming a triangular with the points SI 10 (Nào Shū) and SI 11 (Tiān Zōng).
[Regional Anatomy]	The needle passes through the skin and subcutis and penetrates m. trapezius and m. supraspinatus.
[Acupuncture and Moxibustion]	Insert the needle perpendicularly 0.3~0.5 cun deep and stimulate until there is a sore and numbing sensation in the local area. This point can be moxibusted.
[Indications]	Pain and numbness of the shoulder and arm and inability to raise the arm.

SI 13 – Qǔ Yuán

[Locating]	On the scapula, at the medial end of supraspinous fossa, at the midpoint of the line connecting SI 10 (Nào Shū) to the second thoracic vertebra.
[Regional Anatomy]	The needle passes through the skin and subcutis and penetrates m. trapezius and m. supraspinatus.
[Acupuncture and Moxibustion]	Insert the needle perpendicularly 0.3~0.5 cun deep and stimulate until there is a sore and numbing in the local area. This point can be moxibusted.
[Indications]	Spasm and pain in shoulder and scapula and inability to raise the shoulder.

M. trapezius

M. deltoideus

SI 12

SI 13

Spina scapulae

SI 11

M. teres major

M. infraspinatus

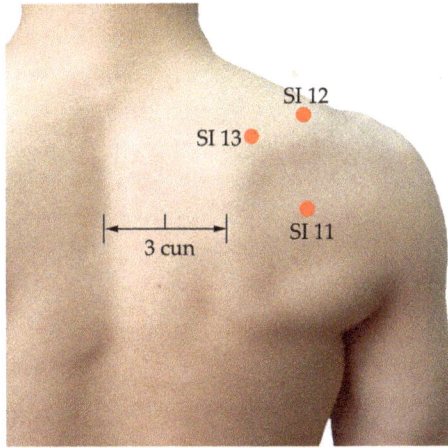

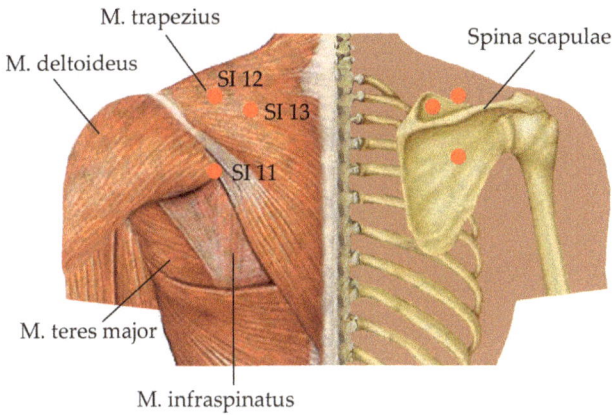

SI 14 – Jiān Wài Shū

[Locating]	The point is located in the sitting or prone position, 3 cun lateral to the posterior middle line, at the level with the medial side of scapula.
[Regional Anatomy]	The needle passes through the skin and subcutis, penetrates m. trapezius and reaches m. levator scapulae.
[Acupuncture and Moxibustion]	Insert the needle obliquely outward 0.3~0.5 cun deep and stimulate until there is a sore and numbing sensation in the local area. This point can be moxibusted.
[Indications]	Pain of the shoulder and back, neck stiffness, and coldness and pain of the arm.
[Note]	Avoid deep puncture to prevent pneumothorax.

SI 15 – Jiān Zhōng Shū

[Locating]	On the upper back, 2 cun lateral from the posterior midline, at the level with the inferior edge of the spinous process of the seventh cervical vertebra.
[Regional Anatomy]	The needle passes through the skin and subcutis and penetrates m. trapezius, m. rhomboideus minor and m. levator scapulae.
[Acupuncture and Moxibustion]	Insert the needle obliquely 0.3~0.5 cun deep and stimulate until there is a sore and numbing sensation in the local area. This point can be moxibusted.
[Indications]	Cough, asthma, pain in the shoulder and back and neck stiffness.
[Note]	Avoid deep puncture to prevent pneumothorax.

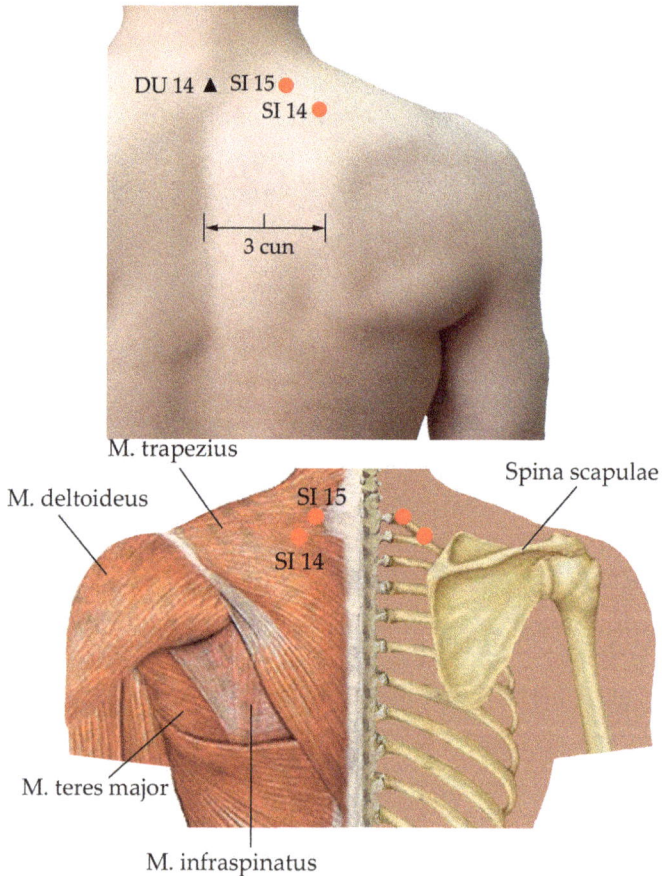

DU 14 ▲ SI 15 ●
SI 14 ●
3 cun

M. trapezius
M. deltoideus
SI 15
SI 14
Spina scapulae
M. teres major
M. infraspinatus

SI 16 – Tiān Chuāng

[Locating]	On the lateral aspect of the neck, on the posterior border of m. sternocleidomastoideus and posterior to LI 18 (Fú Tū), at the level with the Adam's apple.
[Regional Anatomy]	The needle passes through the skin and subcutis and penetrates m. trapezius, m. rhomboideus minor and m. levator scapulae.
[Acupuncture and Moxibustion]	Insert the needle perpendicularly 0.3~0.5 cun deep and stimulate until there is a sore and numbing sensation in the local area radiating to the ear. This point can be moxibusted.
[Indications]	Deafness, tinnitus, sore throat, and sudden loss of voice.

SI 17 – Tiān Róng

[Locating]	The point is located in the sitting or supine position, at the level with the corner of jaw, anterior to the sternocleidomastoid musle, on the inferior border of the posterior m. digastric.
[Regional Anatomy]	The needle passes through the skin and subcutis, penetrates m. stylohyoideus and reaches vagina carotica.
[Acupuncture and Moxibustion]	Insert the needle perpendicularly 0.5~0.8 cun deep and stimulate until there is a sore and numbing sensation in the local area radiating to the base of the tongue or throat. This point can be moxibusted.
[Indications]	Sore throat, tinnitus and deafness.
[Note]	Avoid puncturing the blood vessel.

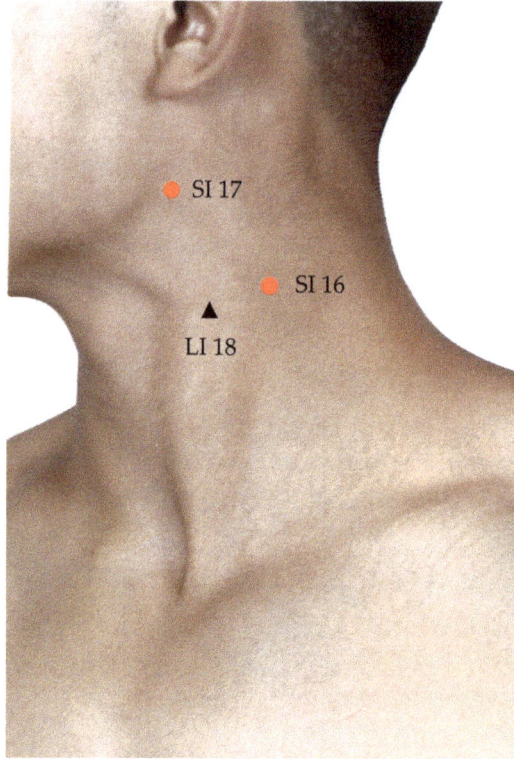

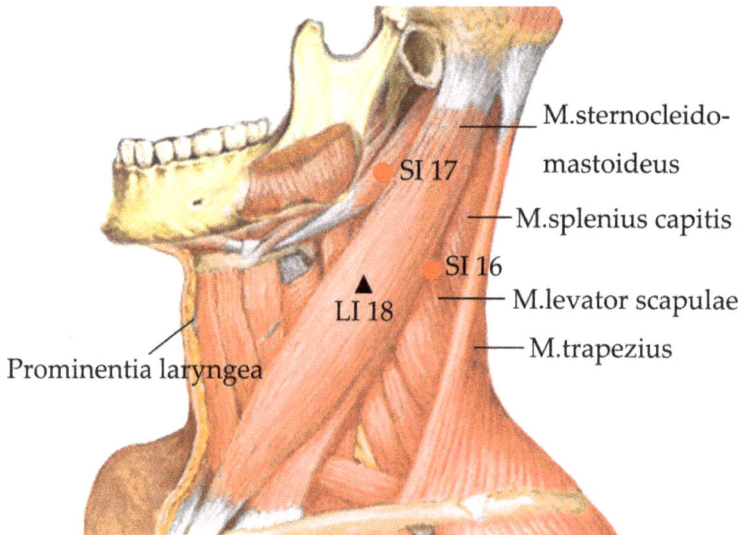

M.sternocleido-
mastoideus

M.splenius capitis

M.levator scapulae

M.trapezius

Prominentia laryngea

SI 18 – Quán Liáo

[Locating]	On the face, inferior to the outer canthus, in the depression at the lower border of the zygomatic bone.
[Regional Anatomy]	The needle passes through the skin and subcutis, penetrates m. zygomaticus (which is innervated by the zygomatic branches of the facial nerve), and enters masseter m. temporalis.
[Acupuncture and Moxibustion]	Insert the needle perpendicularly 0.2~0.3 cun deep and stimulate until there is a sore and numbing sensation in the local area radiating to the lateral side of the face. This point can be moxibusted.
[Indications]	Toothache, swelling of the gum, spasm of the facial muscle, and facial paralysis.

SI 19 – Tīng Gōng

[Locating]	On the face, anterior to the tragus, posterior to the condyloid process of lower jaw bone, in the depression when the mouth is opened.
[Regional Anatomy]	The needle passes through the skin and subcutis and reaches the external meatal cartilage.
[Acupuncture and Moxibustion]	Insert the needle perpendicularly 0.5~1.0 cun deep and stimulate until there is a sore and numbing sensation in the local area radiating to the ear and lateral side of the face, and there might also be a distending sensation in the ear drum. This point can be moxibusted.
[Indications]	Tinnitus, deafness, toothache, loss of voice, epilepsy, and umbago.

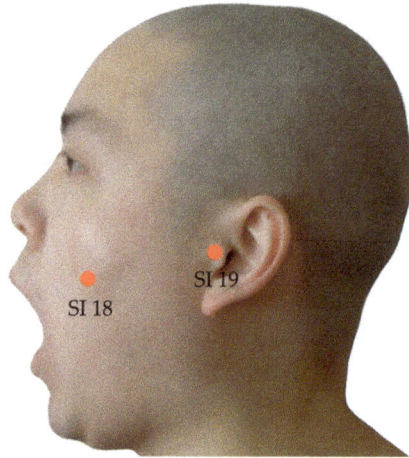

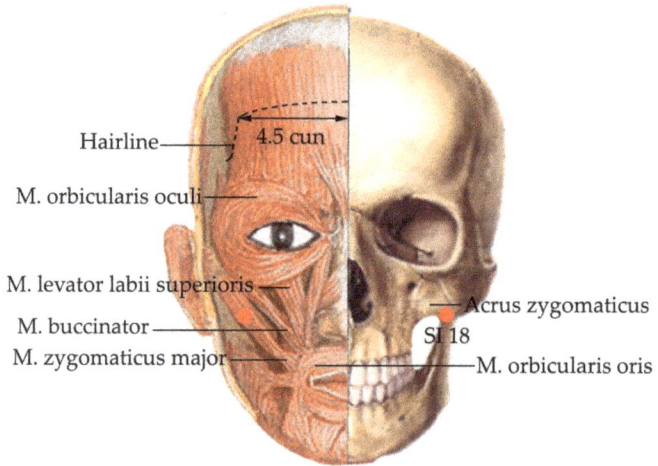

Hairline

4.5 cun

M. orbicularis oculi

M. levator labii superioris

M. buccinator

M. zygomaticus major

Acrus zygomaticus

SI 18

M. orbicularis oris

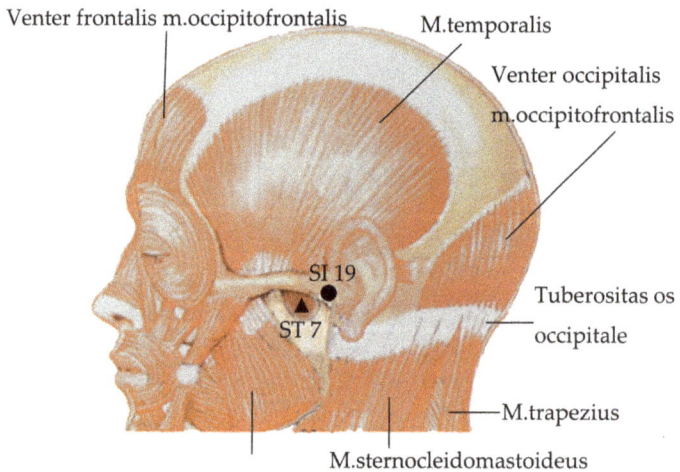

Venter frontalis m.occipitofrontalis

M.temporalis

Venter occipitalis
m.occipitofrontalis

Tuberositas os
occipitale

SI 19

ST 7

M.trapezius

M.sternocleidomastoideus

CHAPTER **8**

Bladder Channel of Foot Taiyang; BL

There are sixty-seven points on the Bladder Channel of Foot *Taiyang* and one hundred and thirty-four in total on both sides. There are forty-nine points on the head and face, neck, back and waist, eighteen points are distributed in the midline behind the lower limbs and the lateral part of the foot. The first point is BL 1 (Jīng Míng) and the last one is BL 67 (Zhì Yīn). The indications for this channel are the diseases of the urinary, reproductive, digestive, circulatory and respiratory systems as well as the syndromes along the course of the channel.

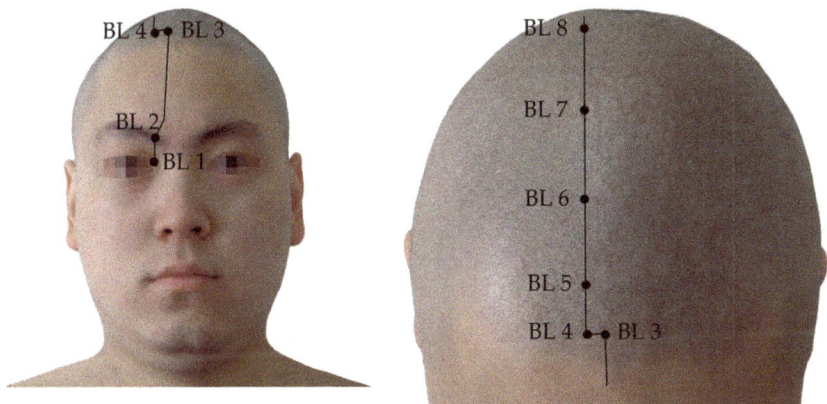

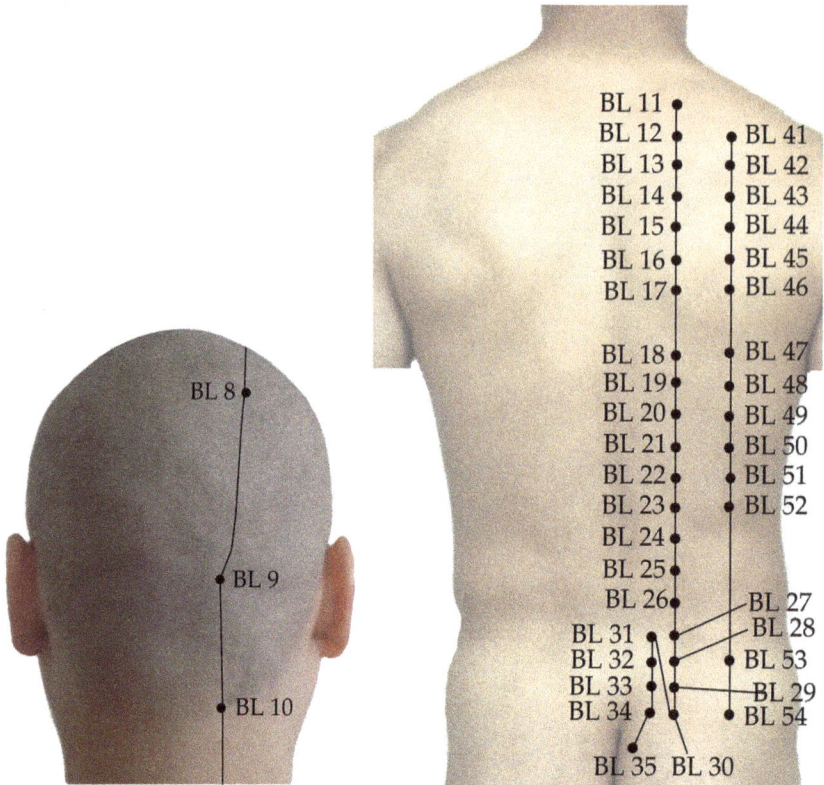

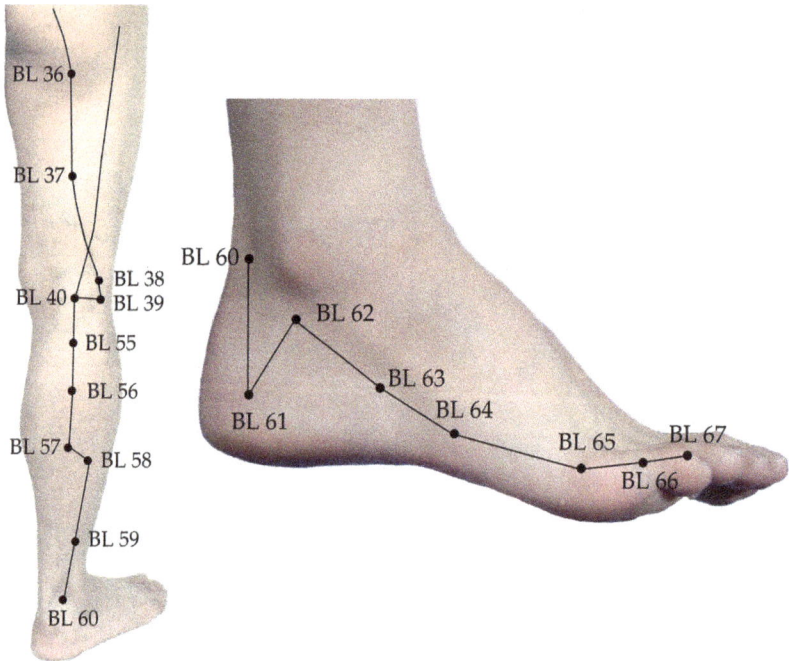

BL 1 – Jīng Míng

[Locating]	The point is located in the sitting position while looking upward or in the supine position, in the depression superior to the inner canthus, 0.1 cun superior to the inner canthus.
[Regional Anatomy]	The needle passes through the skin, subcutaneous tissues and penetrates the orbicularis oculi muscle, above the superior lacrimal canaliculus, and between the medial rectus muscle and ethmoid orbital plate.
[Acupuncture and Moxibustion]	Instruct the patient to close his eyes. the doctor gently pushes the eyeball with his left hand and fixes it to the outside. The right hand holds the needle to puncture the point slowly. The needle sticks 0.3 ~ 0.5 cun deep close to the orbit, without lifting, inserting and turning. There is a sour and distending sensation in the local area radiating to the periphery of the eye. Moxibustion is prohibited.
[Note]	Use a dry cotton ball to press the puncture site for a moment to avoid interal bleeding. The acupuncture at this point should not be too deep.

BL 2 – Cuán Zhú

[Locating]	The point is located in the sitting position while looking upward or in the supine position, in the depression of the medial end of the eyebrow, in the supraorbital notch.
[Regional Anatomy]	The needle passes through the skin, subcutaneous tissues and penetrates the m. occipitofrontalis and m. orbicularis oculi.
[Acupuncture and Moxibustion]	Insert the needle obliquely downwards or transversely towards EX-HN 4 (Yúyāo) 0.5~1.0 cun deep and stimulate until there is a sour and distending sensation around the eye. Moxibustion is prohibited.
[Indications]	Headache, pain in the supraorbital ridge, twitching of the eyelid, deviation of the mouth and eye, redness, swelling and pain of the eye, lacrimation, blurred vision and myopia.

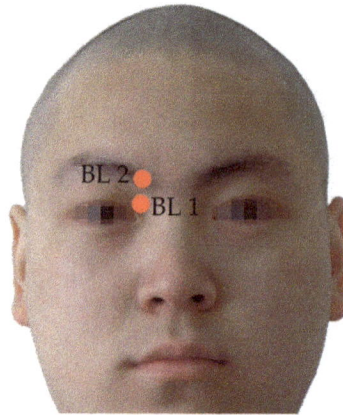

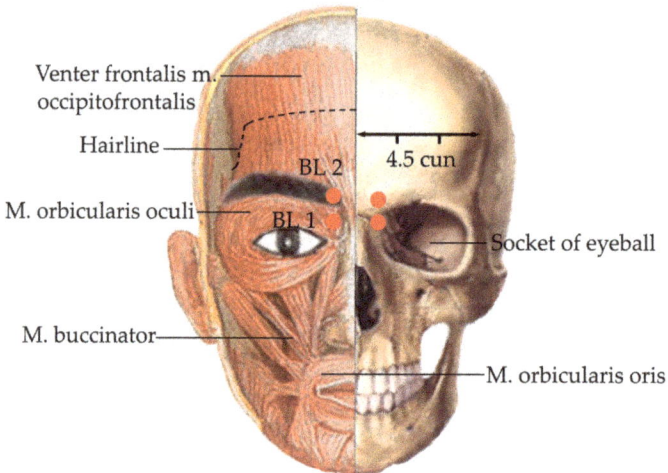

Venter frontalis m. occipitofrontalis

Hairline

M. orbicularis oculi

M. buccinator

BL 2

4.5 cun

BL 1

Socket of eyeball

M. orbicularis oris

BL 3 – Méi Chōng

[Locating]	The point is located in the sitting or supine position, 0.5 cun within the anterior hairline directly above BL 2 (Cuán Zhú).
[Regional Anatomy]	The needle passes through the skin, subcutaneous tissues and penetrates the m. occipitofrontalis. and the connective tissue beneath aponeurosis.
[Acupuncture and Moxibustion]	Insert the needle subcutaneously 0.3~0.5 cun deep and stimulate until there is a sore and distending sensation in the local area. This point can be moxibusted.
[Indications]	Dizziness, headache, nasal obstruction and blurred vision.

BL 4 – Qū Chā

[Locating]	The point is located in the sitting position while looking upward or in the supine position, 0.5 cun within the anterior hairline, 1.5 cun lateral to the midline, at the junction of the medial 1/3 and lateral 2/3 of the line connecting DU 24 (Shéntíng) to ST 8 (Tóuwéi).
[Regional Anatomy]	The needle passes through the skin, subcutaneous tissues and penetrates the m. occipitofrontalis.and the connective tissue beneath aponeurosis.
[Acupuncture and Moxibustion]	Insert the needle subcutaneously 0.3~0.5 cun deep and stimulate until there is a sore and distending sensation in the local area. This point can be moxibusted.
[Indications]	Headache, nasal obstruction, and epistaxis.

BL 5 – Wǔ Chù

[Locating]	The point is located in the sitting position while looking upward or in the supine position, 1.0 cun within the anterior hairline, 1.5 cun lateral to the midline.
[Regional Anatomy]	The needle passes through the skin, subcutaneous tissues and penetrates the m. occipitofrontalis.and the connective tissue beneath aponeurosis.
[Acupuncture and Moxibustion]	Insert the needle subcutaneously 0.3~0.5 cun deep and stimulate until there is a sore and distending sensation in the local area. This point can be moxibusted.
[Indications]	Infantile convulsion, headache, dizziness and blurred vision. 0.3~0.5 cun deep and stimulate until there is a sore and distending sensation in the local area. This point could be moxibusted.
[Indications]	Infantile convulsion, headache, dizziness and blurred vision. Insert the needle subcutaneously

Venter frontalis m. occipitofrontalis — BL 5, BL 4, BL 3

Hairline

4.5 cun

M. buccinator

M. orbicularis oris

ST 8

BL 5

DU 24

BL 4

BL 3

4.5 cun

5.5 cun

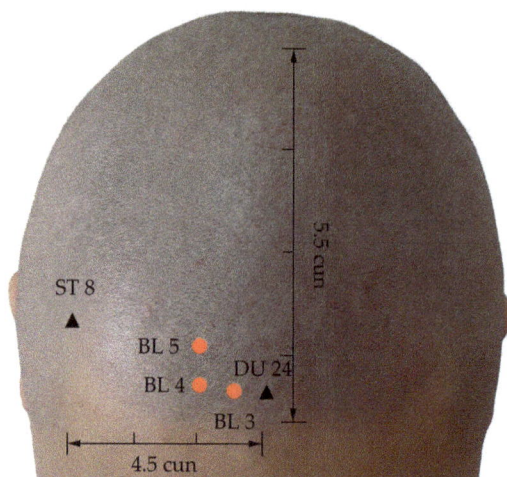

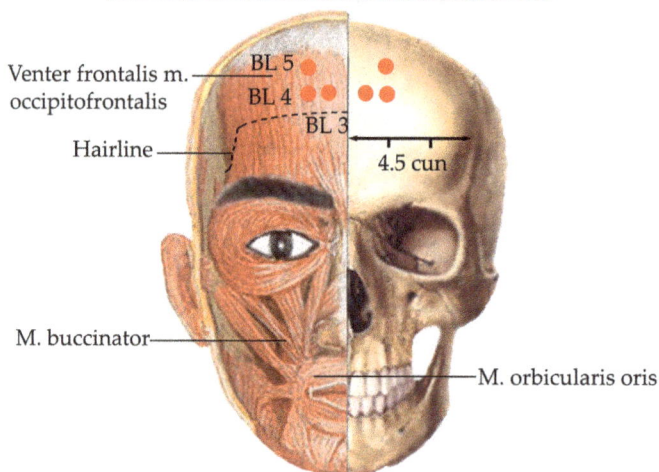

BL 6 – Chéng Guāng

[Locating]	The point is located in the sitting position while looking upward or in the supine position, 2.5 cun within the anterior hairline, 1.5 cun lateral to the midline.
[Regional Anatomy]	The needle passes through the skin subcutaneous tissues and penetrates the galea aponeurotica and the connective tissue beneath the neurosis.
[Acupuncture and Moxibustion]	Insert the needle subcutaneously
[Indications]	Headache, eye pain and blurred vision.

BL 7 – Tōng Tiān

[Locating]	The point is located in the sitting position while look-ing upward, 4.0 cun within the anterior hairline, 1.5 cun lateral to the midline.
[Regional Anatomy]	The needle passes through the skin subcutaneous tis-sues and penetrates the galea aponeurotica and the connective tissue beneath the aponeurosis.
[Acupuncture and Moxibustion]	Insert the needle subcutaneously 0.3~0.5 cun deep and stimulate until there is a sore and distending sen-sation in the local area. This point can be moxibusted.
[Indications]	Headache, and nasal obstruction.

BL 8 – Luò Què

[Locating]	The point is located in the sitting position while look-ing upward, 5.5 cun within the anterior hairline, 1.5 cun lateral to the midline.
[Regional Anatomy]	The needle passes through the skin, subcutaneous tis-sues and penetrates the galea aponeurotica and con-nective tissue beneath aponeurosis.
[Acupuncture and Moxibustion]	Insert the needle subcutaneously 0.3~0.5 cun deep and stimulate until there is a sore and distending sen-sation in the local area. This point can be moxibusted.
[Indications]	Dizziness, nasal obstruction, and epilepsy.

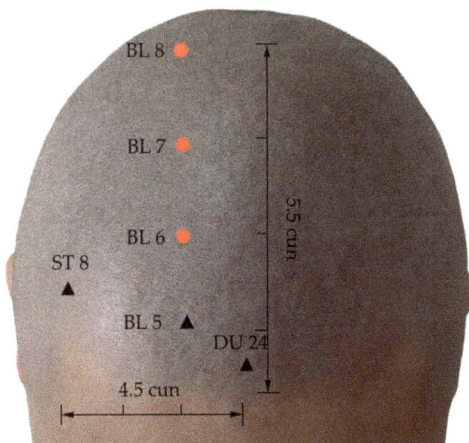

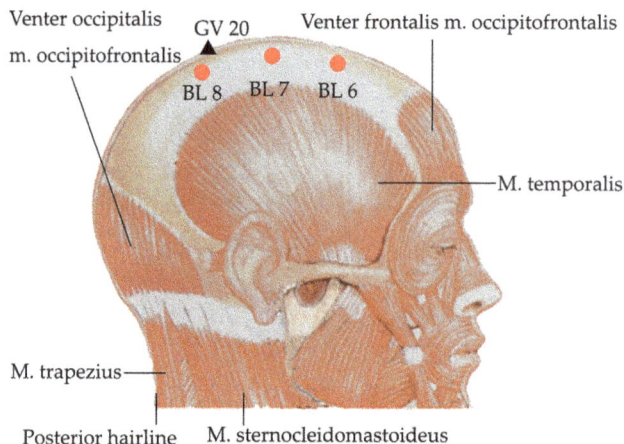

Venter occipitalis m. occipitofrontalis · GV 20 · Venter frontalis m. occipitofrontalis
BL 8 · BL 7 · BL 6
M. temporalis
M. trapezius
Posterior hairline · M. sternocleidomastoideus

BL 9 – Yù Zhěn

[Locating]	DU 17 (Nǎo Hù) is located in the depression superior to the external occipital protuberance. The point is located in the sitting or prone position, 1.3 cun lateral to DU 17 (Nǎo Hù).
[Regional Anatomy]	The needle passes through the skin, subcutaneous tissues and penetrates the galea aponeurotica and connective tissue beneath aponeurosis.
[Acupuncture and Moxibustion]	Insert the needle subcutaneously 0.3~0.5 cun deep and stimulate until there is a sour and distending sensation in the local area. This point can be moxibusted.
[Indications]	Headache, and nasal obstruction.

BL 10 – Tiān Zhù

[Locating]	The point is located in the sitting position with the head bent forward or in the prone position, in the depression on the lateral border of m. trapezius, 0.5 cun superior to the posterior hairline, 1.3 cun lateral to the midline.
[Regional Anatomy]	The needle passes through the, subcutaneous tissues and penetrates the m. trapezius, m. splenius capitis, m. semispinalis capitis and m. rectus capitis posterior major.

[Acupuncture and Moxibustion]	Insert the needle perpendicularly 0.5~0.8 cun deep and stimulate until there is a sour and distending sensation in the local area radiating to the occiput and the eyes. This point can be moxibusted.
[Indications]	Headache and redness, neck stiffness, pain in the shoulder, and back and lumbago.
[Note]	Acupuncture should be straight forward, do not go inward, so as not to penetrate the posterior membrane of the atlantoaxial to enter the spinal canal and damage the medulla oblongata.

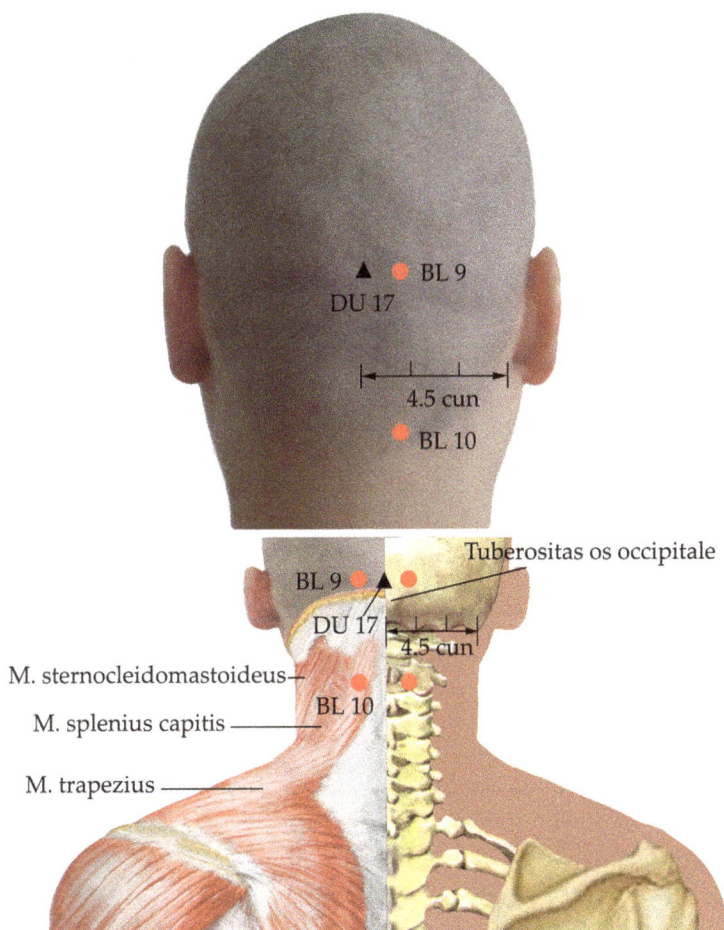

BL 11 – Dà Zhù

[Features]	One of the Eight Influential Point. Influential point of the bone.
[Locating]	The point is located in the sitting position with the head bent forward or in the prone position, on the upper back, at the level with the inferior border of the spinous process of the first thoracic vertebra, 1.5 cun lateral to the posterior midline.
[Regional Anatomy]	The needle passes through the skin, subcutaneous tissues and penetrates m. trapezius, rhomboideus.m serratus posterior superior.m. sacrospinalis and intertransverse muscle.
[Acupuncture and Moxibustion]	Insert the needle obliquely towards the spine 0.5~0.8 cun deep and stimulate until there is a sour and distending sensation in the local area radiating to the intercostal space or the shoulder. This point can be moxibusted.
[Indications]	Neck stiffness, pain in the shoulder and back, cough and tightness in the chest.
[Note]	A deep puncture is contraindicated to avoid damaging the pleura and lung.

BL 12 – Fēng Mén

[Locating]	The point is located in the prone position, on the upper back at the level with the inferior border of the spinous process of the second thoracic vertebra, 1.5 cun lateral to the posterior midline.
[Regional Anatomy]	The needle passes through the skin, subcutaneous tissues and penetrates m. trapezius, rhomboideus,m. serratus posterior superior and m. sacrospinalis.
[Acupuncture and Moxibustion]	Insert the needle obliquely towards the spine 0.5~0.8 cun deep and stimulate until there is a sour and distending sensation in the local area radiating to the intercostal space. This point can be moxibusted.
[Indications]	Cold, cough, nasal obstruction, fever and headache.
[Note]	A deep puncture is contraindicated to avoid damaging the pleura and lung.

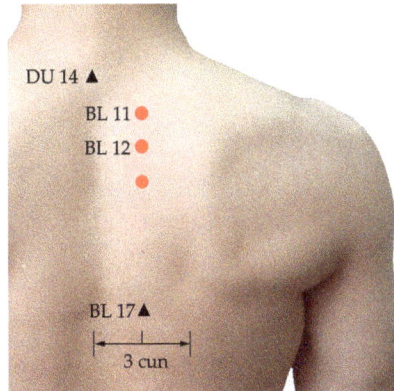

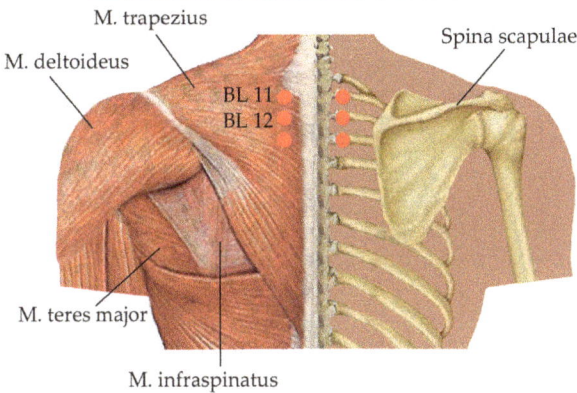

DU 14 ▲
BL 11 ●
BL 12 ●
●

BL 17 ▲
├──────┤
3 cun

M. trapezius
M. deltoideus
Spina scapulae
BL 11 ●
BL 12 ●
M. teres major
M. infraspinatus

BL 13 – Fèi Shū

[Features]	Back-shu point of the lung.
[Locating]	The point is located in the prone position, on the upper back, at the level with the inferior border of the spinous process of the third thoracic vertebra, 1.5 cun lateral to the posterior midline.
[Regional Anatomy]	The needle passes through the subcutaneous tissues and penetrates m.trapezius, rhomboideus and m. sacrospinalis.
[Acupuncture and Moxibustion]	Insert the needle obliquely towards the spine 0.5~0.8 cun deep and stimulate until there is a sour and distending sensation in the local area radiating to the intercostal space. This point can be moxibusted.
[Indications]	Cough, pain in chest and back pain.
[Note]	It is the same as BL11(Dà Zhù).

DU 14 ▲

BL 13●

BL 17▲

3 cun

M. trapezius

M. deltoideus

Spina scapulae

BL 13

M. teres major

M. infraspinatus

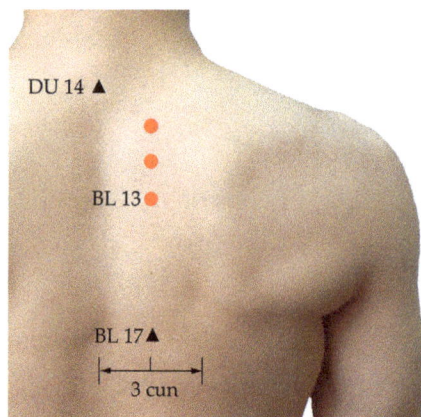

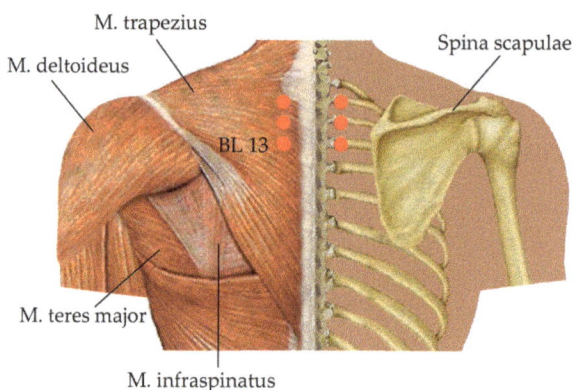

BL 14 – Jué Yīn Shū

[Features]	Back-shu point of the pericardium.
[Locating]	The point is located in the prone position, on the upper back, at the level with the inferior border of the spinous process of the fourth thoracic vertebra, 1.5 cun lateral to the posterior midline.
[Regional Anatomy]	The needle passes through the skin, subcutaneous tissues and penetrates m. trapezius, rhomboideus and m. sacrospinalis.
[Acupuncture and Moxibustion]	Insert the needle obliquely towards the spine 0.5~0.8 cun deep and stimulate until there is a sour and distending sensation in the local area radiating to the intercostal space.
	This point can be moxibusted.
[Indications]	Cardiac pain, palpitation and chest distention .
[Note]	It is the same as BL11(Dà Zhù).

BL 15 – Xīn Shū

[Features]	Back-shu point of the heart.
[Locating]	The point is located in the prone position, on the upper back, at the level with the inferior border of the spinous process of the fifth thoracic vertebra, 1.5 cun lateral to the posterior midline.
[Regional Anatomy]	The needle passes through the subcutaneous tissues and penetrates m. trapezius and m. sacrospinalis.
[Acupuncture and Moxibustion]	Insert the needle obliquely towards the spine 0.5~0.8 cun deep and stimulate until there is a sour and distending sensation in the local area radiating to the intercostal space. This point can be moxibusted.
[Indications]	Cardiac pain, palpitation, chest distention, cough, insomnia, forgetfulness, nocturnal emission, and night sweats.
[Note]	It is the same as BL11 (Dà Zhù).

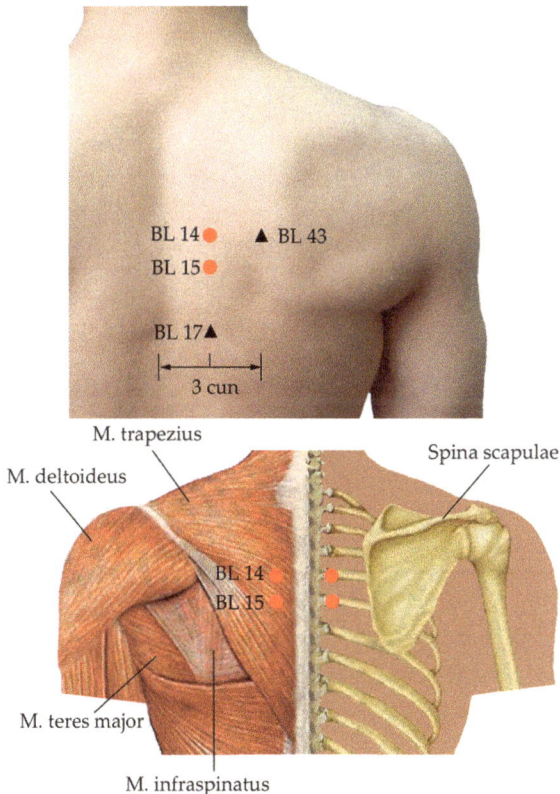

BL 14   ▲ BL 43
BL 15
BL 17▲
3 cun

M. trapezius
M. deltoideus
Spina scapulae
BL 14
BL 15
M. teres major
M. infraspinatus

BL 16 – Dū Shū

[Locating]	The point is located in the prone position, on the upper back, level with the inferior border of the spinous process of the fifth thoracic vertebra, 1.5 cun lateral to the posterior midline.
[Regional Anatomy]	The needle passes through the skin, subcutaneous tissues and penetrates m. trapezius and m. sacrospinalis.
[Acupuncture and Moxibustion]	Insert the needle obliquely towards the spine 0.5~0.8 cun deep and stimulate until there is a sour and distending sensation in the local area radiating to the intercostal space. This point can be moxibusted.
[Indications]	Cardiac pain, abdominal pain, abdominal distention, borborygums and emaciation.
[Note]	It is the same as BL11 (Dà Zhù).

BL 17 – Gé Shū

[Features]	Influential point of the blood.
[Locating]	The point is located in the prone position, on the back, at the level with the inferior border of the spinous process of the seventh thoracic vertebra, 1.5 cun lateral to the posterior midline at the level with the inferior edge of the scapula.
[Regional Anatomy]	The needle passes through the subcutaneous tissues and penetrates m. trapezius, m. latissimus dorsi and m. sacrospinalis.
[Acupuncture and Moxibustion]	Insert the needle obliquely towards the spine 0.5~0.8 cun deep and stimulate until there is a sour and distending sensation in the local area radiating to the intercostal space. This point can be moxibusted.
[Indications]	Cardiac pain, palpitation, vomiting, hiccough, chest pain, hemoptysis and blood in the stools.
[Note]	It is the same as BL11 (Dà Zhù).

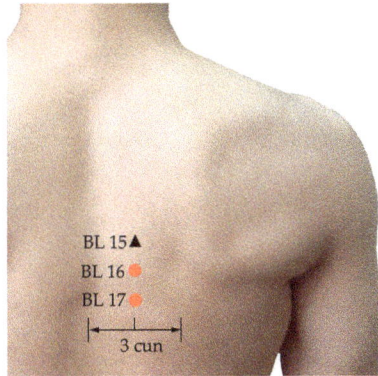

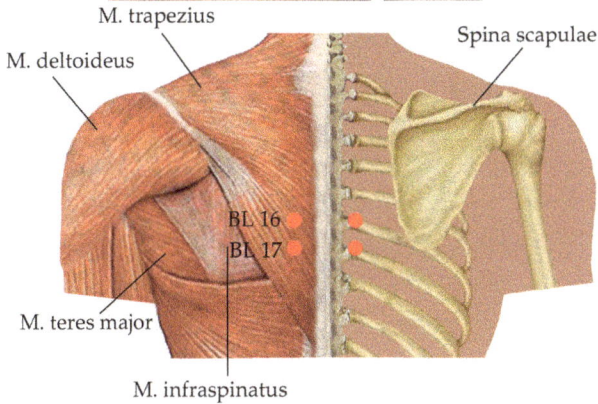

M. trapezius
M. deltoideus
Spina scapulae
BL 15▲
BL 16●
BL 17●
3 cun
BL 16●
BL 17●
M. teres major
M. infraspinatus

BL 18 – Gān Shū

[Features]	Back-shu point of the liver.
[Locating]	The point is located in the prone position, on the back, at the level with the inferior border of the spinous process of the ninth thoracic vertebra, 1.5 cun lateral to the posterior midline.
[Regional Anatomy]	The needle passes through the subcutaneous tissues and penetrates m. trapezius, m. latissimus dorsi and m. sacrospinalis.
[Acupuncture and Moxibustion]	Insert the needle obliquely towards the spine 0.5~0.8 cun deep and stimulate until there is a sour and distending sensation in the local area radiating to the intercostal space. This point can be moxibusted.
[Indications]	Abdominal distention, distension in the chest and hypochondriac rejions, jaundice, hematemesis, irregular menstruation, pain and redness of the eye, pain in the back and lumbar region, and cold hernia.
[Note]	It is the same as BL11 (Dà Zhù).

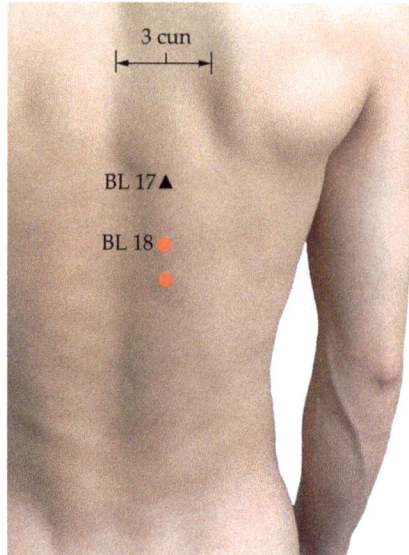

3 cun

BL 17▲

BL 18●

M. trapezius

BL 18●

Processus spinosus
(vertebrae thoracicae XII)

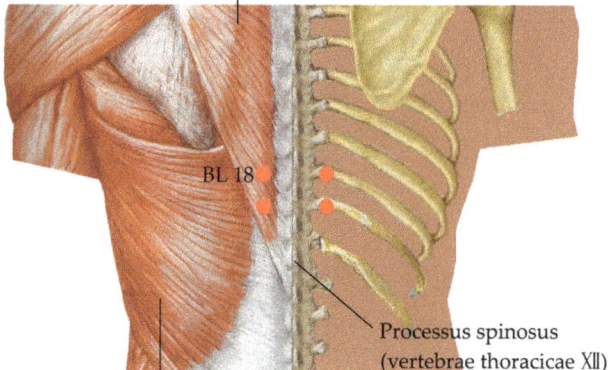

M. latissimus dorsi

BL 19 – Dǎn Shū

[Features]	Back-shu point of the gallbladder.
[Locating]	The point is located in the prone position, on the back, at the level with the inferior border of the spinous process of the tenth thoracic vertebra, 1.5 cun lateral to the posterior midline.
[Regional Anatomy]	The needle passes through the subcutaneous tissues and penetrates m. latissimus, dorsi m. serratus posterior inferior and m. sacrospinalis.

[Acupuncture and Moxibustion]	Insert the needle obliquely towards the spine 0.5~0.8 cun deep and stimulate until there is a sour and distending sensation in the local area radiating to the intercostal space. This point can be moxibusted .
[Indications]	Jaundice, bitter taste in the mouth and pulmonary phthisis.
[Note]	It is the same as BL11 (Dà Zhù).

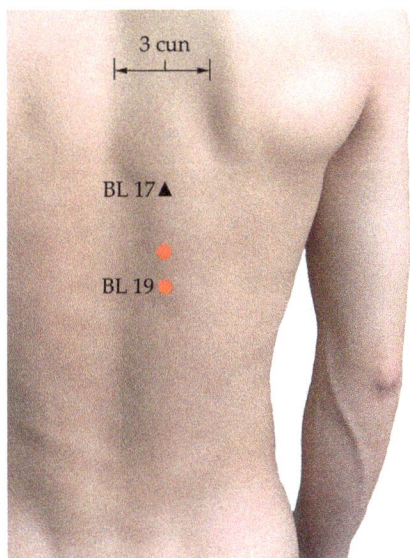

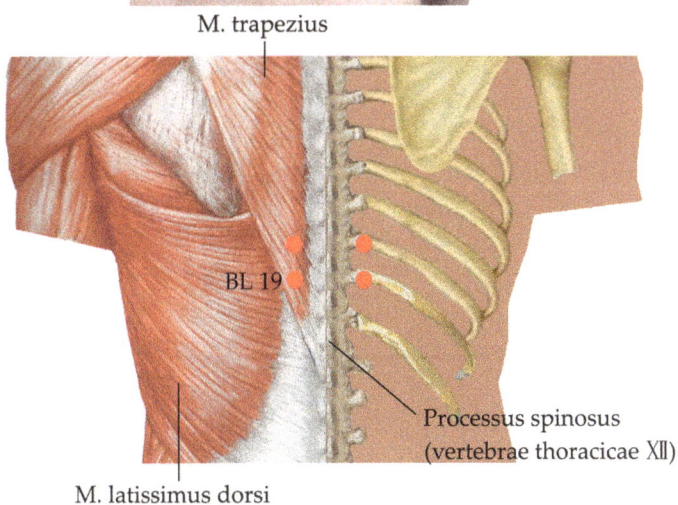

3 cun

BL 17▲

BL 19

M. trapezius

BL 19

Processus spinosus
(vertebrae thoracicae XII)

M. latissimus dorsi

BL 20 - Pí Shū

[Features]	Back-shu point of the spleen.
[Locating]	The point is located in the prone position, on the back at the level with the inferior border of the spinous process of the eleventh thoracic vertebra, 1.5 cun lateral to the posterior midline.
[Regional Anatomy]	The needle passes through the subcutaneous tissues and penetrates m. latissimus dorsi, m. serratus posterior inferior and m. sacrospinalis.
[Acupuncture and Moxibustion]	Insert the needle obliquely towards the spine 0.5~0.8 cun deep and stimulate until there is a sour and distending sensation in the local area radiating to the intercostal space. This point can be moxibusted .
[Indications]	Abdominal pain, vomiting, diarrhea, dysentery and blood in stools and urine.
[Note]	It is the same as BL11 (Dà Zhù).

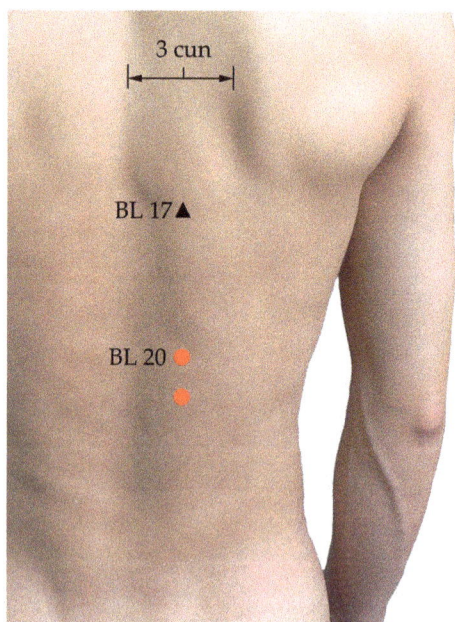

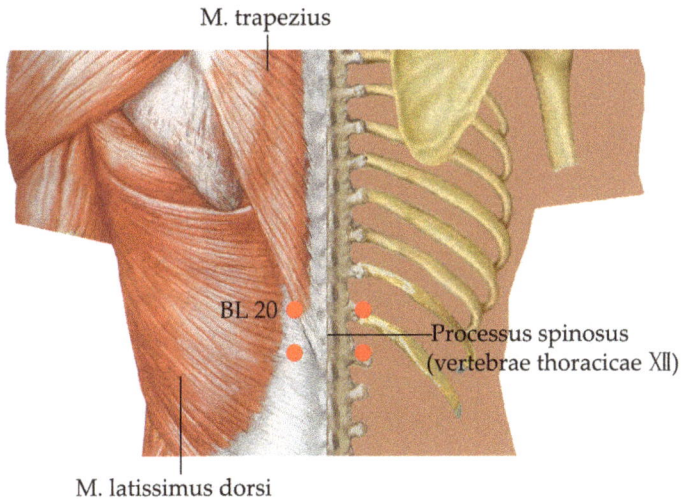

M. trapezius

BL 20

Processus spinosus
(vertebrae thoracicae XII)

M. latissimus dorsi

BL 21 – Wèi Shū

[Features]	Back-shu point of the stomach.
[Locating]	The point is located in the prone position, on the back at the level with the inferior border of the spinous process of the twelfth thoracic vertebra, 1.5 cun lateral to the posterior midline.
[Regional Anatomy]	The needle passes through the skin, subcutaneous tissues and penetrates m. latissimus dorsi m. serratus posterior inferior and m. sacrospinalis.
[Acupuncture and Moxibustion]	Insert the needle perpendicularly 0.5~0.8 cun deep and stimulate until there is a sour and distending sensation in the local area radiating to the abdomen. This point can be moxibusted.
[Indications]	Epigastric pain, vomiting and infantile malnutrition.
[Note]	A deep puncture is contraindicated.

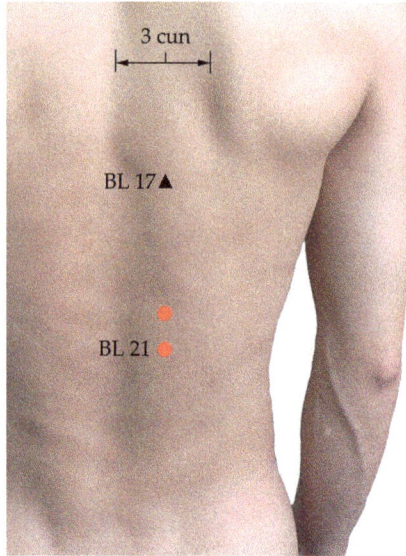

3 cun

BL 17▲

BL 21

M. trapezius

BL 21

Processus spinosus
(vertebrae thoracicae XII)

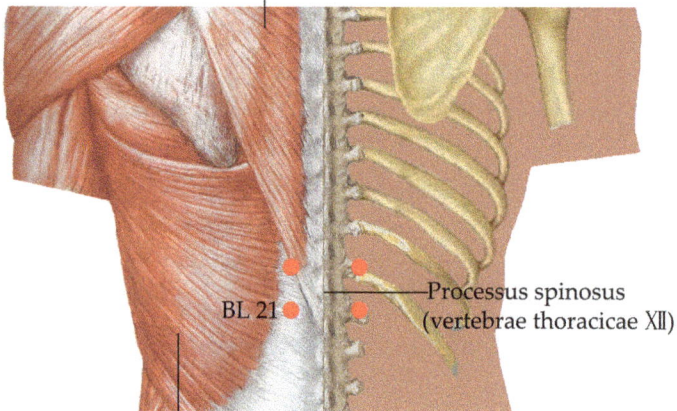

M. latissimus dorsi

BL 22 – Sān Jiāo Shū

[Features]	Back-shu point of the *Sanjiao*.
[Locating]	The point is located in the prone position, on the lower back at the level with the inferior border of the spinous process of the first lumbar vertebra, 1.5 cun lateral to the posterior midline.
[Regional Anatomy]	The needle passes through the skin, subcutaneous tissues and penetrates m. latissimus dorsim, serratus posterior inferior and m. sacrospinalis.

[Acupuncture and Moxibustion]	Insert the needle perpendicularly 0.8~1.0 cun deep and stimulate until there is a sour and distending sensation in the local area radiating to the abdomen.
	The point can be moxibusted.
[Indications]	Edema, dysuria , enuresis, borborygums and diarrhea.
[Note]	Deep puncture to the outside is contraindicated to avoid damaging the kidney by penetrating the posterior wall of abdominal cavity.

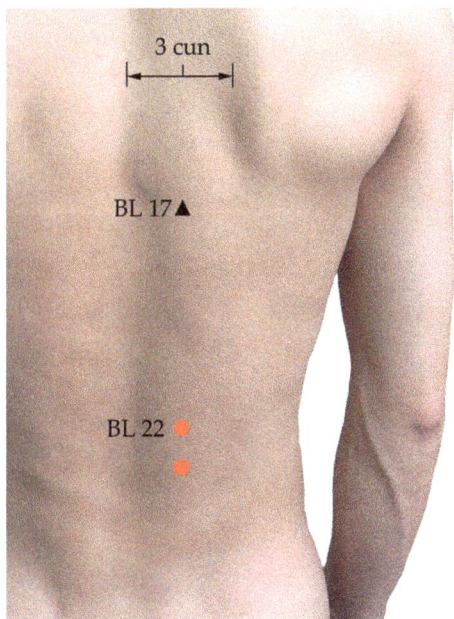

3 cun

BL 17▲

BL 22

M. latissimus dorsi

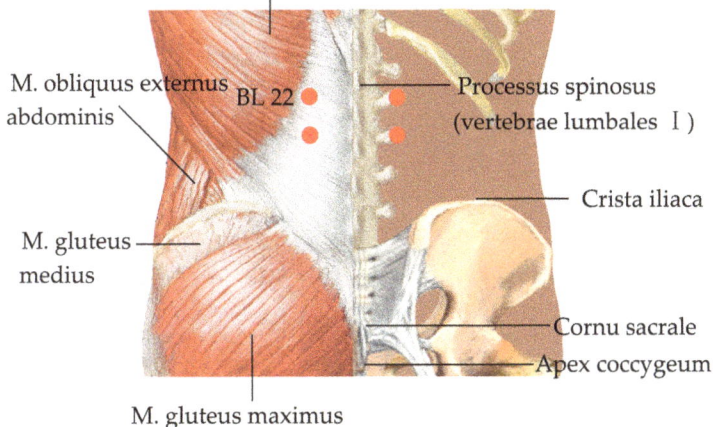

M. obliquus externus abdominis

BL 22

Processus spinosus (vertebrae lumbales Ⅰ)

Crista iliaca

M. gluteus medius

Cornu sacrale

Apex coccygeum

M. gluteus maximus

BL 23 – Shèn Shū

[Features]	Back-shu point of the kidney.
[Locating]	The point is located in the prone position, on the lower back at the level with the inferior border of the spinous process of the second lumbar vertebra, 1.5 cun lateral to the posterior midline.
[Regional Anatomy]	The needle passes through the skin, subcutaneous tissues and penetrates m. latissimus dorsi,m. sacrospinalis m. quadratus lumborum and m. psoas major.
[Acupuncture and Moxibustion]	Insert the needle perpendicularly 08~1.0 cun deep and stimulate until there is a sour and distending sensation in the local area radiating to the hip and down the leg. This point can be moxibusted.
[Indications]	Spermatorrhea, enuresis, edema, impotence, irregular menstruation, blurred vision, tinnitus and deafness, pain and soreness of the lower back and knees.
[Note]	It is the same as BL22 (Sān Jāo Shū).

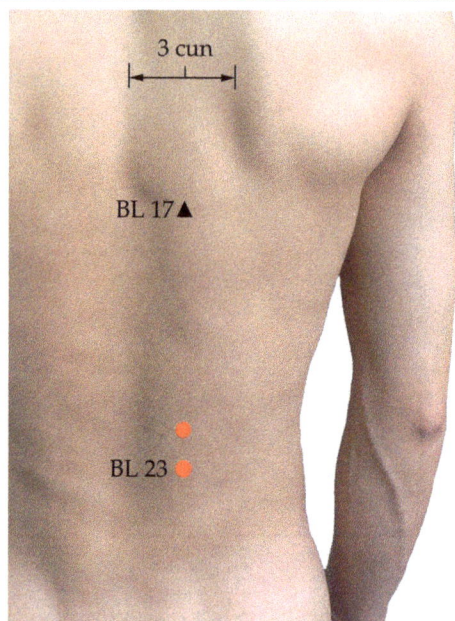

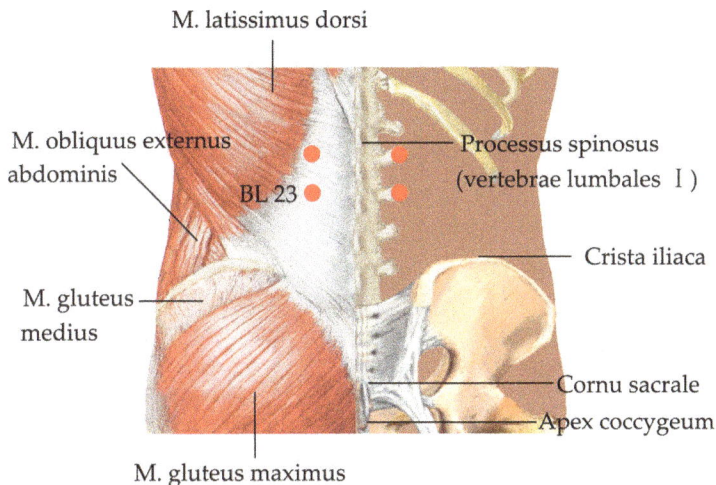

M. latissimus dorsi

M. obliquus externus abdominis

BL 23

Processus spinosus (vertebrae lumbales Ⅰ)

Crista iliaca

M. gluteus medius

Cornu sacrale

Apex coccygeum

M. gluteus maximus

BL 24 – Qì Hǎi Shū

[Locating]	The point is located in the prone position, on the lower back at the level with the inferior border of the spinous process of the third lumbar vertebra, 1.5 cun lateral to the posterior midline.
[Regional Anatomy]	The needle passes through the skin, subcutaneous tissues and penetrates m. latissimus dorsi,m. sacro-spinalism. quadratus lumborum and m. psoas major.
[Acupuncture and Moxibustion]	Insert the needle perpendicularly 0.8~1.0 cun deep and stimulate until there is a sour and distending sensation in the local area radiating to the hip and down the lower limb. This point can be moxibusted.
[Indications]	Dysmenorrhea, anal fistula, lumbago, and rigidity of the lower limbs and knees.

BL 25 – Dà Cháng Shū

[Features]	Back-shu point of the large intestine.
[Locating]	The point is located in the prone position, on the lower back at the level with the inferior border of the spinous process of the fourth lumbar vertebra, 1.5 cun lateral to the posterior middle line.

[Regional Anatomy]	The needle passes through the skin, subcutaneous tissues and penetrates m. latissimus dorsi,m. sacrospinalis m. quadratus lumborum and m. psoas major.
[Acupuncture and Moxibustion]	Insert the needle perpendicularly 0.8~1.0 cun deep and stimulate until there is a sour and distending sensation in the local area radiating to the hips and lower extremities. This point can be moxibusted.
[Indications]	Abdominal pain and distention, diarrhea, constipation, dysentery, stiffness and pain in the lumbar region.

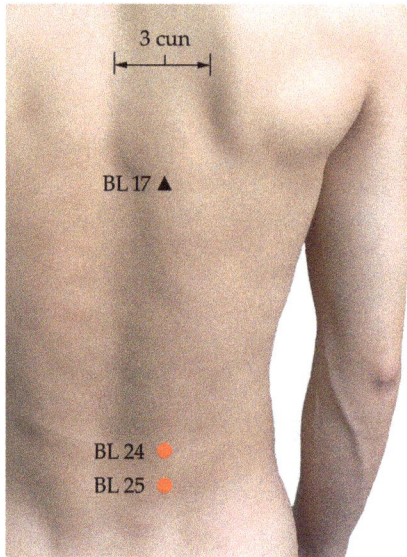

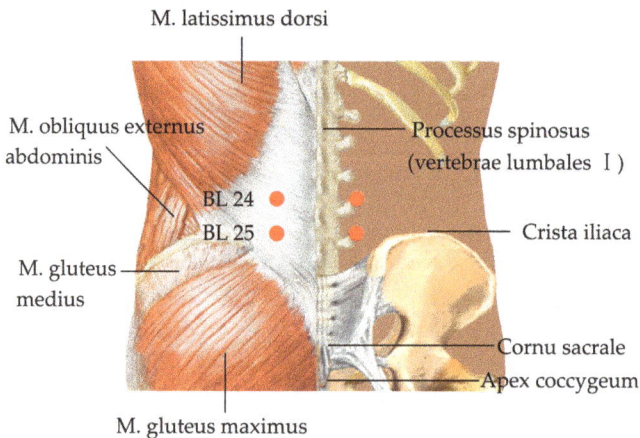

3 cun

BL 17 ▲

BL 24 ●
BL 25 ●

M. latissimus dorsi

M. obliquus externus
abdominis

BL 24 ●
BL 25 ●

Processus spinosus
(vertebrae lumbales Ⅰ)

Crista iliaca

M. gluteus
medius

Cornu sacrale
Apex coccygeum

M. gluteus maximus

BL 26 – Guān Yuán Shū

[Locating]	The point is located in the prone position, on the lower back at the level with the inferior border of the spinous process of the fifth lumbar vertebra, 1.5 cun lateral to the posterior middle line.
[Regional Anatomy]	The needle passes through the skin, subcutaneous tissues and penetrates m. latissimus dorsi,m. sacrospinalis,m. quadratus lumborum and m. psoas major.
[Acupuncture and Moxibustion]	Insert the needle perpendicularly 0.8~1.0 cun deep and stimulate until there is a sour and distending sensation in the local area, with an electric and numbing feeling radiating to the lower. This point can be moxibusted.
[Indications]	Abdominal distention, diarrhea, dysuria, enuresis and lumbago.

BL 27 – Xiǎo Cháng Shū

[Features]	Back-shu point of the small intestine.
[Locating]	The point is located in the prone position, on the lower back at the level with the inferior border of the spinous process of the first sacral vertebra, 1.5 cun lateral to the posterior middle line.
[Regional Anatomy]	The needle passes through the skin, subcutaneous tissues and penetrates m. latissimus dorsi and m. sacrospinalis
[Acupuncture and Moxibustion]	Insert the needle perpendicularly 0.8~1.0 cun deep and stimulate until there is a sour and distending sensation in the local area. This point can be moxibusted.
[Indications]	Dysentery, diarrhea, hernia, and hemorrhoids.

3 cun

DU 3 ▲

● BL 26
● BL 27

M. latissimus dorsi

M. obliquus externus
abdominis

Processus spinosus
(vertebrae lumbales I)

Crista iliaca

M. gluteus
medius

BL 26
BL 27

Cornu sacrale

Apex coccygeum

M. gluteus maximus

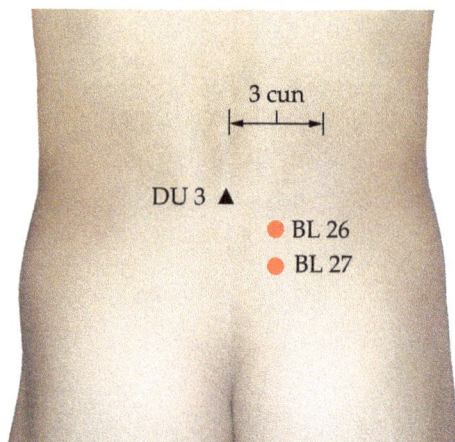

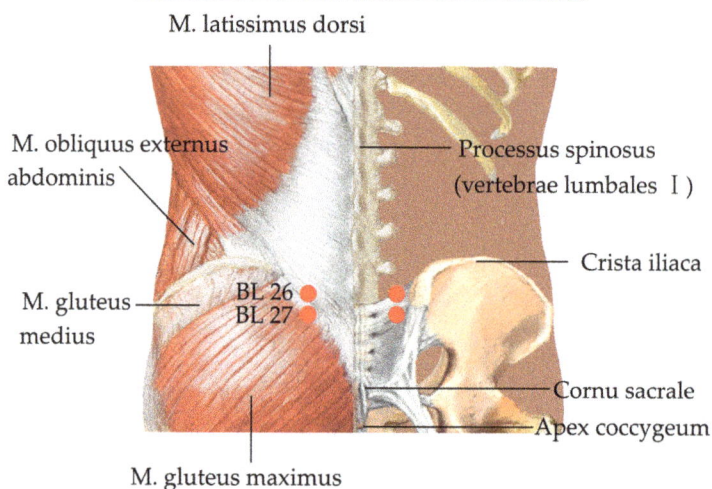

BL 28 – Páng Guāng Shū

[Features]	Back-shu point of the bladder.
[Locating]	The point is located in the prone position, on the sacrum, 1.5 cun lateral to the middle of the sacral crest, at the level with the second posterior sacral foramen.
[Regional Anatomy]	The needle passes through the skin, subcutaneous tissues and penetrates m. latissimus dorsi and m. sacrospinalis.
[Acupuncture and Moxibustion]	Insert the needle perpendicularly 0.8~1.0 cun deep and stimulate until there is a sour and distending sensation in the local area. This point can be moxibusted.
[Indications]	Difficulty and redness of the urination, hesitancy and obstruction, enuresis, and spermatorrhea.

BL 29 – Zhōng Lǚ Shū

[Locating]	The point is located in the prone position, on the sacrum, 1.5 cun lateral to the middle of the sacral crest, at the level with the third posterior sacral foramen.
[Regional Anatomy]	The needle passes through the skin, subcutaneous tissues and penetrates m. gluteus maximus and periosteum of the wing of ililum.
[Acupuncture and Moxibustion]	Insert the needle perpendicularly 0.8~1.0 cun deep and stimulate until there is a sore and numbing sensation in the local area. This point can be moxibusted.
[Indications]	Hernia, dysentery, stiffness and pain in the lower back, and thirst.

BL 30 – Bái Huán Shū

[Locating]	The point is located in the prone position, on the sacrum, 1.5 cun lateral to the middle of the sacrum, at the level with the fourth posterior sacral foramen.
[Regional Anatomy]	The needle passes through the skin, subcutaneous tissues and penetrates m. gluteus maximus and Sacrotuberous ligament.
[Acupuncture and Moxibustion]	Insert the needle perpendicularly 1.0~1.5 cun deep and stimulate until there is a sore and numbing sensation in the local area radiating to the hips. This point can be moxibusted.
[Indications]	Morbid leucorrhea, irregular menstruation, spermatorrhea, and pain in the waist and lower extremities.

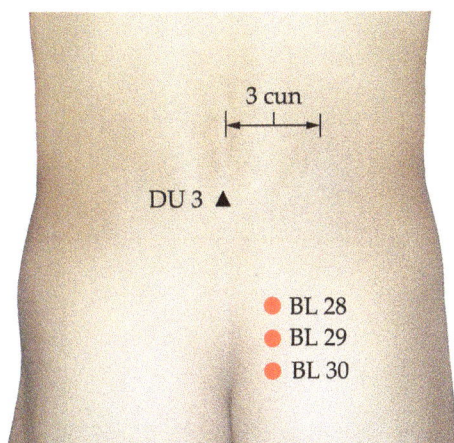

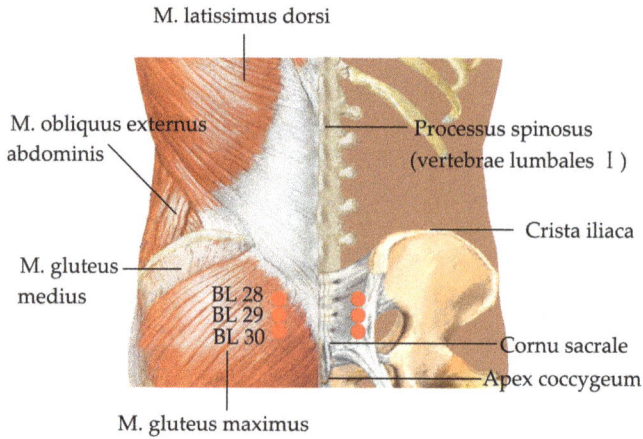

M. latissimus dorsi

M. obliquus externus abdominis

Processus spinosus (vertebrae lumbales I)

Crista iliaca

M. gluteus medius

BL 28
BL 29
BL 30

Cornu sacrale

Apex coccygeum

M. gluteus maximus

BL 31 – Shàng Liáo

[Locating]	The point is located in the prone position, between the line connecting the posterior superior iliac spine and the midline of the back, in the depression of the first posterior sacral foramen..
[Regional Anatomy]	The needle passes through the skin, subcutaneous tissues and penetrates m. sacrospinalis and 1st sacral foramen.
[Acupuncture and Moxibustion]	Insert the needle perpendicularly 0.8~1.0 cun deep and stimulate until there is a sour and distending sensation in the local area radiating to the perineum and the lower extremities. This point can be moxibusted.
[Indications]	Irregular menstruation, dysmenorrhea, spermatorrhea, impotence, prolapse of the uterus, difficulty in urination and defecation, knee soft, and pain in the lower back and sacrum.

BL 32 – Cì Liáo

[Locating]	The point is located in the prone position, medial and superior to the superior iliac spine, in the depression of the second posterior sacral foramen.
[Regional Anatomy]	The needle passes through the skin, subcutaneous tissues and penetrates m. sacrospinalis and 3rd sacral foramen.

[Acupuncture and Moxibustion]	Insert the needle perpendicularly 0.8~1.0 cun deep and stimulate until there is a sour and distending sensation in the local area radiating to the perineum and the lower extremities.
	This point can be moxibusted.
[Indications]	Irregular menstruation, constipation, and pain in the lower back and sacrum.

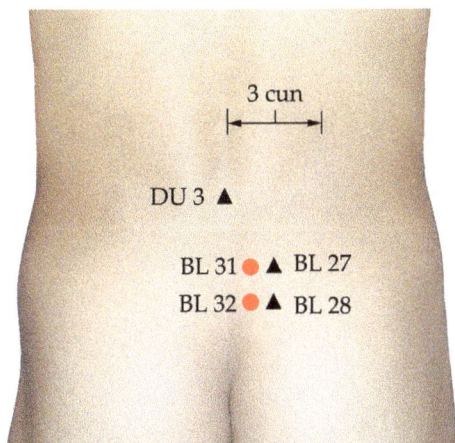

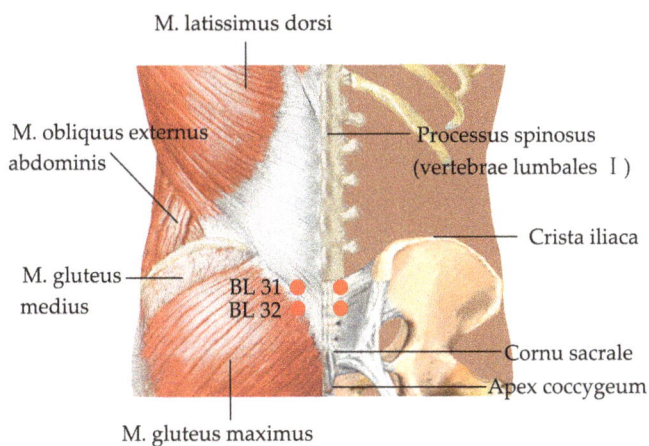

3 cun

DU 3 ▲

BL 31 ● ▲ BL 27
BL 32 ● ▲ BL 28

M. latissimus dorsi

M. obliquus externus abdominis

Processus spinosus (vertebrae lumbales I)

Crista iliaca

M. gluteus medius

BL 31
BL 32

Cornu sacrale

Apex coccygeum

M. gluteus maximus

BL 33 – Zhōng Liáo

[Locating]	The point is located in the prone position, medial and superior to the superior iliac spine, in the depression of the third posterior sacral foramen.
[Regional Anatomy]	The needle passes through the skin, subcutaneous tissues and penetrates m. sacrospinalis and 3rd sacral foramen.
[Acupuncture and Moxibustion]	Insert the needle perpendicularly 0.8~1.0 cun deep and stimulate until there is a sour and distending sensation in the local area radiating to the perineum and the lower extremities. This point can be moxibusted.
[Indications]	Irregular menstruation, constipation, and pain in the lower back and sacrum.

BL 34 – Xià Liáo

[Locating]	The point is located in the prone position, medial and superior to the superior iliac spine, in the depression of the fourth posterior sacral foramen.
[Regional Anatomy]	The needle passes through the skin, subcutaneous tissues and penetrates m. sacrospinalis and 4th sacral foramen.
[Acupuncture and Moxibustion]	Insert the needle perpendicularly 0.8~1.0 cun deep and stimulate until there is a sour and distending sensation in the local area radiating to the perineum and the lower extremities. This point can be moxibusted.
[Indications]	Lower abdominal pain, constipation, difficulty in urination and pain in the lower back and sacrum.

BL 35 – Huì Yáng

[Locating]	The point is located in the prone or kneeling position, in the region of the sacrum, 0.5 cun lateral to the end of the coccyx.
[Regional Anatomy]	The needle passes through the skin, subcutaneous tissues and penetrates m. sacrospinalis.
[Acupuncture and Moxibustion]	Insert the needle perpendicularly 0.8~1.0 cun deep and stimulate until there is a sour and distending sensation in the local area radiating to the perineum. This point can be moxibusted.
[Indications]	Diarrhea, hemorrhoids, blood in the stool, impotence. and morbid leucorrhea.

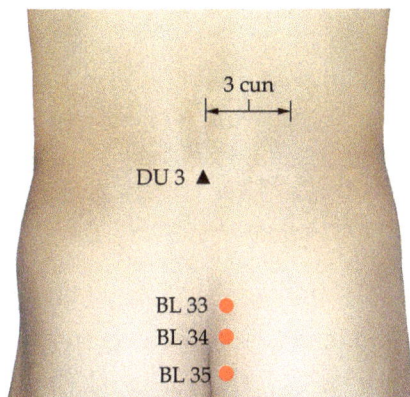

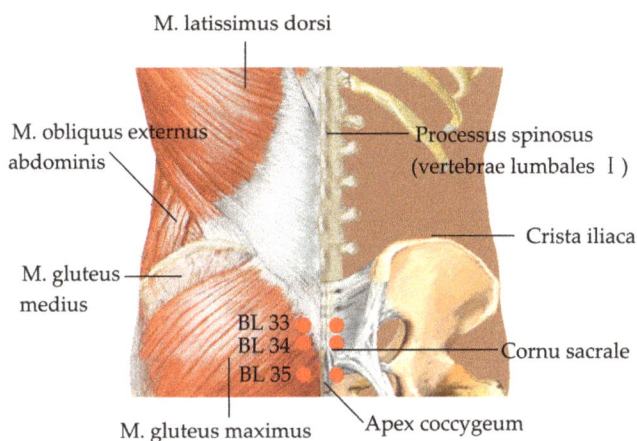

3 cun

DU 3 ▲

BL 33 ●
BL 34 ●
BL 35 ●

M. latissimus dorsi

M. obliquus externus
abdominis

Processus spinosus
(vertebrae lumbales I)

Crista iliaca

M. gluteus
medius

BL 33
BL 34
BL 35

Cornu sacrale

M. gluteus maximus

Apex coccygeum

BL 36 – Chéng Fú

[Locating]	The point is located in the prone position, on the posterior side of the thigh, in the middle of the transverse gluteal fold.
[Regional Anatomy]	The needle passes through the skin, subcutaneous tissues, fascia lata, n. ischiadicus and penetrates the adductor magnus.
[Acupuncture and Moxibustion]	Insert the needle perpendicularly 1.5-2.5 cun deep and stimulate until there is a sour and distending sensation in the local area with an electric sensation radiating to the heel. This point can be moxibusted.
[Indications]	Hemorrhoids, pain and numbness in the lower back and legs.

BL 37 – Yīn Mén

[Locating]	The point is located in prone position, on the posterior aspect of the thigh, 6 cun inferior to BL 36 (Chéng Fú), on the line connecting BL 36 (Chéng Fú) to BL 40 (Wěi Zhōng).
[Regional Anatomy]	The needle passes through the skin, subcutaneous tissues, fascia lata, n. ischiadicus and between the m. biceps femoris and m. semitendinosus.
[Acupuncture and Moxibustion]	Insert the needle perpendicularly 1.5~2.5 cun deep and stimulate until there is a sour and distending sensation in the local area, with an electric sensation radiating to the heel. This point can be moxibusted.
[Indications]	Pain in the lower back and legs.

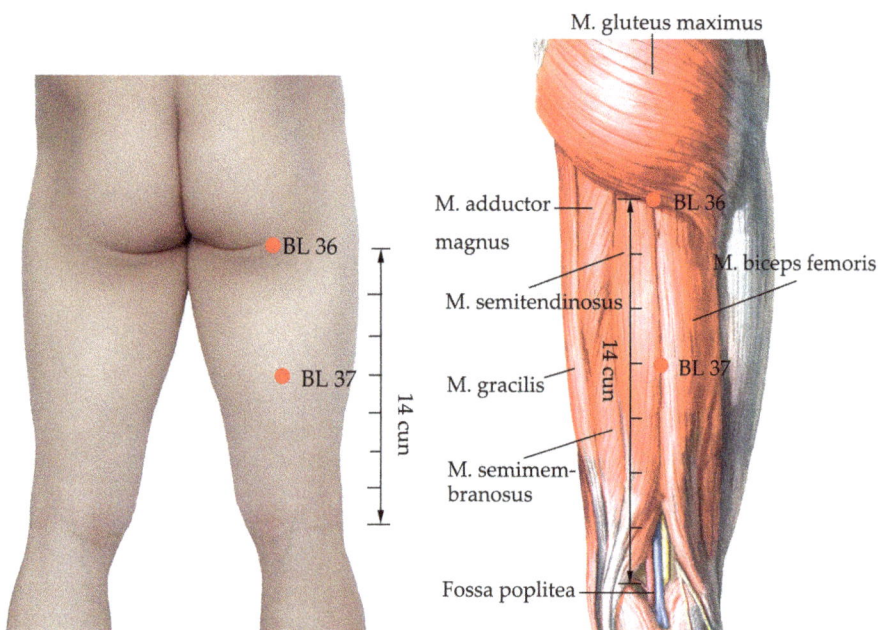

M. gluteus maximus

BL 36

BL 37

14 cun

M. adductor magnus

BL 36

M. biceps femoris

M. semitendinosus

M. gracilis

14 cun

BL 37

M. semimembranosus

Fossa poplitea

BL 38 – Fú Xì

[Locating]	The point is located in the prone position, above popliteal foss, 1 cun above BL 39 (Wěi Yáng), on the medial side of the tendon of the m. biceps femoris.
[Regional Anatomy]	The needle passes through the skin, subcutaneous tissues, popliteal fascia and n. peroneus communispenetrates.
[Acupuncture and Moxibustion]	Insert the needle perpendicularly 0.5~1.0 cun deep and stimulate until there is a sour and distending sensation in the local area, with an electric and numbing sensation radiating to the anterolateral side of the leg. This point can be moxibusted.
[Indications]	Pain and numbness in the lower legs.

BL 39 – Wěi Yáng

[Features]	Lower he-sea point of the Sanjiao.
[Locating]	The point is located in the prone position, on the lateral end of the popliteral transverse crease, on the medial side of the tendon of m. biceps femoris.
[Regional Anatomy]	The needle passes through the skin, subcutaneous tissues, popliteal fascia,n. peroneus communispenetrates, and penetrates the muscle of popliteal fossa.
[Acupuncture and Moxibustion]	Insert the needle perpendicularly 0.5~1.0 cun deep and stimulate until there is a sour and distending sensation in the local area radiating to the calf and thigh. This point can be moxibusted.
[Indications]	Difficulty in urination, enuresis, constipation, and pain in lower limbs.

BL 40 – Wěi Zhōng

[Features]	He-sea point of the Bladder Channel of Foot Taiyang. Lower He-sea point of the Bladder.
[Locating]	The point is located in prone position, at the midpoint of the transverse crease of the popliteal fossa, between the tendon of m. semitendinous and m.biceps femoris.
[Regional Anatomy]	The needle passes through the skin, subcutaneous tissues, popliteal fascia and penetrates the popliteal fossa and oblique popliteal ligament.

[Acupuncture and Moxibustion]	① Insert the needle perpendicularly 0.5~1.0 cun deep stimulate until there is a sore, distending and numbing sensation and radiating to the calf and foot.
	② Prick with a three-edged needle to bleed.
	This point can be moxibusted.
[Indications]	Lumbar pain, joint pain due to stagnation of damp-cold, hemiplegia, furuncle, abdominal pain, vomiting and diarrhea.

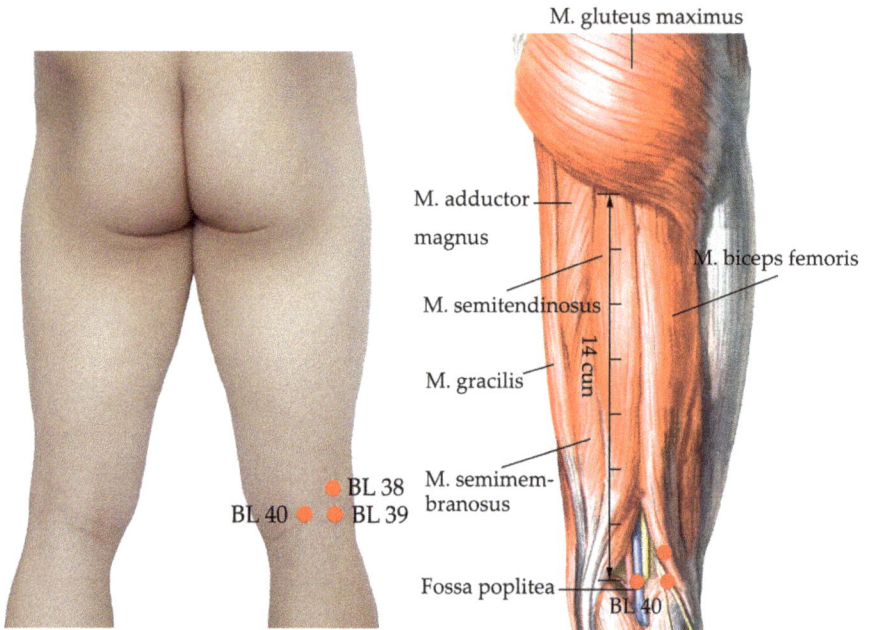

M. gluteus maximus
M. adductor magnus
M. biceps femoris
M. semitendinosus
14 cun
M. gracilis
M. semimem-branosus
BL 38
BL 40   BL 39
Fossa poplitea
BL 40

BL 41 – Fù Fēn

[Locating]	The point is located in prone position, at the level with the lower border of the spinous process of the second thoracic vertebrae, 3 cun lateral to the posterior midline.
[Regional Anatomy]	The needle passes through the skin, subcutaneous tissues and penetrates, m. trapezius, rhomboideus, m. serratus posterior superior and m. sacrospinalis.
[Acupuncture and Moxibustion]	Insert the needle obliquely 0.5~0.8 cun deep and stimulate until there a sour and distending sensation in the local area.
	This point can be moxibusted.

[Indications]	Pain and spasms of the shoulder and back, neck stiff-ness and numbness and pain of the arm and elbow.
[Note]	Avoid deep puncture to prevent pneumothorax

BL 42 – Pò Hù

[Locating]	The point is located in prone position,at the level with the lower border of the spinous process of the third thoracic vertebrae, 3 cun lateral to the posterior midline.
[Regional Anatomy]	The needle passes through the skin, subcutaneous tissues and penetrates,m. trapezius, rhomboideus,m. serratus posterior superior and m. sacrospinalis.
[Acupunc-ture and Moxibustion]	Insert the needle obliquely 0.5~0.8 cun deep and stim-ulate until there is a sour and distending sensation in the local area radiating to the shoulder. This point can be moxibusted.
[Indications]	Cough, asthma, neck stiffness, and pain of the shoul-der and back.
[Note]	It is the same as BL42 (Fùfēn).

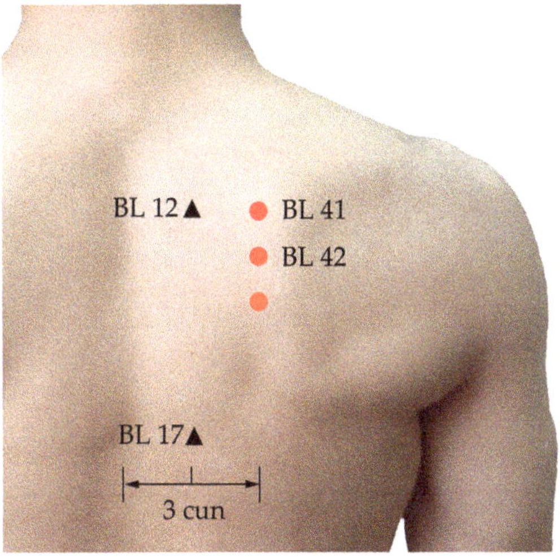

BL 12 ▲ ● BL 41
         ● BL 42
         ●

BL 17 ▲
|← 3 cun →|

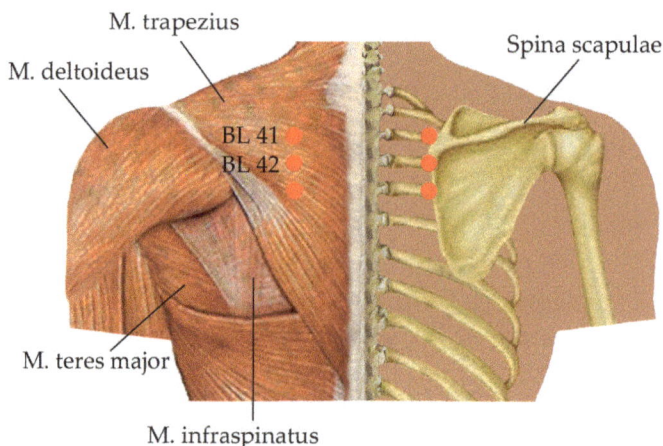

M. trapezius
M. deltoideus
Spina scapulae
BL 41
BL 42
M. teres major
M. infraspinatus

BL 43 – Gāo Huāng

[Locating]	The point is located in prone position, at the level with the lower border of the spinous process of the fourth thoracic vertebrae, 3 cun lateral to the posterior midline.
[Regional Anatomy]	The needle passes through the skin, subcutaneous tissues and penetrates m. trapezius, rhomboideus and m. sacrospinalis.
[Acupuncture and Moxibustion]	Insert the needle obliquely 0.5~0.8 cun deep and stimulate until there is a sour and distending sensation in the local area radiating to the shoulder.

This point can be moxibusted. |
| [Indications] | Cough, asthma, night sweating, amnesia, spermatorrhea, chronic weakness and diarrhea with undigested food. |
| [Note] | It is the same as BL42 (Fù Fēn). |

BL 12 ▲
BL 43
BL 17 ▲
3 cun

M. trapezius
M. deltoideus
Spina scapulae
BL 43
M. teres major
M. infraspinatus

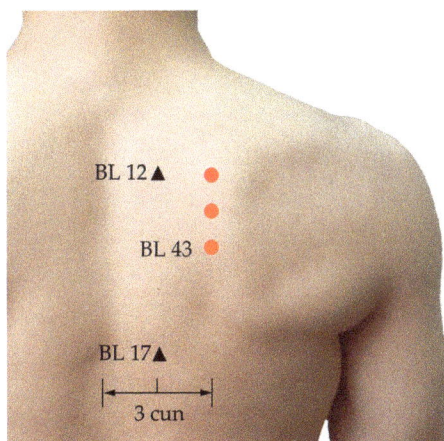

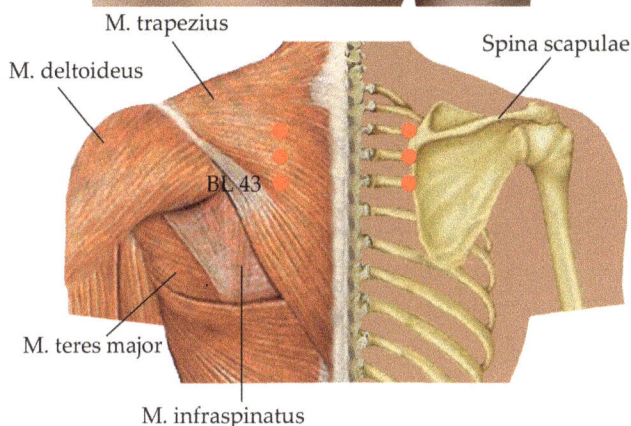

BL 44 – Shén Táng

[Locating]	The point is located in prone position, at the level with the lower border of the spinous process of the fifth thoracic vertebrae, 3 cun lateral to the posterior midline.
[Regional Anatomy]	The needle passes through the skin, subcutaneous tissues and penetrates m. trapezius, rhomboideus and m. sacrospinalis.
[Acupuncture and Moxibustion]	Insert the needle obliquely 0.5~0.8 cun deep and stimulate until there is a sour and distending sensation in the local area radiating to the shoulder. This point can be moxibusted.
[Indications]	Cardiac pain, palpitation, insomnia and depressive disorder.
[Note]	It is the same as BL42 (Fù Fēn).

BL 45 – Yì Xĭ

[Locating]	The point is located in prone position, at the level with the lower border of the spinous process of the sixth thoracic vertebrae, 3 cun lateral to the posterior midline.
[Regional Anatomy]	The needle passes through the skin, subcutaneous tissues and penetrates m. trapezius, rhomboideus and m. sacrospinalis.
[Acupuncture and Moxibustion]	Insert the needle obliquely 0.5~0.8 cun deep and stimulate until there is a sour and distending sensation in the local area radiating to the shoulder. This point can be moxibusted.
[Indications]	Cough, asthma, pain of the shoulder, back and costal region.
[Note]	It is the same as BL42 (Fù Fēn).

BL 46 – Gé Guān

[Locating]	The point is located in prone position, at the level with the lower border of the spinous process of the seventh thoracic vertebrae, 3 cun lateral to the posterior midline.
[Regional Anatomy]	The needle passes through the skin, subcutaneous tissues and penetrates m. latissimus dorsi and m. sacrospinalis.
[Acupuncture and Moxibustion]	Insert the needle obliquely 0.5~0.8 cun deep and stimulate until there is a sour and distending sensation in the local area. This point can be moxibusted.
[Indications]	a, vomiting, hiccupand, stiffness and pain in the back and choking sensation in chest.

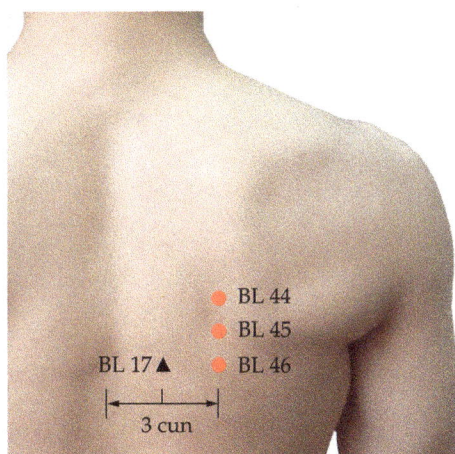

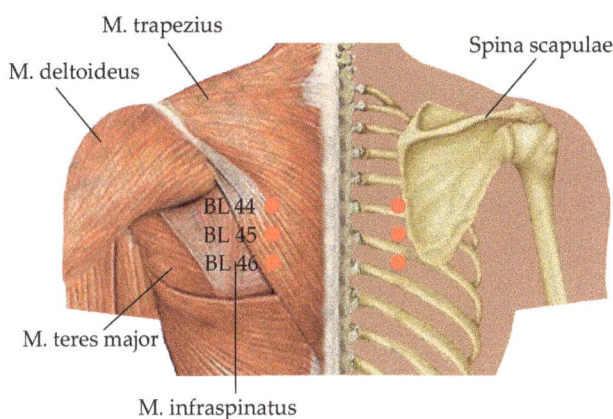

M. trapezius

M. deltoideus

Spina scapulae

BL 44
BL 45
BL 46

M. teres major

M. infraspinatus

BL 44
BL 45
BL 46

BL 17 ▲

3 cun

BL 47 – Hún Mén

[Locating]	The point is located in prone position, at the level with the lower border of the spinous process of the ninth thoracic vertebrae, 3 cun lateral to the posterior midline.
[Regional Anatomy]	The needle passes through the skin, subcutaneous tissues and penetrates m. latissimus dorsi,m. serratus posterior inferior and m. sacrospinalis.
[Acupuncture and Moxibustion]	Insert the needle obliquely 0.5~0.8 cun deep and stimulate until there is a sour and distending sensation in the local area. This point can be moxibusted.
[Indications]	Pain and distention of the chest, dysphagia, vomiting, pain in shoulder and back.
[Note]	It is the same as BL42 (Fù Fēn).

BL 48 – Yáng Gāng

[Locating]	The point is located in prone position, at the level with the lower border of the spinous process of the tenth thoracic vertebrae, 3 cun lateral to the posterior midline.
[Regional Anatomy]	The needle passes through the skin, subcutaneous tissues and penetrates m. latissimus dorsi,m. serratus posterior inferior and m. sacrospinalis.
[Acupuncture and Moxibustion]	Insert the needle obliquely 0.5~0.8 cun deep and stimulate until there is a sour and distending sensation in the local area. This point can be moxibusted.
[Indications]	Diarrhea, jaundice, abdominal pain, borborygums and diadetes.
[Note]	It is the same as BL42(Fù Fēn).

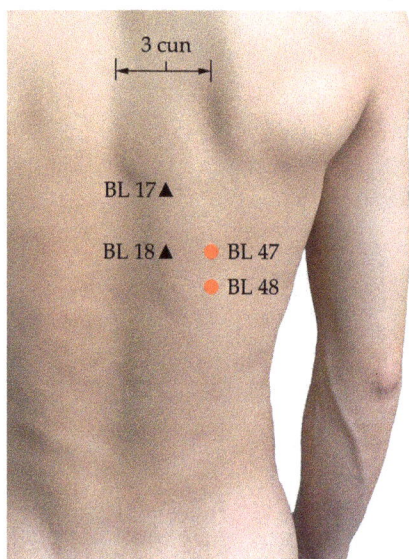

3 cun

BL 17▲

BL 18▲   ● BL 47
         ● BL 48

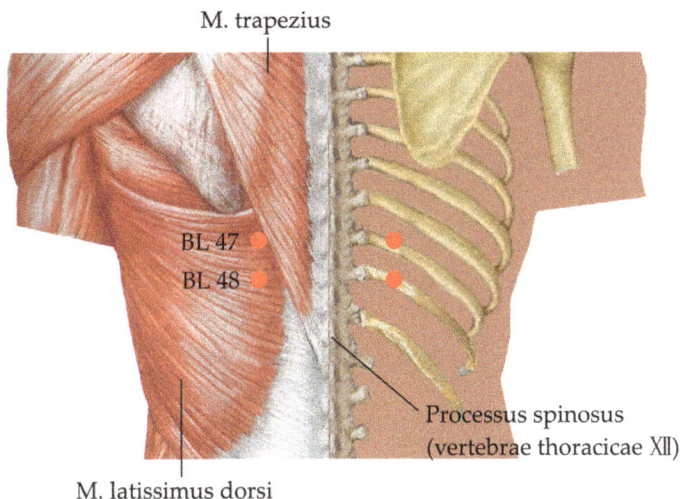

M. trapezius

BL 47
BL 48

Processus spinosus
(vertebrae thoracicae XⅡ)

M. latissimus dorsi

BL 49 – Yì Shè

[Locating]	The point is located in prone position, at the level with the lower border of the spinous process of the eleventh thoracic vertebrae, 3 cun lateral to the posterior midline.
[Regional Anatomy]	The needle passes through the skin, subcutaneous tissues and penetrates m. latissimus dorsi, m. serratus posterior inferior and m. sacrospinalis.
[Acupuncture and Moxibustion]	Insert the needle obliquely 0.5~0.8 cun deep and stimulate until there is a sour and distending sensation in the local area. This point can be moxibusted.
[Indications]	Abdominal distention, diarrhea, vomiting and anorexia.
[Note]	This point lies below the lower border of the lung, above the lower border of the pleura, the two come close when breathing deeply. So that a deep puncture is contraindicated to avoid damaging the pleura and the lung.

BL 50 – Wèi Cāng

[Locating]	The point is located in prone position at the level with the lower border of the spinous process of the twelfth thoracic vertebrae, 3 cun lateral to the posterior mid-line.
[Regional Anatomy]	The needle passes through the skin, subcutaneous tissues and penetrates m. latissimus dorsi.m. serratus posterior inferior and m. sacrospinalis.
[Acupuncture and Moxibustion]	Insert the needle obliquely 0.5~0.8 cun deep and stimulate until there is a sour and distending sensation in the local area. This point can be moxibusted.
[Indications]	Stomach ache, childhood malnutrition, abdominal distention, and pain in the back.
[Note]	Avoid deep puncture to prevent pneumothorax and injury to the viscera.

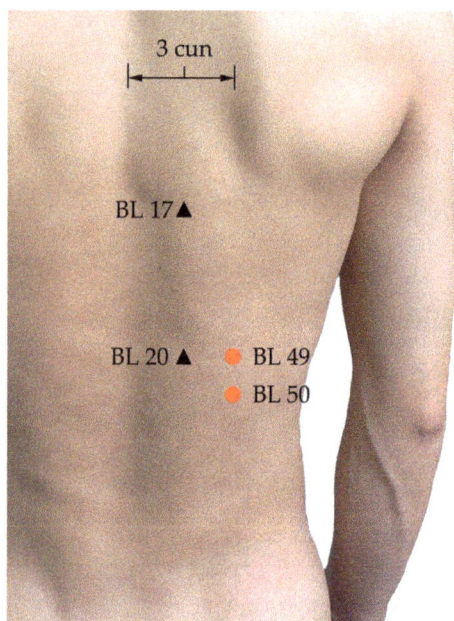

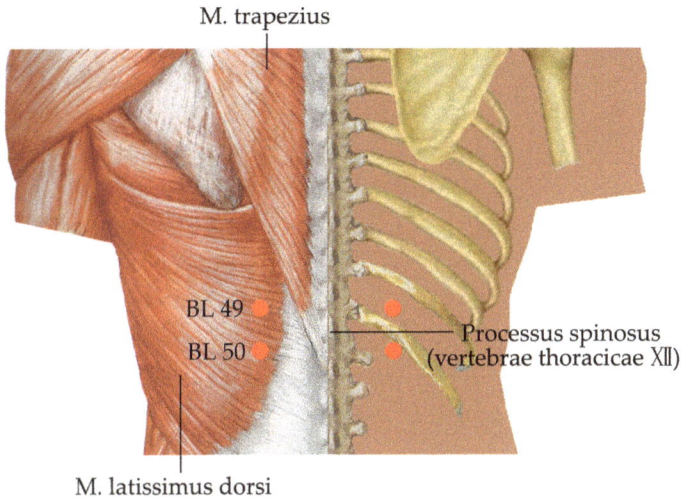

M. trapezius

BL 49
BL 50

Processus spinosus
(vertebrae thoracicae XII)

M. latissimus dorsi

BL 51 – Huāng Mén

[Locating]	The point is located in prone position, at the level with the lower border of the spinous process of the first lumbar vertebrae.3 cun lateral to the posterior midline.
[Regional Anatomy]	The needle passes through the skin, subcutaneous tissues and penetrates m. latissimus dorsi,m. serratus posterior inferior and m. sacrospinalis.
[Acupuncture and Moxibustion]	Insert the needle perpendicularly 0.8~1.0 cun deep and stimulate until there is a sour and distending sensation in the local area radiating to the ipsilateral waist. This point can be moxibusted.
[Indications]	Breast lumps, abdominal pain, and constipation.
[Note]	Avoid deep puncture to prevent pneumothorax and injury to the viscera.

BL 52 – Zhì Shì

[Locating]	The point is located in prone position, at the level with the lower border of the spinous process of the second lumbar vertebrae.3 cun lateral to the posterior midline.
[Regional Anatomy]	The needle passes through the subcutaneous tissues and penetrates m. latissimus dorsi,m. sacrospinalis,m. quadratus lumborum and m. quadratus lumborum.

[Acupuncture and Moxibustion]	Insert the needle perpendicularly 0.8~1.0 cun deep and stimulate until there is a sour and distending sensation in the local area radiating to the hips.
	This point can be moxibusted.
[Indications]	Nocturnal emission, impotence, enuresis, frequent urination and dysuria, and stiffness and pain in the lumbar region.

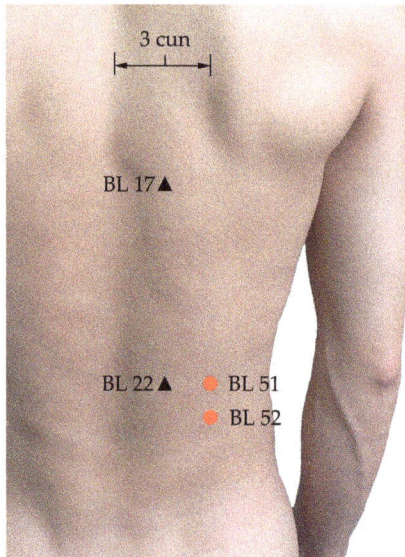

M. latissimus dorsi

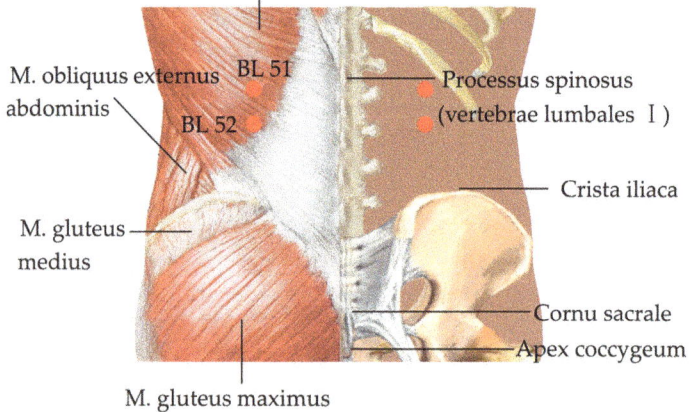

M. obliquus externus abdominis

M. gluteus medius

M. gluteus maximus

Processus spinosus (vertebrae lumbales I)

Crista iliaca

Cornu sacrale

Apex coccygeum

BL 53 – Bāo Huāng

[Locating]	The point is located in prone position, on the lower back, 3 cun lateral to the middle sacral crest, at the level with the second posterior sacral foramen.
[Regional Anatomy]	The needle passes through the skin, subcutaneous tissues and penetrates m. gluteus maximus and m. gluteus medius.
[Acupuncture and Moxibustion]	Insert the needle perpendicularly 0.8~1.0 cun deep and stimulate until there is a sour and distending sensation in the local area radiating to the lower abdomen and hips. This point can be moxibusted.
[Indications]	Dysuria, stiffness and pain of the lower back, abdominal distention, borborygums and constipation.

BL 54 – Zhì Biān

[Locating]	The point is located in prone position, on the lower back, 3 cun lateral to the middle sacral creast, at the level with the fourth posterior sacral foramen.
[Acupuncture and Moxibustion]	Insert the needle perpendicularly 1.5~3 cun deep and stimulate until there is a sour and distending sensation in the local area with an electric and numbing feeling radiating to the lower extremities. This point can be moxibusted.
[Regional Anatomy]	The needle passes through the skin, subcutaneous tissues and penetrates m. gluteus maximus.
[Indications]	Lumbosacral pain, paralysis or muscular atrophy of the lower extremities, hemorrhoids, dysuria, constipation, impotency and irregular menstruation.

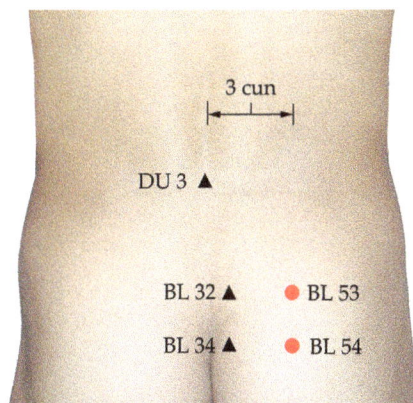

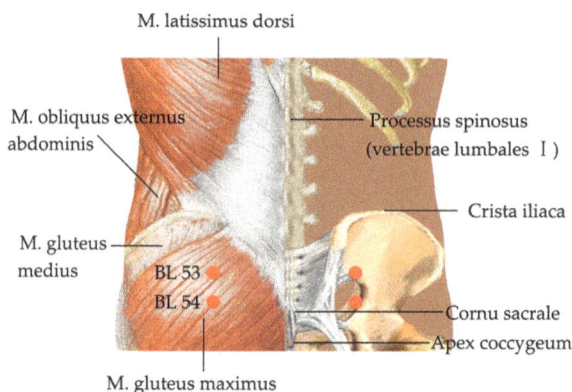

M. latissimus dorsi

M. obliquus externus abdominis

Processus spinosus (vertebrae lumbales Ⅰ)

Crista iliaca

M. gluteus medius

BL 53
BL 54

Cornu sacrale

Apex coccygeum

M. gluteus maximus

BL 55 – Hé Yáng

[Locating]	The point is located in prone position, 2 cun inferior to BL 40 (Wěi Zhōng), on the line connecting BL 57 (Chéng Shān) to BL 40 (Wěi Zhōng).
[Regional Anatomy]	The needle passes through the skin, subcutaneous tissues and penetrates m. triceps surae, m. plantaris and m. popliteus.
[Acupuncture and Moxibustion]	Insert the needle perpendicularly 0.5~1.0 cun deep and stimulate until there is a sour and distending sensation in the local area with an electric and numbing sensation radiating to the sole of the foot. This point can be moxibusted.
[Indications]	Paralysis or muscular atrophy of the lower extremities, metrorrhagia and morbid leucorrhea.

BL 56 – Chéng Jīn

[Locating]	The point is located in prone position, at the midpoint of the line connecting BL 55 (Hé Yang) to BL 57 (Chéng Shān), in the center of the m. gastrocnemius, 5 cun inferior to BL 40 (Wěi Zhōng).
[Regional Anatomy]	The needle passes through the skin, subcutaneous tissues and penetrates m. triceps surae and m. tibialis posterior.
[Acupuncture and Moxibustion]	Insert the needle perpendicularly 0.5~1.0 cun deep and stimulate until there is a sour and distending sensation in the local area radiating to the sole of the foot. This point can be moxibusted.
[Indications]	Spasm of the gastrocnemius and hemorrhoids.

BL 57 – Chéng Shān

[Locating]	The point is located in prone position, in the depression of the belly of the m. gastrocnemius when the toes are extended or the heel is lifted from the ground.
[Regional Anatomy]	The needle passes through the skin, subcutaneous tissues and penetrates m. triceps surae, m. flexor hallucis longus and m. tibialis posterior.
[Acupuncture and Moxibustion]	Insert the needle perpendicularly 1.0~1.5 cun deep and stimulate until there is a sour and distending sensation in the local area radiating to the popliteal space, or an electric and numbing sensation radiating to the sole of the foot. This point can be moxibusted
[Indications]	Hemorrhoids, constipation, abdominal pain, and pain in the lower back and legs.

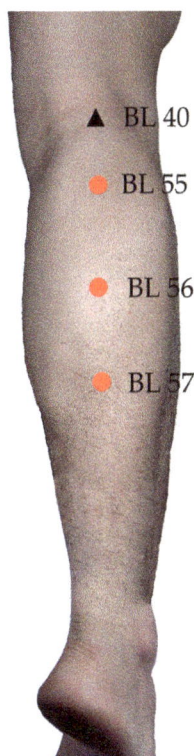

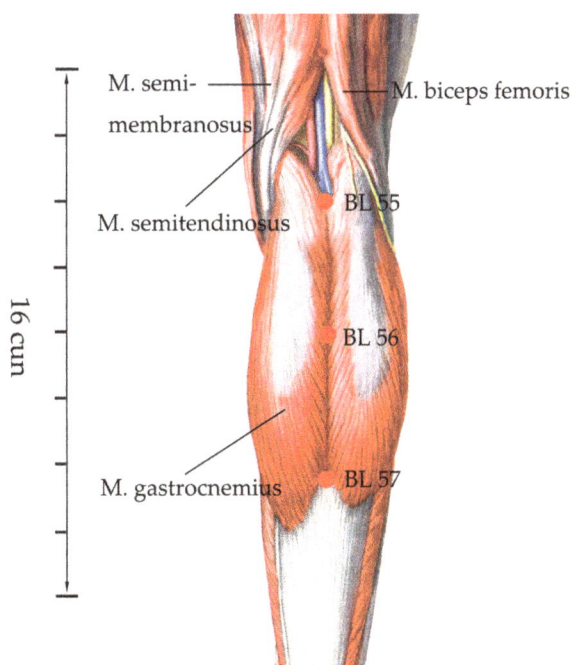

BL 58 – Fēi Yáng

[Features]	Luo-connecting point of the Bladder Channel of Foot *Taiyang*.
[Locating]	The point is located in prone position,7 cun superior to BL 60 (Kūn Lún), 1 cun inferior and lateral to BL 57 (Chéng Shān).
[Regional Anatomy]	The needle passes through the subcutaneous tissues and penetrates m. triceps suraem and tibialis posterior.
[Acupuncture and Moxibustion]	Insert the needle perpendicularly 0.7~1.0 cun deep and stimulate until there is a sour, distending and numbing sensation in the local area radiating to the lower. This point can be moxibusted.
[Indications]	Headache, nasal obstruction, weakness of the knees, and sore legs.

BL 59 – Fū Yáng

[Features]	Xi-cleft point of the Yang Motility Vessel.
[Locating]	The point is located in the sitting position with the foot resting on the ground, posterior to the external mallelous, 3 cun superior to BL 60 (Kūn Lún), between the fibula and the tendon calcaneus.
[Regional Anatomy]	The needle passes through the skin, subcutaneous tissues and penetrates m. peroneus brevis and m. flexor hallucis longus.
[Acupuncture and Moxibustion]	Insert the needle perpendicularly 0.5~1.0 cun deep and stimulate until there is a sour and distending sensation in the local area radiating to the heel. This point can be moxibusted.
[Indications]	Headache, pain of the lower back, and paralysis or muscular atrophy of the lower extremities.

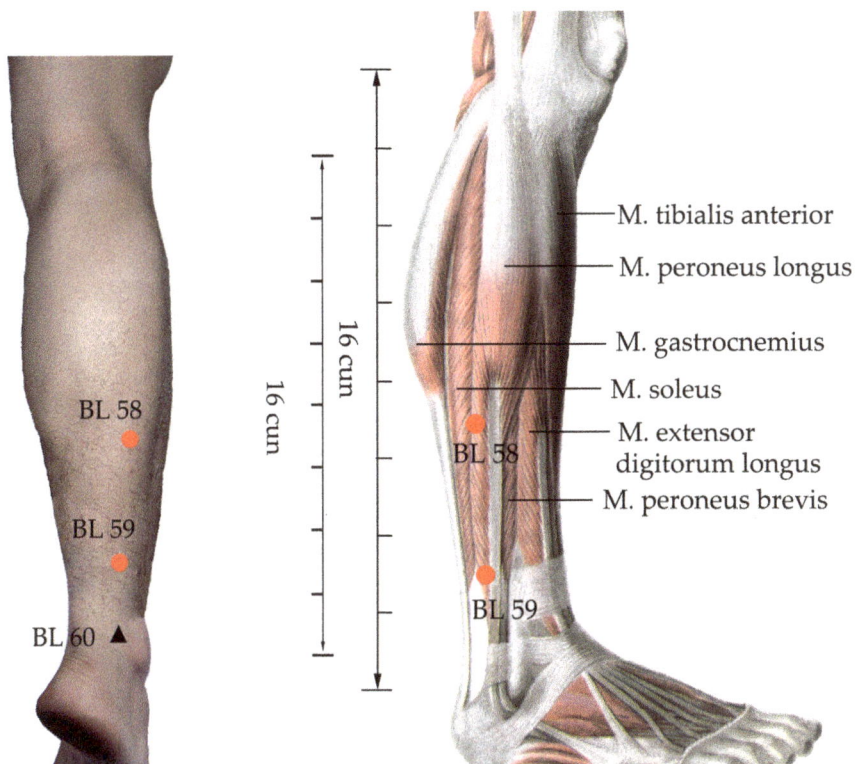

M. tibialis anterior
M. peroneus longus
M. gastrocnemius
M. soleus
M. extensor digitorum longus
M. peroneus brevis

BL 58
BL 59
BL 60 ▲

16 cun
16 cun

BL 60 – Kūn Lún

[Features]	Jing-river point of the Bladder Channel of Foot *Tai-yang*.
[Locating]	The point is located in the sitting position with the foot resting on the ground, in the depression between the tip of the external mallelous and tendon calcaneus.
[Regional Anatomy]	The needle passes through the skin, subcutaneous tissues and penetrates m. peroneus longus and m. peroneus brevis.
[Acupuncture and Moxibustion]	Insert the needle perpendicularly 0.5~1.0 cun deep and stimulate until there is a sour and distending sensation in the local area radiating to the toe. This point can be moxibusted.
[Indications]	Headache, neck stiffness, lumbosacral pain, and epilepsia.

BL 61 – Pú Cān

[Locating]	The point is located in the sitting position with the foot resting on the ground, on the lateral side of the foot, posterior and inferior to the external malleolus, 2 cun inferior to BL 60 (Kūn Lún), lateral to the calcaneum at the junction of the red and white skin.
[Regional Anatomy]	The needle passes through the skin, subcutaneous tissues and penetrates calcaneofibular ligament.
[Acupuncture and Moxibustion]	Insert the needle perpendicularly 0.3~0.5 cun deep and stimulate until there is a sour and distending sensation in the local area.
	This point can be moxibusted.
[Indications]	Weakness of the lower extremities and pain of the heel.

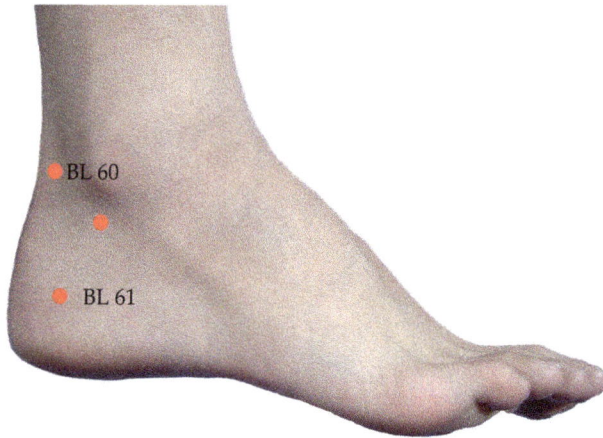

BL 60

BL 61

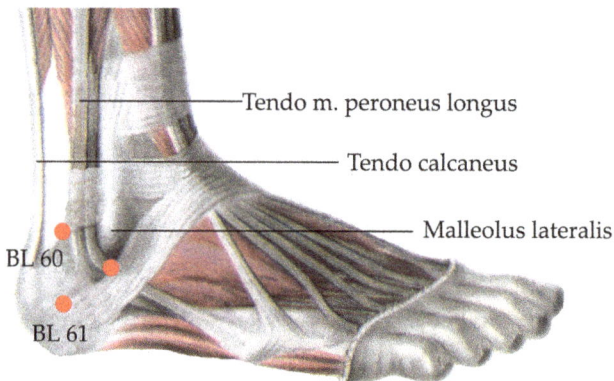

Tendo m. peroneus longus

Tendo calcaneus

Malleolus lateralis

BL 60

BL 61

BL 62 – Shēn Mài

[Features]	One of the Eight Confluent points associating with the Yang Motility Vessel.
[Locating]	The point is located in the sitting or prone position with the foot resting on the ground, on the lateral side of the foot, in the depression directly below the tip of the external malleolus, between the inferior border of the external malleolus and the tendon calcaneus.
[Regional Anatomy]	The needle passes through the skin, subcutaneous tissues and penetrates m. peroneus longus and peroneus brevis.
[Acupuncture and Moxibustion]	Insert the needle perpendicularly 0.2~0.3 cun deep and stimulate until there is a sour and distending sensation in the local area. This point can be moxibusted.
[Indications]	Headache, dizziness, insomnia, and epilepsy.

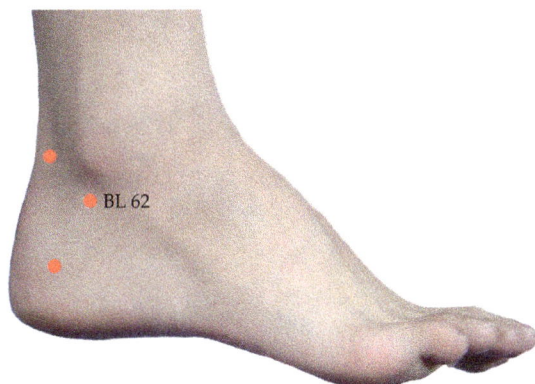

BL 62

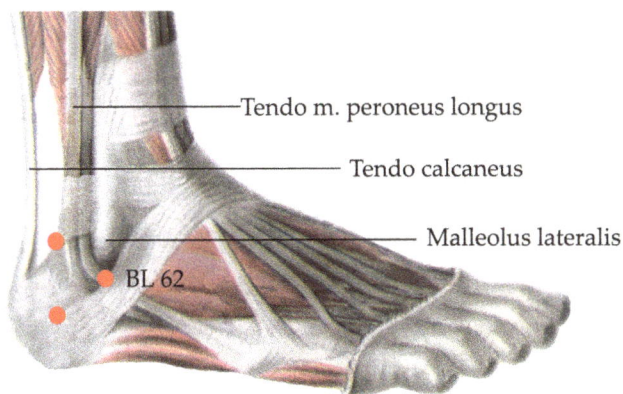

Tendo m. peroneus longus

Tendo calcaneus

Malleolus lateralis

BL 62

BL 63 – Jīn Mén

[Features]	Xi-cleft point of the Bladder Channel of Foot *Taiyang*.
[Locating]	The point is located in the supine position, on the lateral side of the foot, anterior and inferior to BL 62 (Shēn Mài), in the depression lateral to the cuboid bone.
[Regional Anatomy]	The needle passes through the skin, subcutaneous tissues and penetrates m. abductor digiti minimi pedis.
[Acupuncture and Moxibustion]	Insert the needle perpendicularly 0.3~0.5 cun deep and stimulate until there is a sour and distending sensation in the local area. This point can be moxibusted.
[Indications]	Epilepsy, infantile convulsions, headache, lumbar pain, and foot sprain.

BL 64 – Jīng Gǔ

[Features]	Yuan-source point of the Bladder Channel of the Foot *Taiyang*.
[Locating]	The point is located in the sitting or prone position with the foot resting on the ground, on the lateral side of the foot, anterior and inferior to the tuberosity of the fifth metatarsal bone, at the junction of the red and white skin.
[Regional Anatomy]	The needle passes through the skin, subcutaneous tissues and penetrates m. abductor digiti minimi pedis.
[Acupuncture and Moxibustion]	Insert the needle perpendicularly 0.3~0.5 cun deep and stimulate until there is a sour and distending sensation in the local area radiating to the sole of the foot. This point can be moxibusted.
[Indications]	Headache, dizziness, and pain in the lower back and legs.

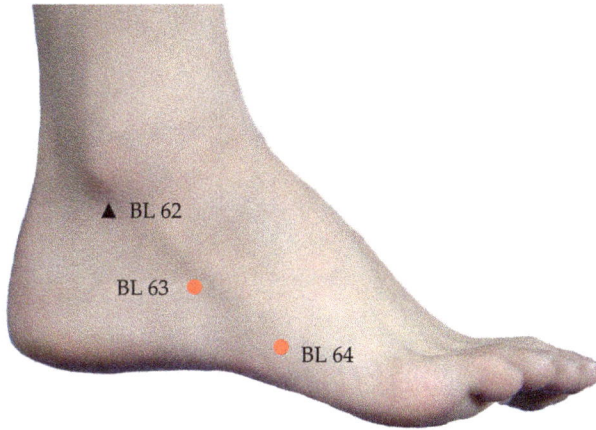

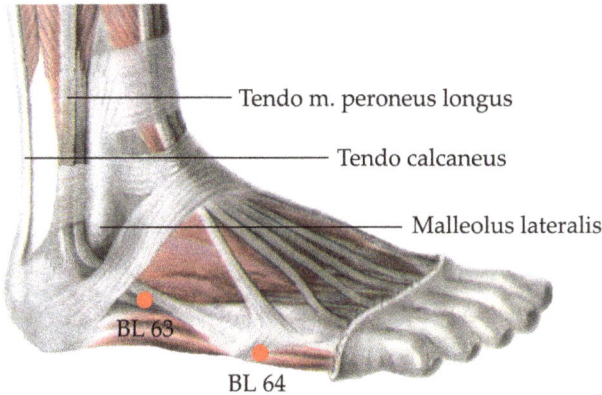

Tendo m. peroneus longus

Tendo calcaneus

Malleolus lateralis

BL 63

BL 64

BL 65 – Shù Gǔ

[Features]	Shu-stream point of the Bladder Channel of Foot *Tai-yang*.
[Locating]	The point is located in the sitting or prone position with the foot resting on the ground, lateral and posterior to the fifth metatarsophalangeal joint, at the junction of the red and white skin.
[Regional Anatomy]	The needle passes through the skin, subcutaneous tissues and penetrates m. abductor digiti minimi pedis.
[Acupuncture and Moxibustion]	Insert the needle perpendicularly 0.3~0.5 cun deep and stimulate until there is a sour and distending sensation in the local area. This point can be moxibusted.
[Indications]	Headache, redness and pain of the eye, hemorrhoids, and pain in the posterior side of the lower extremities.

BL 66 – Zú Tōng Gǔ

[Features]	Ying-spring point of the Bladder Channel of Foot *Tai-yang*.
[Locating]	The point is located in the sitting or prone position with the foot resting on the ground, lateral and anterior to the fifth metatarsophalangeal joint, at the junction of the red and white skin.
[Regional Anatomy]	The needle passes through the skin, subcutaneous tissues and penetrates tendo m. flexor digitorum brevis.
[Acupuncture and Moxibustion]	Insert the needle perpendicularly 0.2~0.3 cun deep and stimulate until there is a sour and distending sensation in the local area. This point can be moxibusted.
[Indications]	Headache, neck pain, and epistaxis.

BL 67 – Zhì Yīn

[Features]	Jing-well point of the Bladder Channel of Foot *Tai-yang*.
[Locating]	The point is located in the sitting or prone position with the foot resting on the ground, on the lateral border of the end of small toe, on the line crossing the lateral border and the base of the nail of the small toe, 0.1 cun from the lateral corner of the nail.
[Regional Anatomy]	① The needle passes through the skin, subcutaneous tissues and stimulate until there is a sore and numbing sensation in the local area. ② Prick with the three-edged needle to bleed. This point can be moxibusted.
[Indications]	Headache, nasal obstruction, malposition of the fetus and difficult labor.

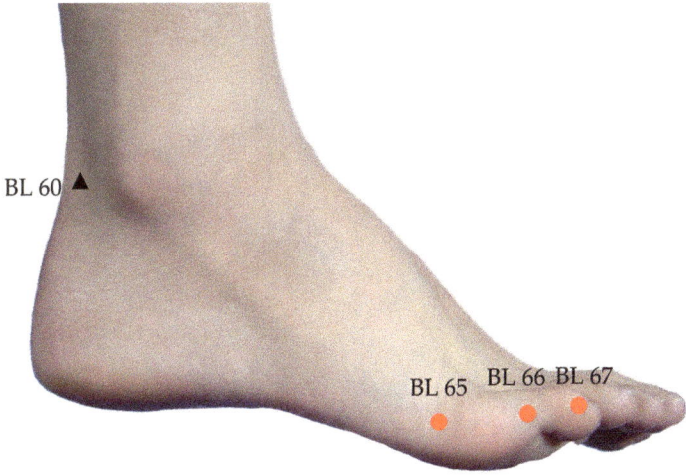

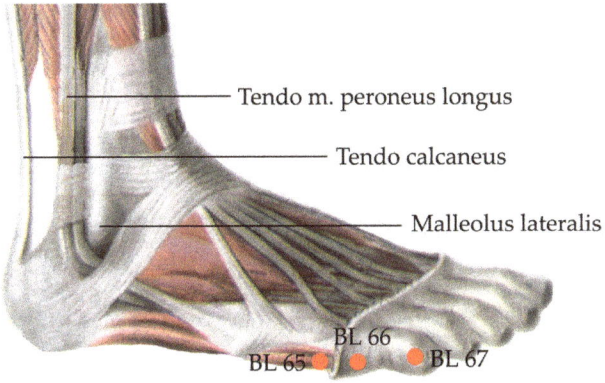

Tendo m. peroneus longus

Tendo calcaneus

Malleolus lateralis

CHAPTER 9

Kidney Channel of Foot Shaoyin; KI

There are twenty-seven acupuncture points in the Kidney Channel of Foot Shaoyin, and fifty-four points in total on both sides. There are ten points on the posterior and interior part of the lower extremities and seventeen are distributed on the chest and abdomen. The first point is KI 1 (Yŏng Quán) and the last point is KI 27 (Shū Fŭ). The indications for this channel are diseases of the urogenital, digestive, respiratory, circulatory systems and the symptoms along the course of the channel.

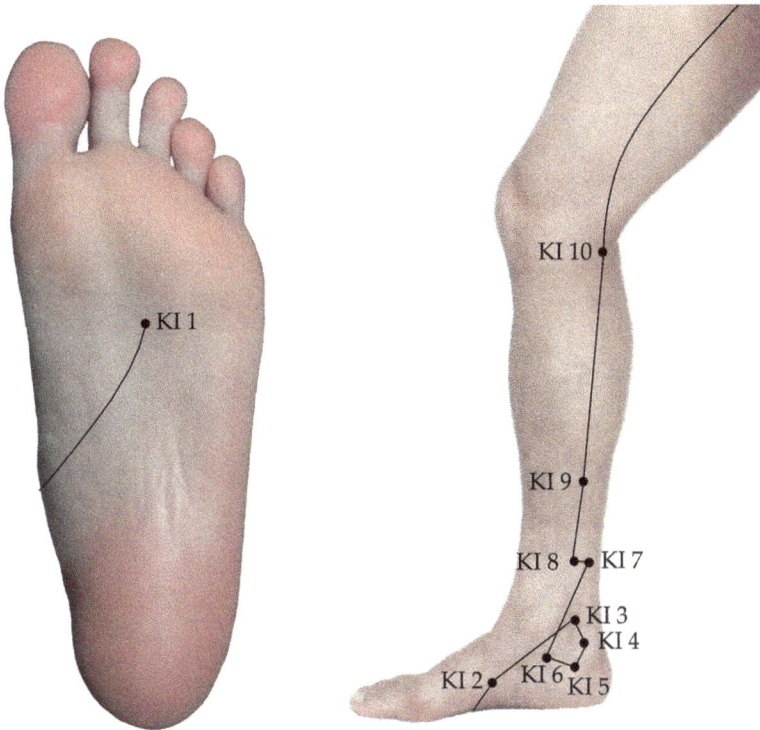

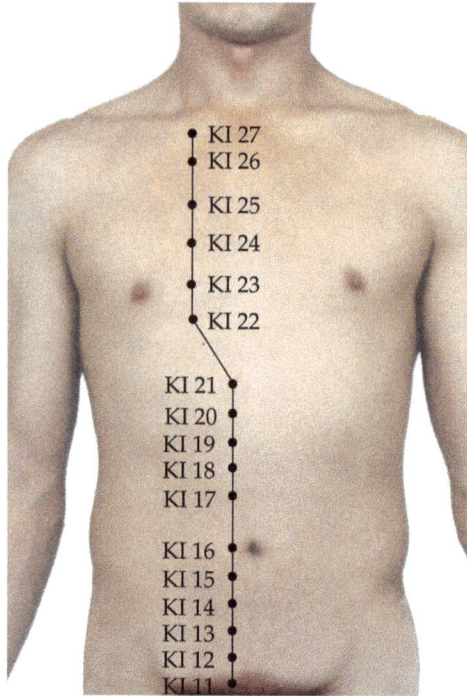

KI 27
KI 26
KI 25
KI 24
KI 23
KI 22
KI 21
KI 20
KI 19
KI 18
KI 17
KI 16
KI 15
KI 14
KI 13
KI 12
KI 11

KI 1 – Yŏng Quán

[Features]	Jing-well point of the Kidney Channel of Foot *Shaoyin*.
[Locating]	The point is located in the supine position when the foot is flexing, on the anterior 1/3 and posterior 2/3 of the sole, on the line connecting the web between the second and the third toes to the back of the heel.
[Regional Anatomy]	The needle passes through the skin and subcutaneous tissues, penetrates the m. flexor digitorum brevis, second lumbrical muscles,m. adductoris hallucis and metatarsal interosseous muscles.
[Acupuncture and Moxibustion]	Insert the needle perpendicularly 0.5~1.0 cun deep and stimulate until there is a sore and distending sensation in the local area spreading around the sole of the foot. This point can be moxibusted.
[Indications]	Epilepsy, infantile convulsion, headache, sore throat, asthma, difficulty in micturition, and difficulty in labor.

KI 2 – Rán Gǔ

[Features]	Ying-spring point of the Kidney Channel of Foot *Shaoyin*.
[Locating]	The point is located in the sitting or supine position, anterior and inferior to the internal mallelous, in the depression inferior to the tuberosity of the navicular bone, at the junction of the red and white skin.
[Regional Anatomy]	The needle passes through the skin, subcutaneous tissues and penetrates the m. abductor hallucis and m. flexor hallucis longus.
[Acupuncture and Moxibustion]	Insert the needle perpendicularly 0.5~1.0 cun deep and stimulate until there is a sore and distending sensation in the local area spreading around the sole of the foot. This point can be moxibusted.
[Indications]	Irregular menstruation, Swelling pain in chest and hypochondrium in chest, and hypochondrium.

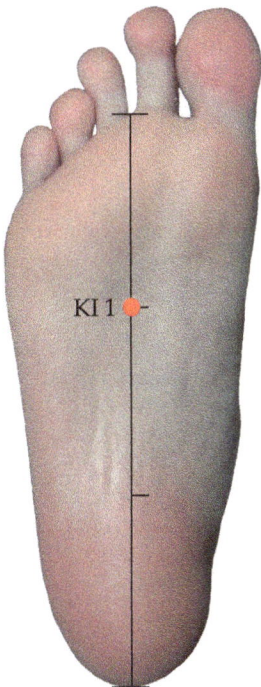

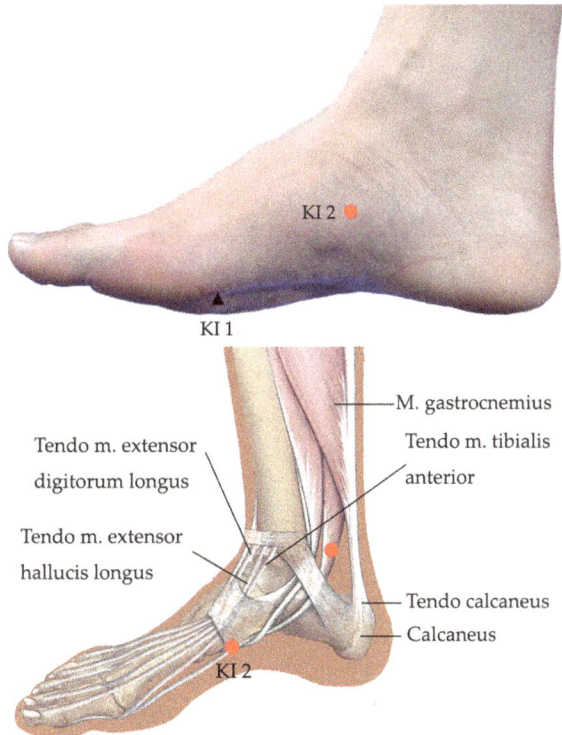

KI 3 – Tài Xī

[Features]	Shu-stream and yuan-source points of the Kidney Channel of Foot *Shaoyin*.
[Locating]	The point is located in the sitting or supine position, posterior to the medial mallelous, in the depression between the tip of the medial malleolus and the tendon calcaneus.
[Regional Anatomy]	The needle passes through the skin and subcutaneous tissues, tendo m. flexor digitorum longus, tendo m. plantaris, penetrates m. tibialis posterior and m. flexor pollicis longus and runs between the inner ankle and tendo calcaneus.
[Acupuncture and Moxibustion]	Insert the needle perpendicularly 0.5~1.0 cun deep and stimulate until there is a sore and distending sensation in the local area, with a numbing and electric sensation spreading around the sole of the foot. This point can be moxibusted.
[Indications]	Enuresis, difficulty in urination, spermatorrhea, impotence, edema irregular menstruation, insomnia, amnesia, dizziness, headache, toothache, tinnitus and weakness, drinking and urine isues, soreness and swelling of the internal malleolus, and pain of the heel.

KI 4 – Dà Zhōng

[Features]	Luo-connecting point of the Kidney Channel of Foot *Shaoyin*.
[Locating]	The point is located in the sitting or supine position, posterior and inferior to the medial mallelous, 0.5 cun inferior to KI 3 (Tài Xī), in the depression anterior to the anterior border of the tendon calcaneus.
[Regional Anatomy]	The needle passes through the skin and subcutaneous fascia, penetrates the deep crural fascia and runs between the tendo calcaneus and the trunk of n. tibialis.
[Acupuncture and Moxibustion]	Insert the needle perpendicularly 0.3~0.5 cun deep and stimulate until there is a sour and distending sensation in the local area. This point can be moxibusted.
[Indications]	Swelling and pain in the throat, and pain and stiffness in the lower back.

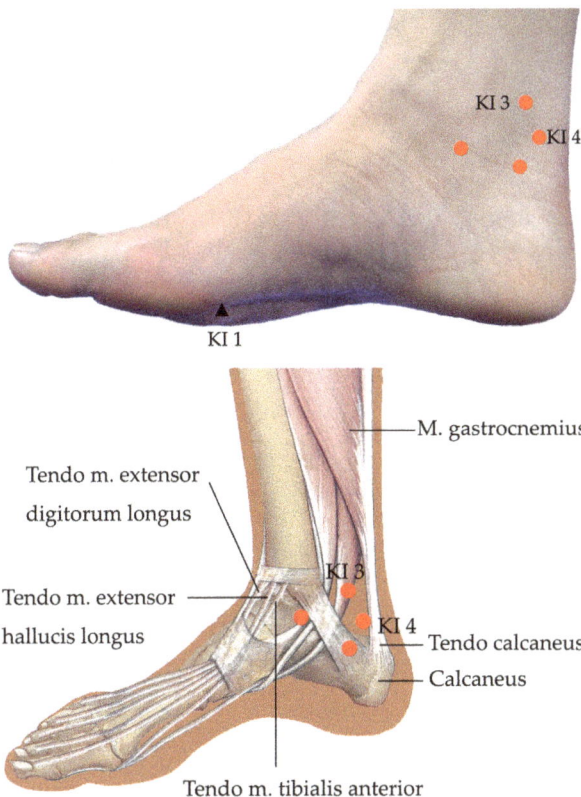

KI 3
KI 4
KI 1

M. gastrocnemius

Tendo m. extensor digitorum longus

Tendo m. extensor hallucis longus

KI 3
KI 4

Tendo calcaneus

Calcaneus

Tendo m. tibialis anterior

KI 5 – Shuǐ Quán

[Features]	Xi-cleft point of the Kidney Channel of Foot *Shaoyin*.
[Locating]	The point is located in the sitting or supine position, on the medial side of the foot, posterior and inferior to the medial mallelous, 1 cun directly inferior to KI 3 (Tài Xī), in the depression anterior to the tuberosity of the calcaneum.
[Regional Anatomy]	The needle passes through the skin and subcutaneous fascia, penertrates the deep crural fascia, runs between the inner aspect of the ankle and tendo calcaneus and enters the tarsal tunnel.
[Acupuncture and Moxibustion]	Insert the needle perpendicularly 0.3~0.5 cun deep and stimulate until there is a sour and distending sensation in the local area.
	This point can be moxibusted.
[Indications]	Difficulty in urination, and pain in heel.

KI 6 – Zhào Hǎi

[Features]	One of the Eight Confluent Points associated with the Yin Motility Vessel.
[Locating]	The point is located in the sitting or supine position, on the medial side of the foot, in the depression inferior to the tip of the medial malleous, 0.4 cun inferior to the lower border of the medial malleous.
[Regional Anatomy]	The needle passes through the skin and subcutaneous fascia and penertrates the m. tibialis posterior near the inner malleolar rete.
[Acupuncture and Moxibustion]	Insert the needle perpendicularly 0.5~0.8 cun deep and stimulate until there is a sour and numbing sensation in the local area radiating to the whole ankle.
[Indications]	Swelling and pain in the throat, cardialgia, irregular menstruation, epilespy happening at night, constipation, dysmenorrhea, and enuresis.

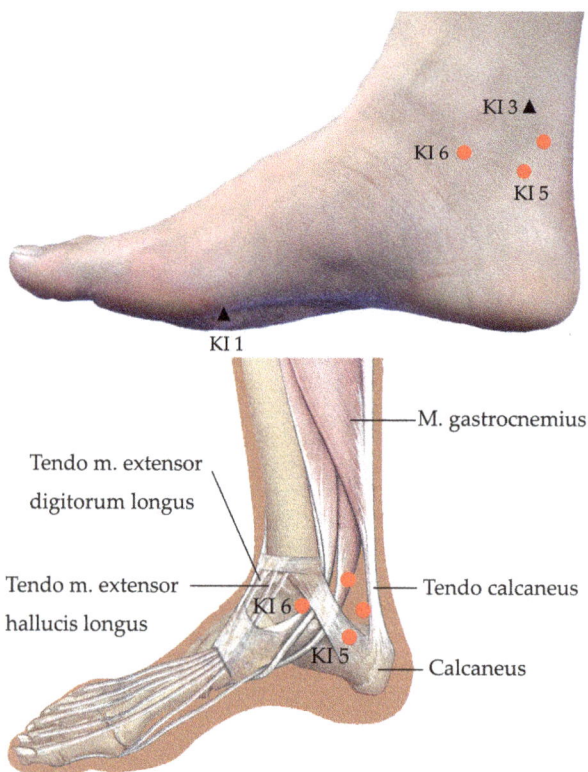

KI 7 – Fù Liū

[Features]	Jing-river point of the Kidney Channel of Foot *Shao-yin*.
[Locating]	The point is located in the sitting or supine position, on the medial aspect of the lower leg, 2 cun directly superior to the tip of the medial malleous, anterior to the tendon calcaneus.
[Regional Anatomy]	The needle passes through the skin and subcutaneous fascia and penetrates m. flexor digitorum longus and m. tibialis posterior.
[Acupuncture and Moxibustion]	Insert the needle perpendicularly 0.8~1.0 cun deep and stimulate until there is a sour and numbing sensation in the local area, or a numbing and electric feeling radiating to the sole of the feet. This point can be moxibusted.
[Indications]	Edema, abdominal distension, stiffness and pain in lower back, and night sweats and self-sweat.

KI8 – Jiāo Xìn

[Features]	Xi-cleft point of the Yin Motility Vessel.
[Locating]	The point is located the sitting position, on the medial aspect of the lower leg, 2 cun superior to the medial malleous, between the medial border of the tibia and KI 7 (Fù Liū).
[Regional Anatomy]	The needle passes through the skin and subcutaneous fascia and penetrates m. tibialis posterior, m. flexor digitorum longus, and m. flexor hallucis longus.
[Acupuncture and Moxibustion]	Insert the needle perpendicularly 0.8~1.0 cun deep and stimulate until there is a sour and distending sensation in the local area radiating to the sole of the feet. This point can be moxibusted.
[Indications]	Irregular menstruation, difficulty in stool, and dysentery.

KI 9 – Zhù Bīn

[Features]	Xi-cleft point of the Yin Linking Vessel.
[Locating]	The point is located in the sitting or supine position, on the line connecting KI 10 (Yīn Gǔ) and KI 3 (Tài Xī), 5 cun superior to the tip of the medial malleous, medial and inferior to the belly of m. gastrocnemius.
[Regional Anatomy]	The needle passes through the skin and subcutaneous fascia and penetrates m. triceps surae and m. flexor digitorum longus.
[Acupuncture and Moxibustion]	Insert the needle perpendicularly 0.5~0.8 cun deep and stimulate until there is a sore and numbing sensation in the local area radiating to the sole of the feet. This point can be moxibusted.
[Indications]	Epilepsy, vomiting, Lower limb weakness and pain on the medial aspect of the lower limbs.

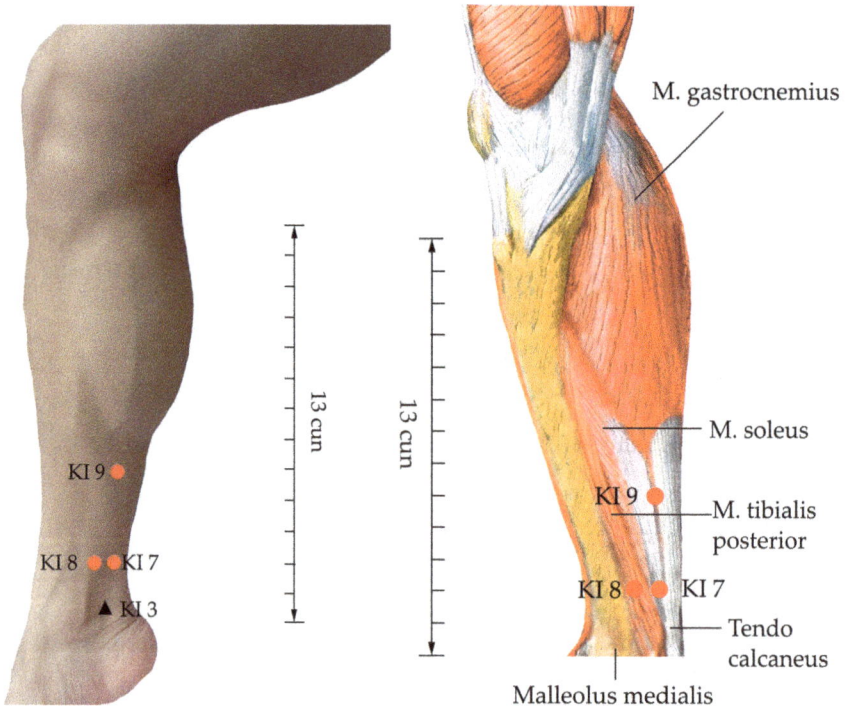

KI 10 – Yīn Gǔ

[Features]	He-sea point of the Kidney Channel of Foot *Shaoyin*.
[Locating]	The point is located in the sitting position when the knee is flexed, on the medial aspect of the popliteal fossa, in the depression between the tendons of m. semitendinusus and semimembranosus.
[Regional Anatomy]	The needle passes through the skin and subcutaneous tissue, penetrates the medial aspect of the popliteal fascia, enters caput mediale m. gastrocnemii along the lateral aspect of the tendons of m. semitendinosus and m. semimembranosus and reaches the periost of condylus medialis of the femur.
[Acupuncture and Moxibustion]	Insert the needle perpendicularly 0.8~1.2 cun deep and stimulate until there is a distending and numbing sensation in the local area radiating to the popliteal fascia, sometimes to the heel. This point can be moxibusted.
[Indications]	Spermatorrhea, impotence, irregular menstruation, and difficulty in urination.

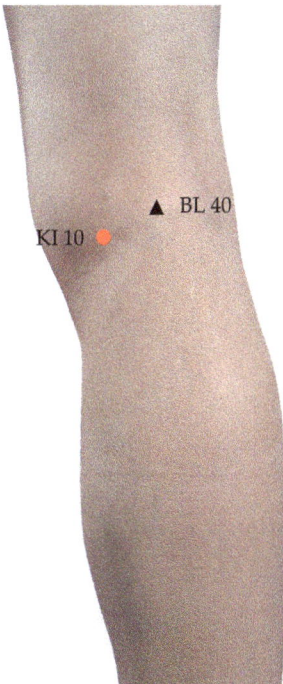

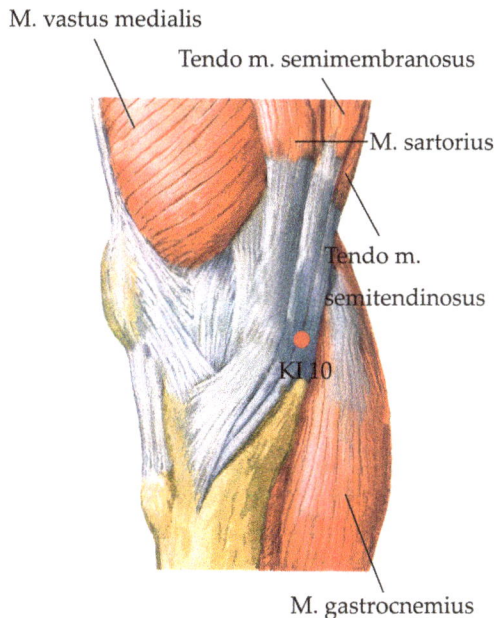

M. vastus medialis
Tendo m. semimembranosus
BL 40
M. sartorius
KI 10
Tendo m. semitendinosus
KI 10
M. gastrocnemius

KI 11 – Héng Gǔ

[Locating]	The point is located in the supine position, on the lower abdomen, 5 cun inferior to the umbilicus, 0.5 cun lateral to the anterior midline.
[Regional Anatomy]	The needle passes through the skin and subcutaneous tissue, penetrates the anterior layer of sheath of m. rectus abdomini, enters m. pyramidalis and m. rectus abdomini, and reaches the parietal peritoneum.
[Acupuncture and Moxibustion]	Insert the needle perpendicularly 0.8~1.2 cun deep and stimulate until there is a sour and distending sensation in the local area. This point can be moxibusted.
[Indications]	Pain and distention in the lower abdomen, diarrhea and constipation.
[Note]	Request the patient empty their bladder before needling to prevent injury to the bladder.

KI 12 – Dà Hè

[Locating]	The point is located in the supine position, on the lower abdomen, 4 cun inferior to the umbilicus, 0.5 cun lateral to the anterior midline.
[Regional Anatomy]	The needle passes through the skin and subcutaneous tissue, penetrates the anterior layer of sheath of m. rectus abdomini, enters m. rectus abdomini and reaches the parietal peritoneum.
[Acupuncture and Moxibustion]	Insert the needle perpendicularly 0.8~1.2 cun deep and stimulate until there is a sour and distending sensation in the local area. This point can be moxibusted.
[Indications]	Spermatorrhea, irregular menstruation, prolapse uterus, dysmenorrhea, infertility, and morbid leucorrhea.
[Note]	It is the same as KL 11 (Héng Gǔ).

KI 13 – Qì Xué

[Locating]	The point is located in the supine position, on the lower abdomen, 3 cun inferior to the umbilicus, 0.5 cun lateral to the anterior midline.
[Regional Anatomy]	The needle passes through the skin and subcutaneous tissue, penetrates the anterior layer of sheath of m. rectus abdomini, enters m. rectus abdomini and reaches the parietal peritoneum.
[Acupuncture and Moxibustion]	Insert the needle perpendicularly 0.8~1.2 cun deep and stimulate until there is a sour and distending sensation in the local area. This point can be moxibusted.
[Indications]	Dysmenorrhea, morbid leucorrhea, retention of urine, spermatorrhea, and impotence.

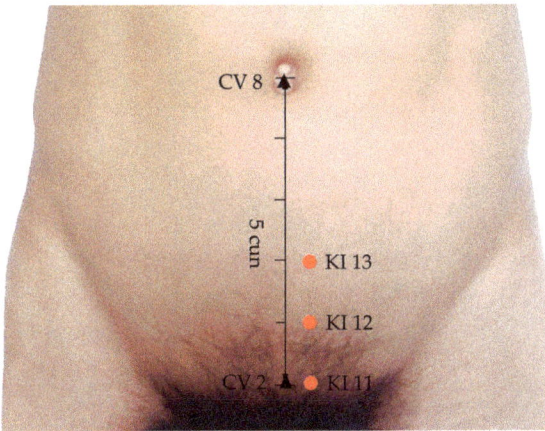

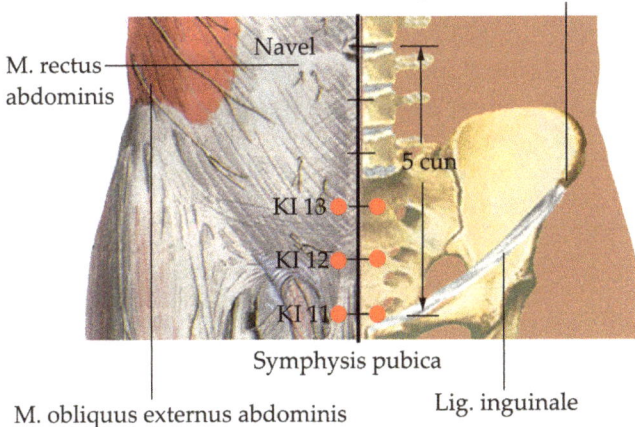

KI 14 – Sì Mǎn

[Locating]	The point is located in the supine position, on the lower abdomen, 2 cun inferior to the umbilicus, 0.5 cun lateral to the anterior midline.
[Regional Anatomy]	The needle passes through the skin and subcutaneous tissue, penetrates the anterior layer of sheath of m. rectus abdomini, enters m. rectus abdomini, penetrates the posterior layer of sheath of m. rectus abdomini and reaches the parietal peritoneum.
[Acupuncture and Moxibustion]	Insert the needle perpendicularly 0.8~1.2 cun deep and stimulate until there is a sour and distending sensation in the local area. This point can be moxibusted.
[Indications]	Irregular menstruation, enuresis, spermatorrhea, edema, lower abdominal pain, and constipation

KI 15 – Zhōng Zhù

[Locating]	The point is located in the supine position, on the lower abdomen, 1 cun inferior to the umbilicus, 0.5 cun lateral to the anterior midline.
[Regional Anatomy]	The needle passes through the skin and subcutaneous tissue, penetrates the anterior layer of sheath of m. rectus abdomini, enters m. rectus abdomini, penetrates the posterior layer of sheath of m. rectus abdomini and reaches the parietal peritoneum.
[Acupuncture and Moxibustion]	Insert the needle perpendicularly 0.8~1.2 cun deep and stimulate until there is a sour and distending sensation in the local area. This point can be moxibusted.
[Indications]	Abdominal distention, vomiting, diarrhea, and dysentery.

KI 16 – Huāng Shū

[Locating]	The point is located in the supine position, on the lower abdomen, at the level with the umbilicus, 0.5 cun lateral to the anterior midline.
[Regional Anatomy]	The needle passes through the skin and subcutaneous tissue, penetrates the fascia transversalis and reaches the subperitoneal fascia.

[Acupuncture and Moxibustion]	Insert the needle perpendicularly 0.8~1.2 cun deep.
[Indications]	Abdominal pain around the umbilicus, abdominal distention, vomiting, diarrhea and constipation.

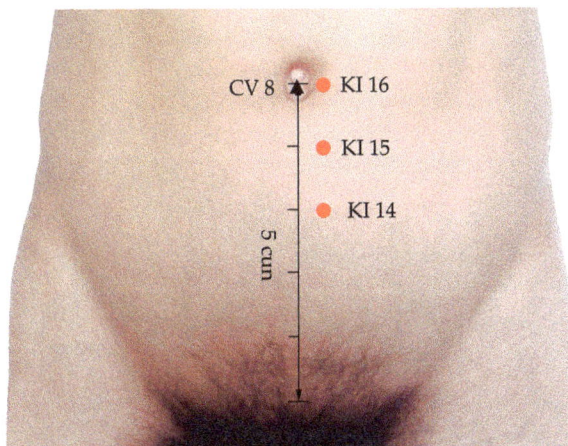

CV 8 ● KI 16
● KI 15
● KI 14
5 cun

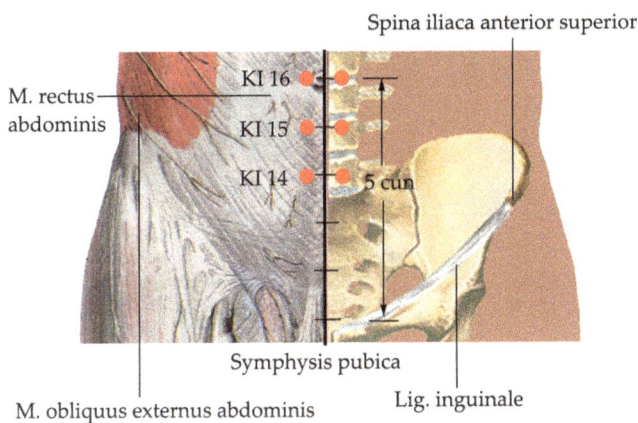

Spina iliaca anterior superior
M. rectus abdominis — KI 16
KI 15
KI 14 — 5 cun
M. obliquus externus abdominis
Symphysis pubica
Lig. inguinale

KI 17 Shāng Qū

[Locating]	The point is located in the supine position, on the upper abdomen, 2 cun superior to the umbilicus, 0.5 cun lateral to the anterior midline.
[Regional Anatomy]	The needle passes through the skin and subcutaneous tissue, penetrates m. rectus abdomini, and reaches the subperitoneal fascia.

[Acupuncture and Moxibustion]	Insert the needle perpendicularly 0.5~0.8 cun deep and stimulate until there is a sour and distending sensation in the local area radiating to the upper abdomen.This point can be moxibusted.
[Indications]	Abdominal distention, vomiting and diarrhea.

KI 18 – Shí Guān

[Locating]	The point is located in the supine position, on the upper abdomen, 3 cun superior to the umbilicus, 0.5 cun lateral to the anterior midline.
[Regional Anatomy]	The needle passes through the skin and subcutaneous tissue, penetrates m. rectus abdomini and reaches the subperitoneal fascia.
[Acupuncture and Moxibustion]	Insert the needle perpendicularly 0.5~0.8 cun deep and stimulate until there is a sour and distending sensation in the local area radiating to the upper abdomen. This point can be moxibusted.
[Indications]	Amenorrhea, morbid leucorrhea, and postpartum lochia.

KI 19 – Yīn Dū

[Locating]	The point is located in the supine position, on the upper abdomen, 4 cun superior to the umbilicus, 0.5 cun lateral to the anterior midline.
[Regional Anatomy]	The needle passes through the skin and subcutaneous tissue, penetrates m. rectus abdomini and reaches the subperitoneal fascia.
[Acupuncture and Moxibustion]	Insert the needle perpendicularly 0.5~0.8 cun deep and stimulate until there is a sour and distending sensation in the local area radiating to the upper abdomen. This point can be moxibusted.
[Indications]	Abdominal distention, borborygmus, abdominal pain, constipation, and infertility.

CV 16

8 cun

KI 19
KI 18
KI 17

CV 8

Joint of corpus sterni and processus xiphoideus

M. serratus anterior

KI 19
KI 18
KI 17

8 cun

M. rectus abdominis

Navel

M. obliquus externus abdominis

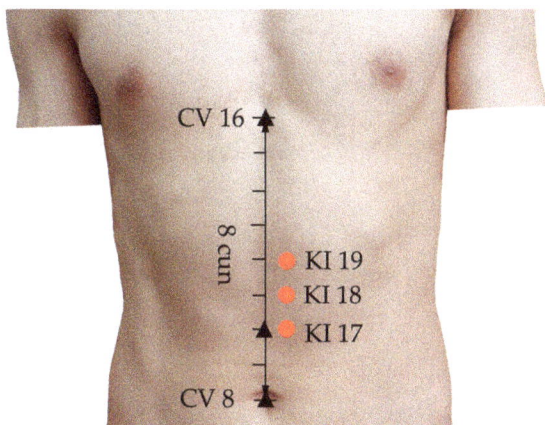

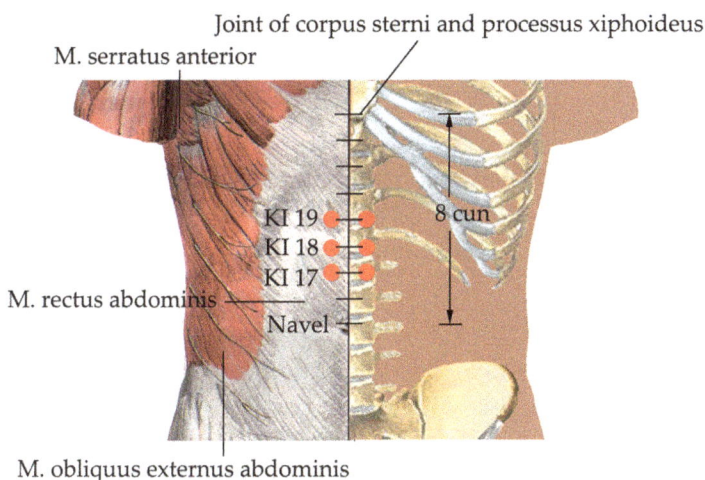

KI 20 – Fù Tōng Gǔ

[Locating]	The point is located in the supine position, on the upper abdomen, 5 cun superior to the umbilicus, 0.5 cun lateral to the anterior midline.
[Regional Anatomy]	The needle passes through the skin and subcutaneous tissue, penetrates m. rectus abdomini, and reaches the subperitoneal fascia.
[Acupuncture and Moxibustion]	Insert the needle perpendicularly 0.5~0.8 cun deep and stimulate until there is a sour and distending sensation in the local area radiating to the upper abdomen. This point can be moxibusted.
[Indications]	Abdominal pain and distention, vomiting, chest pain, cardiac pain, and palpitation.

KI 21 – Yōu Mén

[Locating]	The point is located in the supine position, on the upper abdomen, 6 cun superior to the umbilicus, 0.5 cun lateral to the anterior midline.
[Regional Anatomy]	The needle passes through the skin and subcutaneous tissue, penetrates m. rectus abdomini and reaches the subperitoneal fascia.
[Acupuncture and Moxibustion]	Insert the needle perpendicularly 0.5~0.8 cun deep and stimulate until there is a sour and distending sensation in the local area radiating to the upper abdomen. This point can be moxibusted.
[Indications]	Abdominal pain, vomiting, indigestion, diarrhea and dysentery.

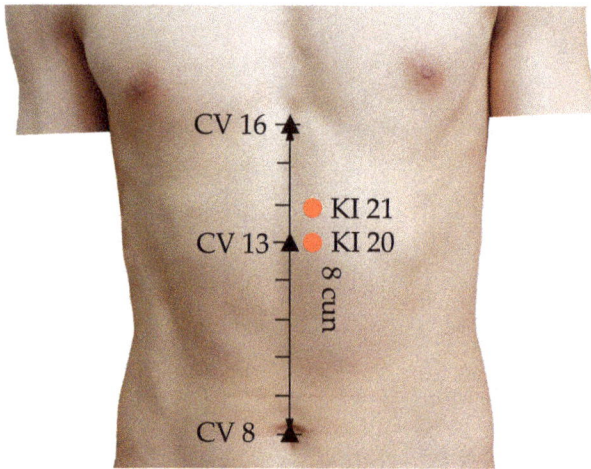

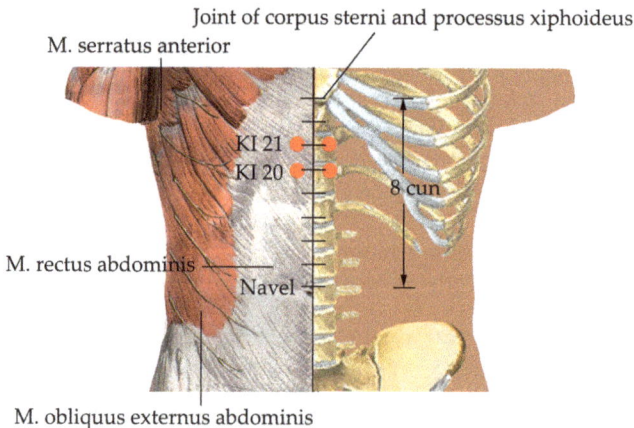

KI 22 – Bù Láng

[Locating]	The point is located in the supine position, on the chest, in the fifth intercostal space, 2 cun lateral to the anterior midline.
[Regional Anatomy]	The needle passes through the skin and subcutaneous tissue, penetrates m. pectoralis major, m. intercostales externi, m. intercostales interni and reaches before the endothoracic fascia.
[Acupuncture and Moxibustion]	Insert the needle obliquely or subcutaneously 0.5~0.8 cun deep and stimulate until there is a sour and numbing sensation in the local area. This point can be moxibusted.
[Indications]	Cough, chest pain, asthma, and acute mastitis.
[Note]	Avoid deep puncture to prevent pneumothorax

KI 23 – Shén Fēng

[Locating]	The point is located in the supine position, on the the chest, in the fourth intercostal space, 2 cun lateral to the anterior midline.
[Regional Anatomy]	The needle passes through the skin and subcutaneous tissue, penetrates m. pectoralis major, m. intercostales externi, m. intercostales interni and reaches before the endothoracic fascia.
[Acupuncture and Moxibustion]	Insert the needle obliquely or subcutaneously 0.5~0.8 cun deep and stimulate until there is a sour and numbing sensation in the local area. This point can be moxibusted.
[Indications]	Cough, asthma, chest pain, and acute mastitis.
[Note]	It is the same as KL 22(Bù Láng)

KI 24 – Líng Xū

[Locating]	The point is located in the supine position, on the chest, in the third intercostal space, 2 cun lateral to the anterior midline.
[Regional Anatomy]	The needle passes through the skin and subcutaneous tissue, penetrates m. pectoralis major,m.intercostales externi,m.intercostales interni and reaches before the endothoracic fascia.
[Acupuncture and Moxibustion]	Insert the needle obliquely or subcutaneously 0.5~0.8 cun deep and stimulate until there is a sour and numbing sensation in the local area. This point can be moxibusted.
[Indications]	Cough, asthma, chest pain, palpitation, and acute mastitis.
[Note]	It is the same as KL 22(Bù Láng)

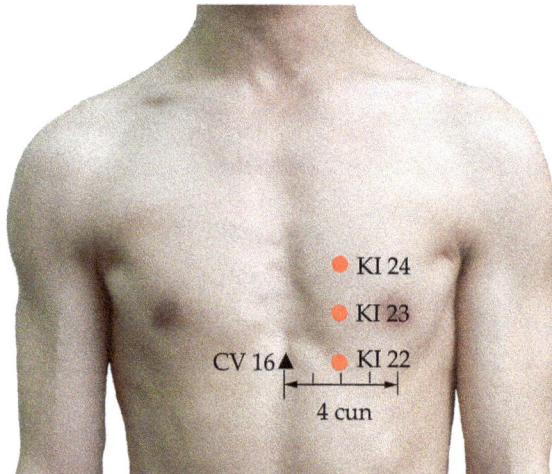

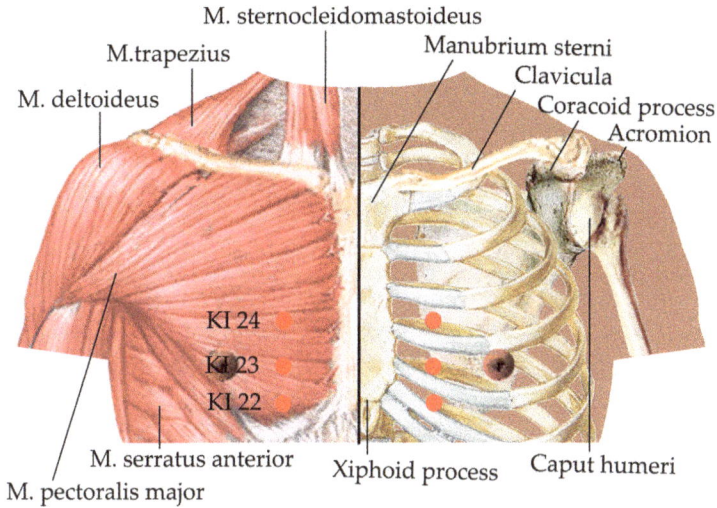

M. sternocleidomastoideus
M.trapezius
M. deltoideus
Manubrium sterni
Clavicula
Coracoid process
Acromion
KI 24
KI 23
KI 22
M. serratus anterior
M. pectoralis major
Xiphoid process
Caput humeri

KI 25 – Shén Cáng

[Locating]	The point is located in the supine position, on the chest, in the second intercostal space, 2 cun lateral to the anterior midline.
[Regional Anatomy]	The needle passes through the skin and subcutaneous tissue, penetrates m. pectoralis major, m. intercostales externi, m. intercostales interni and reaches before the endothoracic fascia.
[Acupuncture and Moxibustion]	Insert the needle obliquely or subcutaneously 0.5~0.8 cun deep and stimulate until there is a sour and numbing sensation in the local area. This point can be moxibusted.
[Indications]	Cough, asthma, and chest pain.
[Note]	It is the same as KL 22(Bù Láng)

KI 26 – Yù Zhōng

[Locating]	The point is located in the supine position, on the chest, in the first intercostal space, 2 cun lateral to the anterior midline.
[Regional Anatomy]	The needle passes through the skin and subcutaneous tissue, penetrates m. pectoralis major, m. intercostales externi, m. intercostales interni and reaches before the endothoracic fascia.
[Acupuncture and Moxibustion]	Insert the needle obliquely or subcutaneously 0.5~0.8 cun deep and stimulate until there is a sour and numbing sensation in the local area. This point can be moxibusted.
[Indications]	Cough, asthma, distending pain in the chest and hypochondriac regions.
[Note]	It is the same as KL 22(Bù Láng).

KI 27 – Shū Fǔ

[Locating]	The point is located in the supine position, on the chest, on the lower border of the clavicle, 2 cun lateral to the anterior midline.
[Regional Anatomy]	The needle passes through the skin and subcutaneous tissue, and penetrates m. pectoralis major and m. subclavius.
[Acupuncture and Moxibustion]	Insert the needle obliquely or subcutaneously 0.5~0.8 cun deep and stimulate until there is a sour and numbing sensation in the local area. This point can be moxibusted.
[Indications]	Cough, asthma, vomiting, distention in the chest, and hypochondriac regions and anorexia.
[Note]	It is the same as KL 22(Bù Láng).

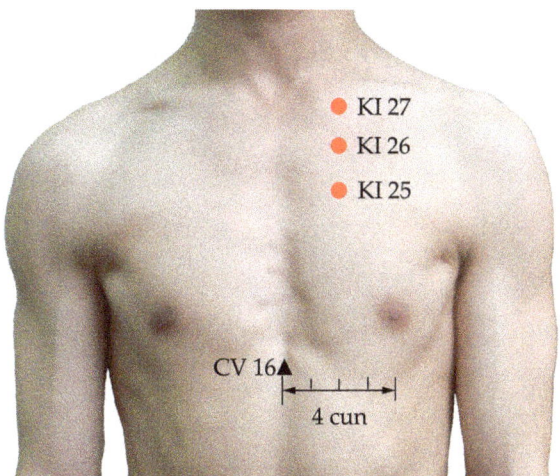

KI 27
KI 26
KI 25

CV 16
4 cun

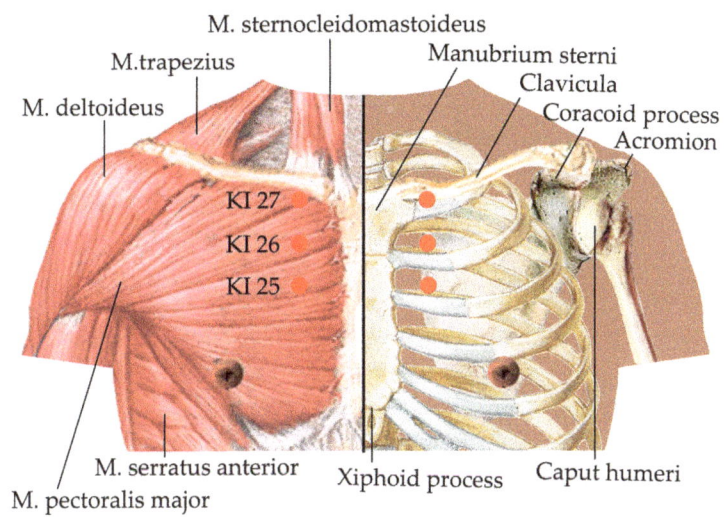

M. sternocleidomastoideus

M.trapezius

M. deltoideus

Manubrium sterni

Clavicula

Coracoid process

Acromion

KI 27

KI 26

KI 25

M. serratus anterior

M. pectoralis major

Xiphoid process

Caput humeri

CHAPTER 10

Pericardium Channel of Hand Jueyin; PC

There are nine points on the Pericardium Channel of the Hand *Jueyin*, eighteen points in total on both sides. There are eight points on the interior midline of the upper extremities and one point is on the chest. The first point is PC 1 (Tiān Chí) and the last point is PC 9 (Zhōng Chōng). The indications for this channel are mental diseases and diseases of the nervous and circulatory systems and the symptoms along the course of the channel.

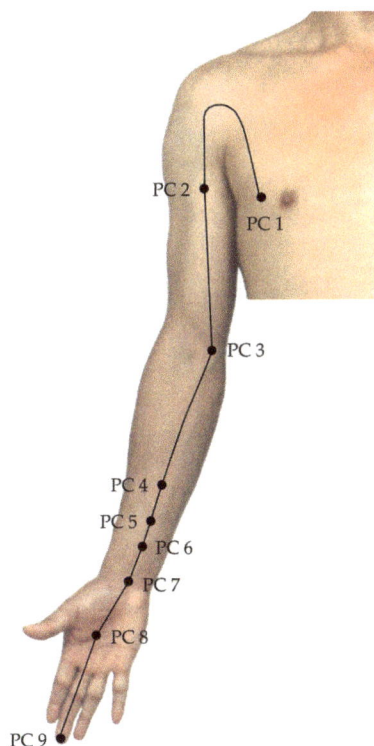

PC 2

PC 1

PC 3

PC 4

PC 5

PC 6

PC 7

PC 8

PC 9

PC 1 – Tiān Chí

[Locating]	On the chest, in the fourth intercostal space, 1 cun lateral to the nipple, 5 cun lateral to the anterior midline.
[Regional Anatomy]	The needle passes through the skin and subcutaneous fascia, penetrates m. pectoralis major and m. serratus anterior. M. pectoralis major and m. serratus anterior are innervated by the anterior thoracic nerve and long thoracic nerve.
[Acupuncture and Moxibustion]	Insert the needle perpendicularly or obliquely 0.3~0.8 cun deep and stimulate until there is a sore and numbing sensation in the local area radiating to the chest. This point can be moxibusted.
[Locating]	Congestion and pain of the chest and insufficient lactation.
[Note]	Avoid deep insertion to prevent pneumothorax.

PC 2 – Tiān Quán

[Locating]	On the medial aspect of the upper arm, 2 cun inferior to the anterior axillary fossa, between the heads of m. biceps brachii longus and brevis.
[Regional Anatomy]	The needle passes through the skin and subcutaneous fascia, penetrates brachia fascia, and enters m. biceps brachii and m. coracobrachialis.
[Acupuncture and Moxibustion]	Insert the needle perpendicularly or obliquely 0.5~0.8 cun deep and stimulate until there is a sore and numbing sensation in the local area radiating to the shoulder. This point can be moxibusted.
[Indications]	Pain of the medial side of the upper arm, back and chest.

PC 3 – Qū Zé

[Features]	He-sea point of the Pericardium Channel of the Hand *Jueyin*.
[Locating]	On the transverse crease of the elbow, on the ulnar side of the tendon of m. biceps brachii.

[Regional Anatomy]	The needle passes through skin and subcutaneous fascia, pierces the anterior cubital fascia between v. basilica and intermedian cubital vein, reaches the trunk of n. medianus and m. brachialis at the medial side of the brachial artery.
[Acupuncture and Moxibustion]	Insert the needle perpendicularly 0.5~1.0 cun deep and stimulate until there is a numbing and distending sensation in the local area the the middle finger. This point can be moxibusted.
[Indications]	Cardiac pain, palpitation, irritability, spasm and pain in the elbow and arm.

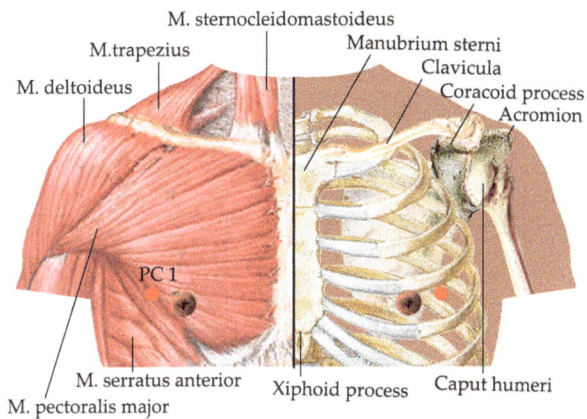

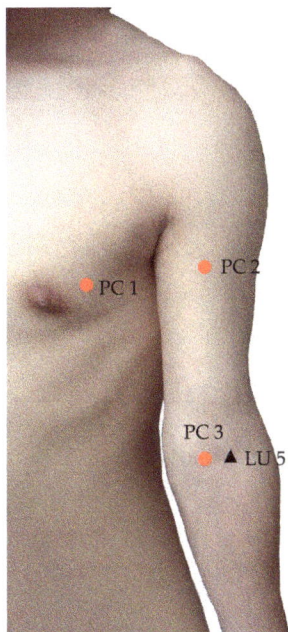

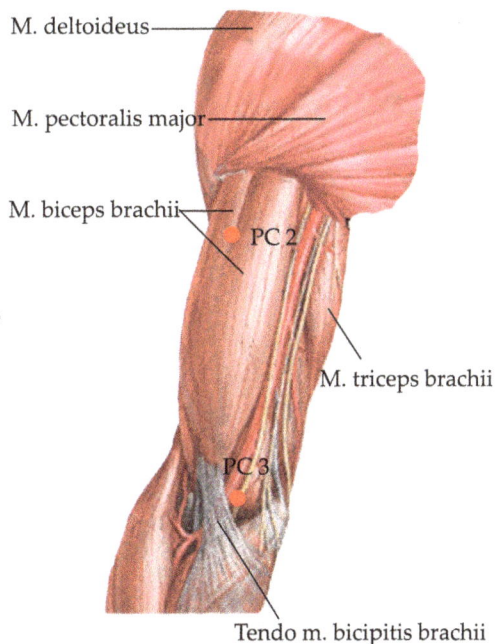

PC 4 – Xì Mén

[Features]	Xi-cleft point of the Pericardium Channel of the Hand *Jueyin*.
[Locating]	The point is located when the arm is stretched forward with palm upward and the elbow flexed, 5 cun above the midpoint of the transverse crease of the wrist, between the tendon of m.palmaris longus and m. flexor carpi radialis.
[Regional Anatomy]	The needle passes through the skin and subcutaneous fascia, penetrates the deep brachial fascia and the muscular layer, and reaches membrana interossea antebrachii.
[Acupuncture and Moxibustion]	Insert the needle perpendicularly 0.5~0.8 cun deep and stimulate until there is a sore and numbing sensation in the local area radiating to the finger. This point can be moxibusted.
[Indications]	Cardiac pain and palpitation.

PC 5 – Jiān Shǐ

[Features]	Jing-river point of the Pericardium Channel of the Hand *Jueyin*.
[Locating]	The point is located the arm is stretched forward with palm upward and the elbow flexed, 3 cun superior to the midpoint of the transverse crease of the wrist, between the tendon of m.palmaris longus and m. flexor carpi radialis.
[Regional Anatomy]	The needle passes through the skin and subcutaneous fascia, penetrates m. flexor digitorum superficialis between m. palmaris longus and m. flexor carpi radialis, enters m. flexor digitorum profundus and m. pronator quadratus.
[Acupuncture and Moxibustion]	Insert the needle perpendicularly towards SJ 6 (Zhīgōu) 0.5~0.8 cun deep and stimulate until there is a sore and numbing sensation in the local area with an electric shock sensation radiating to the finger. This point can be moxibusted.
[Indications]	Malaria.

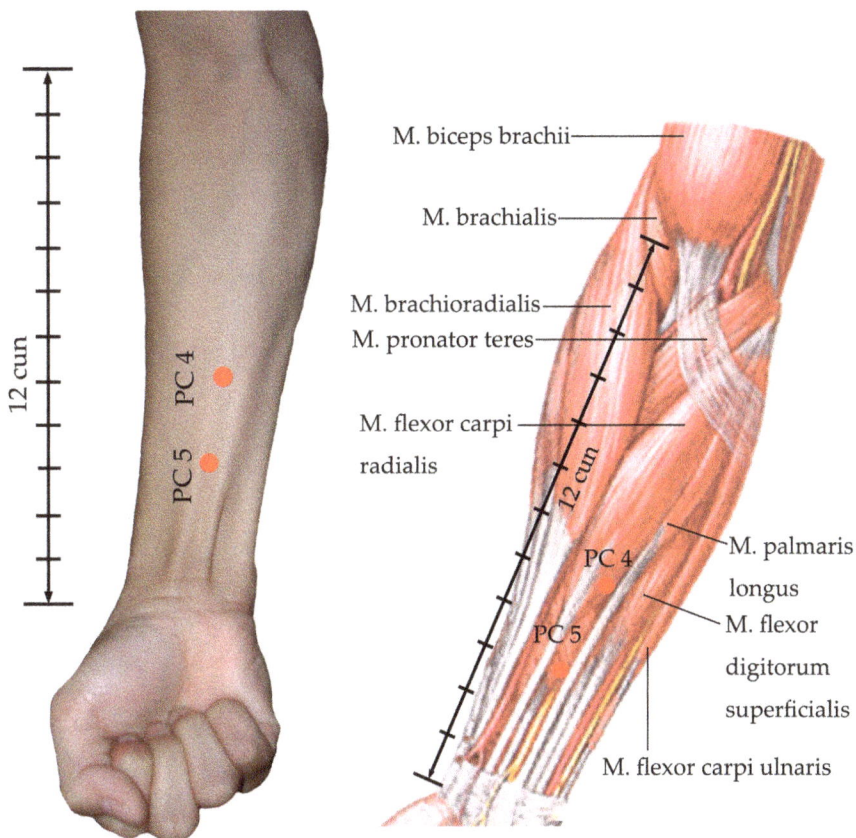

M. biceps brachii

M. brachialis

M. brachioradialis

M. pronator teres

M. flexor carpi radialis

12 cun

PC 4

PC 5

M. palmaris longus

M. flexor digitorum superficialis

M. flexor carpi ulnaris

12 cun

PC 4

PC 5

PC 6 – Nèi Guān

[Features]	Luo-connecting point of the Pericardium Channel of the Hand *Jueyin*; Confluent points of the yang linking vessel.
[Locating]	The point is located on the forearm with the palm upward and the wrist slightly flexed, 2 cun superior to the midpoint of the transverse crease of the wrist, between the tendon of m. palmaris longus and m. flexor carpi radialis.
[Regional Anatomy]	The needle passes through the skin and subcutaneous fascia, pierces the deep brachial fascia, reaches m. flexor digitorum superficialis between m. palmaris longus and m. flexor carpi radialis, enters m. flexor digitorum profundus and m. pronator quadratus.

[Acupuncture and Moxibustion]	Insert the needle perpendicularly 0.5~1.0 cun deep and stimulate until there is a sore and numbing sensation in the local area with an electric sensation radiating to the finger tip. This point can be moxibusted.
[Indications]	Cardiac pain, palpitation and insomnia, stomach ache, vomiting and hiccough.

PC 7 – Dà Líng

[Features]	Shu-stream and yuan-source point of the Pericardium Channel of the Hand *Jueyin*.
[Locating]	The point is located when the arm is stretched forward with palm upward and the elbow flexed, in the midpoint of the transverse crease of the wrist, between the tendon of m.palmaris longus and m. flexor carpi radialis.
[Regional Anatomy]	The needle passes through the skin and subcutaneous fascia, penetrates the deep brachial fascia and reaches intercarpal joint capsule.
[Acupuncture and Moxibustion]	Insert the needle perpendicularly 0.3~0.5 cun deep and stimulate until there is a sore and numbing sensation in the local area with an electric sensation radiating to the finger tip. This point can be moxibusted.
[Indications]	Cardiac pain, palpitation, irritability, stomach ache, vomiting, and hematemesis.

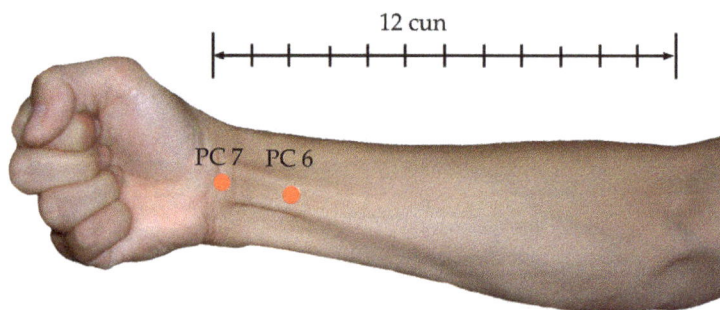

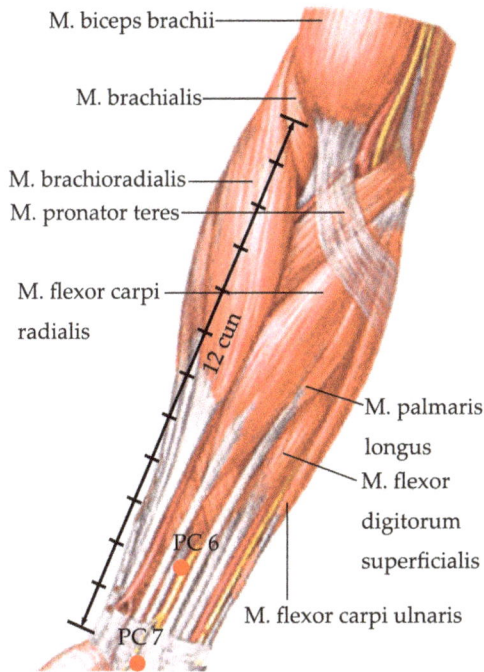

M. biceps brachii

M. brachialis

M. brachioradialis
M. pronator teres

M. flexor carpi
radialis

12 cun

M. palmaris
longus

M. flexor
digitorum
superficialis

PC 6

M. flexor carpi ulnaris

PC 7

PC 8 – Láo Gōng

[Features]	Ying-spring point of the Pericardium Channel of the Hand *Jueyin*.
[Locating]	In the center of the palm, between the second and the third metacarpal bones, closer to the third metacarpal bone, when the fist is clenched, under the tip of the third finger.
[Regional Anatomy]	The needle passes through the skin and subcutaneous fascia, pierces aponeurosis palmaris and m. lumbricales II, enters m. adductor pollicis, and reaches the interosseous muscles between the 2nd and 3rd metacarpal bones.
[Acupuncture and Moxibustion]	Insert the needle perpendicularly 0.3~0.5 cun deep and stimulate until there is a sore and numbing sensation in the local area radiating to the palm. This point can be moxibusted.
[Indications]	Hyperactivity, epilepsy, childhood convulsion, irritability and halitosis.

PC 9 – Zhōng Chōng

[Features]	Jing-well point of the Pericardium Channel of the Hand *Jueyin*.
[Locating]	In the center of the tip of the distal phalanx of the middle finger.
[Regional Anatomy]	The needle passes through the skin and subcutaneous fascia, pierces digital tendon sheath and tendo m. flexor digitorum profundus.
[Acupuncture and Moxibustion]	① Insert the needle 0.1~0.2 cun deep and stimulate until there is a sore and distending sensation in the local area. ② Prick with the three-edged needle to bleed. This point can be moxibusted.
[Indications]	Cardiac pain, irritability, stroke, febrile diseases without sweating, heatstroke, redness of eye and tongue, and night cry during childhood.

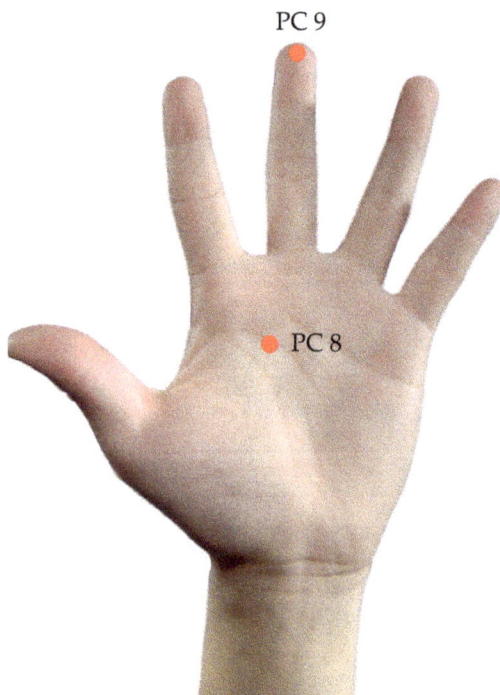

PC 9

PC 8

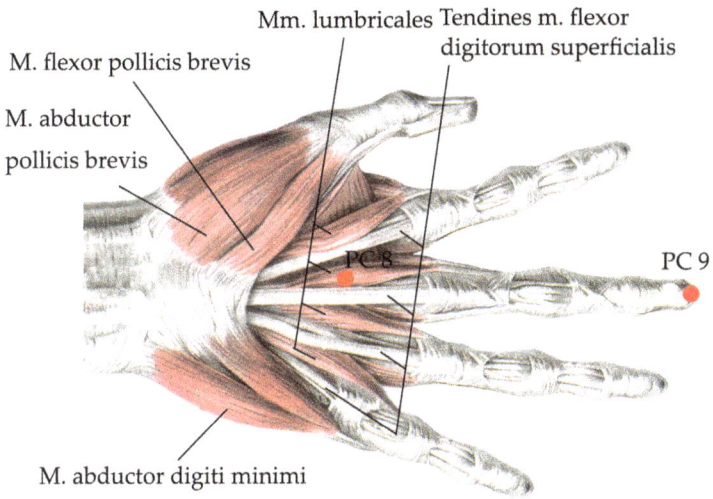

M. flexor pollicis brevis

M. abductor
pollicis brevis

Mm. lumbricales

Tendines m. flexor
digitorum superficialis

PC 8

PC 9

M. abductor digiti minimi

Sanjiao Channel of Hand Shaoyang; TE

There are twenty-three acupuncture points in the *Sanjiao* Channel of Hand *Shaoyang* and forty-six points in total on both sides. There are thirteen points on the lateral side of the upper extremities and ten points distributed on the neck and head. The first point is TE 1 (Guān Chōng) and the last is TE 23 (Sī Zhú Kōng). The indications are diseases of the chest and hypochondriac region, head, ears, eyes, throat, febrile diseases and the symptoms along the course of the channel.

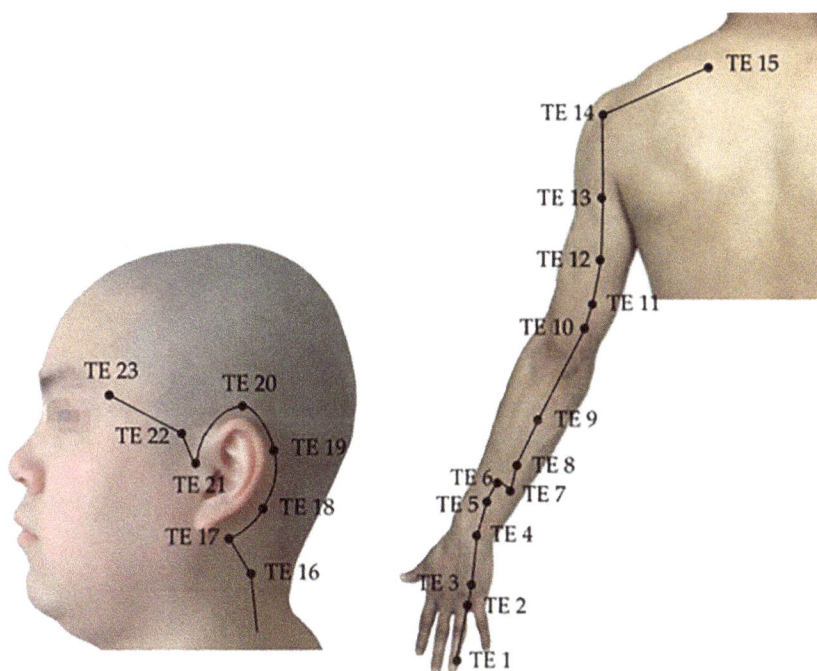

TE 1 – Guān Chōng

[Features]	Jing-well point of the *Sanjiao* Channel of Hand *Shaoyang*.
[Locating]	The point is located when the hand is in a loose fist and the palm is facing upward, on the line crossing the ulnar border and the base of the nail of the ring finger, 0.1 cun lateral to the ulnar side of the corner of the nail on the ring finger.
[Regional Anatomy]	The needle passes through the skin and subcutaneous fascia and penetrates the digital tendon sheath.
[Acupuncture and Moxibustion]	① Insert the needle perpendicularly 0.1~0.3 cun deep and stimulate until there is a sore and distending sensation in the local area radiating to the palm. ② Prick with a three-edged needle to bleed. This point can be moxibusted.
[Indications]	Headache, febrile diseases.

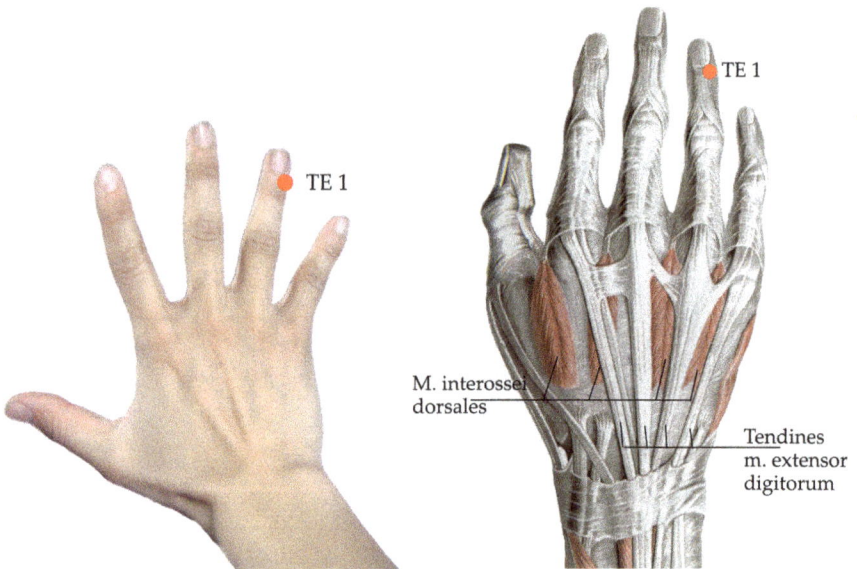

TE 1

TE 1

M. interossei dorsales

Tendines m. extensor digitorum

TE 2 – Yè Mén

[Features]	Ying-spring point of the *Sanjiao* Channel of Hand *Shaoyang*.
[Locating]	The point is located on the dorsum aspect of the hand when the palm faces downwards, in the depression between the anterior border of the fourth and fifth metacarpophalangeal joint.
[Regional Anatomy]	The needle passes through the skin and subcutaneous tissue, penetrates the m . interossei dorsales.
[Acupuncture and Moxibustion]	Insert the needle perpendicularly 0.3~0.5 cun deep and stimulate until there is a sore and distending sensation in the local area radiating to the dorsum of the hand. This point can be moxibusted.
[Indications]	Headache, tinnitus, sore throat, and helopyra.

TE 3 – Zhōng Zhǔ

[Features]	Shu-stream points of the *Sanjiao* Channel of Hand *Shaoyang*.
[Locating]	The point is located on the dorsum aspect of the hand when the palm faces downwards, in the depression between the posterior border of the fourth and fifth metacarpophalangeal joint.
[Regional Anatomy]	The needle passes through the skin and subcutaneous tissue, penetrates the m . interossei dorsales.
[Acupuncture and Moxibustion]	Insert the needle perpendicularly 0.3~0.5 cun deep and stimulate until there is a sore and distending sensation in the local area radiating to the dorsum of the hand. This point can be moxibusted.
[Indications]	Tinnitus, febrile diseases, and inability to flex and extend the fingers.

TE 4 – Yáng Chí

[Features]	Yuan-source point of the *Sanjiao* Channel of Hand *Shaoyang*.
[Locating]	On the dorsum aspect of the transverse wrist crease, in the depression on the ulnar side of the tendon of m. extensor digitorum communis.
[Regional Anatomy]	The needle passes through the skin and subcutaneous fascia, penetrates dorsal carpal ligament.
[Acupuncture and Moxibustion]	Insert the needle perpendicularly 0.3~0.5 cun deep and stimulate until there is a sore and distending sensation in the local area radiating to the middle finger. This point can be moxibusted.
[Indications]	Tinnitus, diabetes, and pain in the wrist.

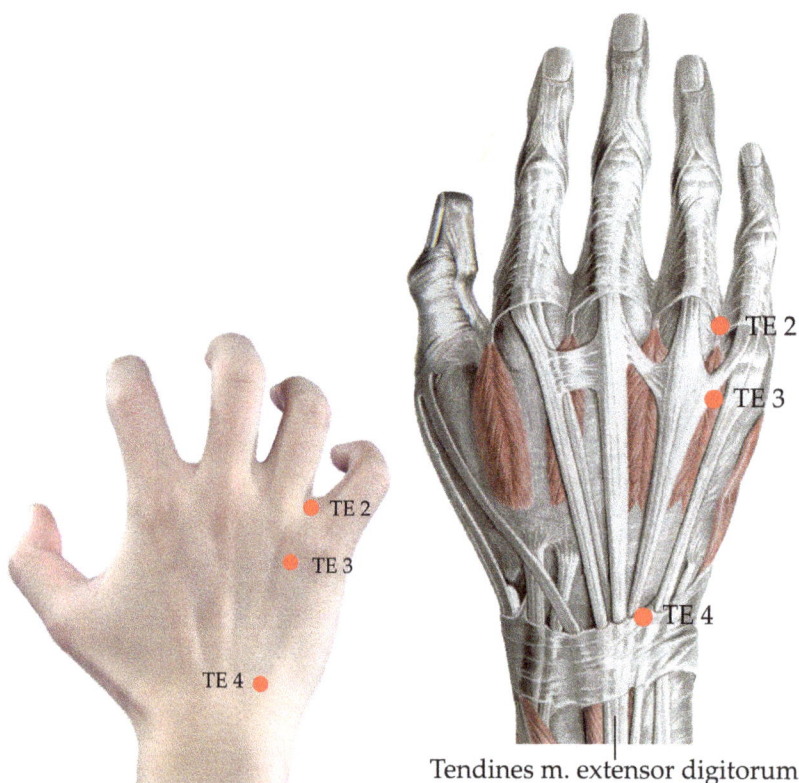

TE 2
TE 3
TE 4

TE 2
TE 3
TE 4

Tendines m. extensor digitorum

TE 5 – Wài Guān

[Features]	Luo-connecting point of the *Sanjiao* Channel of Hand *Shaoyang*. One of the Eight Confluent Points associating with the Yang Linking Vessel.
[Locating]	The point is located on the forearm when the arm is stretched with the palm facing down, 2 cun superior to SJ 4 (Yang Chí), in the depression between the ulna and radius.
[Regional Anatomy]	The needle passes through the skin and subcutaneous fascia, penetrates the deep brachial fascia, enters m. extensor digiti minimi from the radial side of m. extensor digitorum, and finally penetrates m. extensor indicis.
[Acupuncture and Moxibustion]	Insert the needle perpendicularly 0.5~1.0 cun deep and stimulate until there is a sore and distending sensation in the local area radiating to the tip of the finger. This point can be moxibusted.
[Indications]	Febrile diseases, headache, tinnitus, headache, infantile convulsions and pain in the chest and hypochondriac region.

TE 6 – Zhī Gōu

[Features]	Jing-river point of the *Sanjiao* Channel of Hand *Shaoyang*.
[Locating]	The point is located on the forearm when the arm is stretched with the palm facing down, 3 cun superior to SJ 4 (Yang Chí), between the ulna and radius.
[Regional Anatomy]	The needle passes through the skin and subcutaneous fascia, pierces the antebrachial deep fascia, enters m. extensor digiti minimi, and reaches m. extensor pollicis longus.
[Acupuncture and Moxibustion]	Insert the needle perpendicularly 0.5~1.0 cun deep and stimulate until there is a sore and distending sensation in the local area radiating to the upper and lower. This point can be moxibusted.
[Indications]	Constipation and chest and hypochondriac pain.

TE 7 – Huì Zōng

[Features]	Xi-cleft point of the *Sanjiao* Channel of Hand *Shaoyang*.
[Locating]	Stretch the arm with palm down, 3 cun superior to SJ 4 (Yang Chí), in the depression between the ulna and radius, on the ulnar side of SJ 6 (Zhī Gōu) and radial side of the ulna.
[Regional Anatomy]	The needle passes through the skin and subcutaneous fascia, penetrates m. extensor carpi ulnaris and m. extensor indicis.
[Acupuncture and Moxibustion]	Insert the needle perpendicularly 0.5~1.0 cun deep and stimulate until there is a sore and distending sensation in the local area. This point can be moxibusted.
[Indications]	Headache, tinnitus, cough, and asthma.

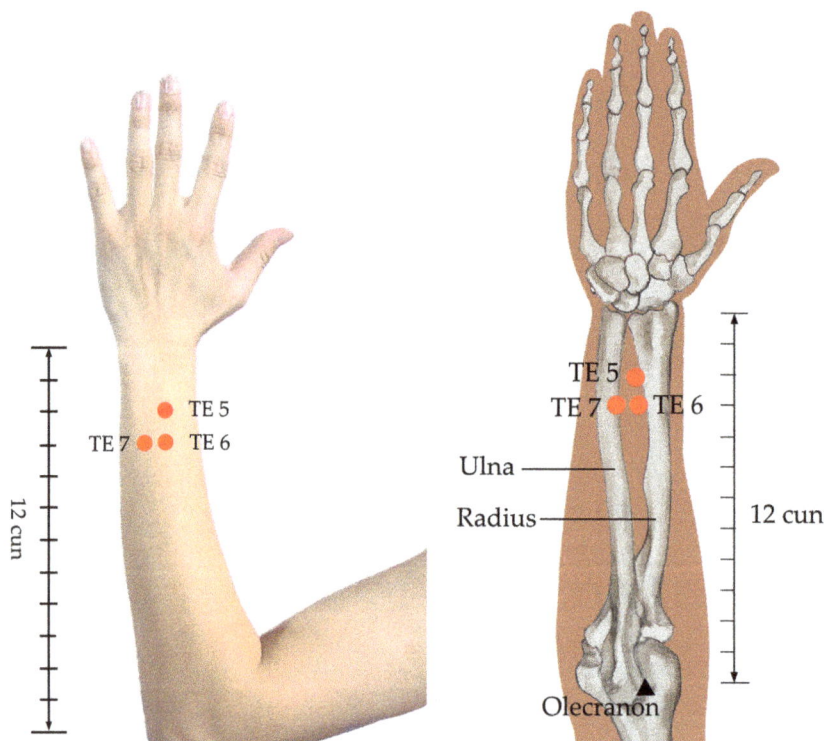

TE 8 – Sān Yáng Luò

[Locating]	The point is located when the arm is stretched with palm facing down, 4 cun superior to SJ 4 (Yang Chí), in the depression between the ulna and radius.
[Regional Anatomy]	The needle passes through the skin and subcutaneous tissue, penetrates m. extensor digitorum, m. abductor pollicis longus and m. abductor pollicis brevis.
[Acupuncture and Moxibustion]	Insert the needle perpendicularly 0.5~1.0 cun deep and stimulate until there is a sore and distending sensation in the local area radiating to the elbow. This point can be moxibusted.
[Indications]	Sudden loss of voice, deafness, and pain of the arm.

TE 9 – Sì Dú

[Locating]	The point is located when the elbow is flexed slightly with the palm facing down, 7 cun superior to SJ 4 (Yang Chí), in the depression between the ulna and radius.
[Regional Anatomy]	The needle passes through the skin and subcutaneous tissue, penetrates m. extensor carpi ulnaris and m. abductor pollicis brevis.
[Acupuncture and Moxibustion]	Insert the needle perpendicularly 0.5~1.0 cun deep and stimulate until there is a sore and distending sensation in the local area radiating to the elbow. This point can be moxibusted.
[Indications]	Sudden loss of voice, tinnitus, and toothache.

TE 10 – Tiān Jǐng

[Features]	He-sea point of the *Sanjiao* Channel of Hand *Shaoyang*.
[Locating]	The point is located by standing with arm on hips and elbow extending outward, 1 cun posterior and superior to the tip of the elbow.
[Regional Anatomy]	The needle passes through the skin and subcutaneous bursa of olecranon, penetrates m. triceps brachii

[Acupuncture and Moxibustion]	Insert the needle perpendicularly 0.5~1.0 cun deep and stimulate until there is a sour and distending sensation in the local area.
	This point can be moxibusted.
[Indications]	Sudden loss of voice, and eye disease.

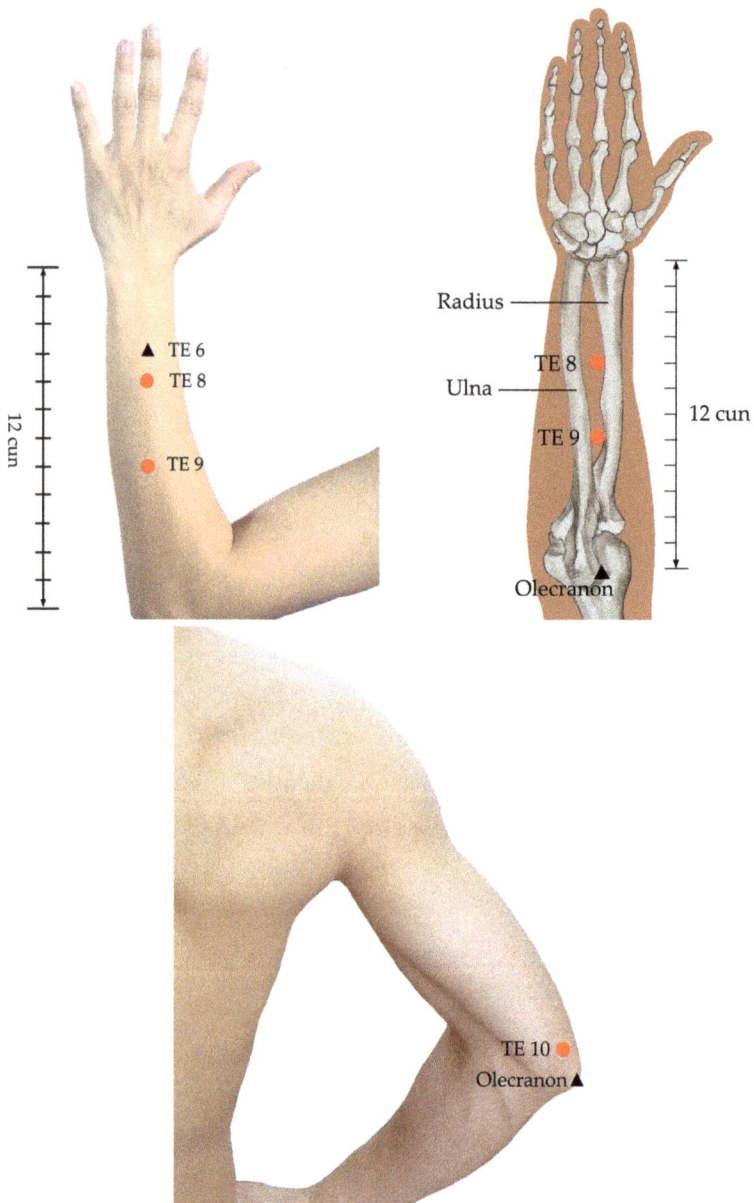

TE 11 – Qīng Líng Yuān

[Locating]	The point is located by standing with arm on hips and elbow extending outward, on the lateral aspect of the arm when the elbow is flexed, on the line connecting the tip of the elbow and the TE 14 (Jiān Liáo), 2 cun superior to the tip of the elbow.
[Regional Anatomy]	The needle passes through the skin and subcutaneous fascia, penetrates posterior cubital deep fascia, enters tendo m. triceps brachii, and reaches the periost of humerus.
[Acupuncture and Moxibustion]	Insert the needle perpendicularly 0.5~1.0 cun deep and stimulate until there is a sour and distending sensation in the local area. This point can be moxibusted.
[Indications]	Diseases of the eye, and pain in the arm and neck.

TE 12 – Xiāo Luò

[Locating]	The point is located in the sitting position with the arm adducted, on the line connecting the tip of the elbow and the TE 14 (Jiānl Láo), in the midpoint on the line connecting TE 11 (Qīng Líng Yuān) to TE 13 (Nào Huì).
[Regional Anatomy]	The needle passes through the skin and subcutaneous fascia, penetrates posterior cubital deep fascia, enters tendo m. triceps brachii, and reaches the periost of humerus.
[Acupuncture and Moxibustion]	Insert the needle perpendicularly 0.8~1.2 cun deep and stimulate until there is a sour and distending sensation in the local area.
[Indications]	Stiffness and pain of the neck and head, and arm pain.

TE 13 – Nào Huì

[Locating]	The point is located when the arm is adducted, on the line connecting the tip of the elbow and SJ 14 (Jiān Liáo), 3 cun inferior to TE 14 (Jiān Liáo), on the posterior and inferior border of m. deltoideus.
[Regional Anatomy]	The needle passes through the skin and subcutaneous fascia, penetrates posterior cubital deep fascia, enters tendo m. triceps brachii, and reaches the periost of humerus. Figure 11-40

[Acupuncture and Moxibustion]	Insert the needle perpendicularly 1.0~1.5 cun deep and stimulate until there is a sour and distending sensation in the local area radiating to the shoulder.
	This point can be moxibusted.
[Indications]	Swelling and pain of the shoulder, and arm and scrofula.

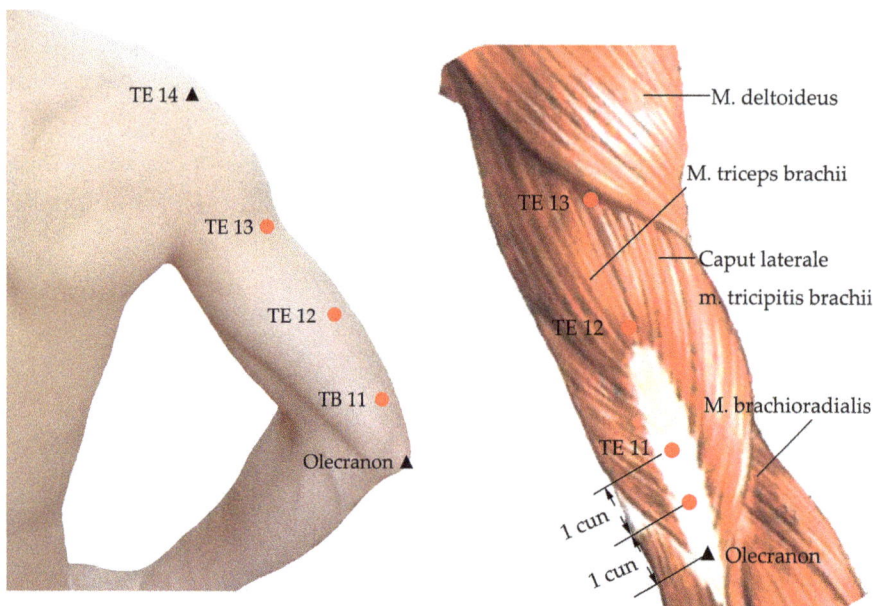

TE 14 – Jiān Liáo

[Locating]	When the arm is abducted, posterior and inferior to the acromion, in the depression posterior to the shoulder joint.
[Regional Anatomy]	The needle passes through the skin and subcutaneous fascia, penetrates m. deltoideus, enters m.teres minor and m. teres major.
[Acupuncture and Moxibustion]	Insert the needle perpendicularly 0.5~1.0 cun deep and stimulate until there is a sour and distending sensation in the local area.
	This point can be moxibusted.
[Indications]	Swelling and pain of the shoulder and scapular.

Acromion

TE 14

Clavicula

Coracoid process

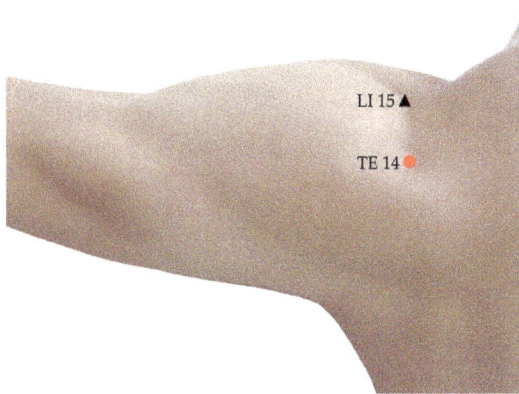

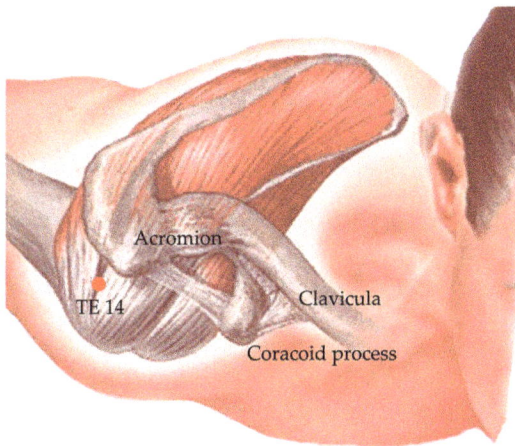

TE 15 – Tiān Liáo

[Locating]	The point is located in the sitting or prone position, on the superior and medial angle of the scapular, in the midpoint of the line connecting GB 21 (Jiān Jǐng) to SI 13 (Qū Yuán).
[Regional Anatomy]	The needle passes through the skin and subcutaneous fascia, penetrates m. trapezius and enters m. supraspinatus.
[Acupuncture and Moxibustion]	Insert the needle perpendicularly 0.5~0.8 cun deep and stimulate until there is a sour and distending sensation in the local area radiating to the shoulder and scapular. This point can be moxibusted.
[Indications]	Distention of the chest, pain of the shoulder and arm and neck stiffness.

TE 16 Tiān Yŏu

[Locating]	The point is located in the sitting or prone position, inferior and posterior to the mastoid process, at the level of the angle of the mandible, on the posterior border of m. sternocleidomastoideus.
[Regional Anatomy]	The needle passes through the skin and subcutaneous fascia, pierces fascia of nape, enters m. splenius capitis and m. semispinalis capitis.
[Acupuncture and Moxibustion]	Insert the needle perpendicularly 0.5~1.0 cun deep and stimulate until there is a sour and distending sensation in the local area radiating to the ear. This point can be moxibusted.
[Indications]	Headache, sudden deafness and neck stiffness.

TE 17 – Yì Fēng

[Locating]	The point is located in the sitting by folding the lobule of the ear, in the depression anterior to the mastoid process.
[Regional Anatomy]	The needle passes through the skin and subcutaneous fascia, penetrates the masseteric fascia of parotid, and finally reaches the retromandibular prognathism of parotid.
[Acupuncture and Moxibustion]	Insert the needle perpendicularly 0.8~1.2 cun deep and stimulate until there is a sour and distending sensation in the local area radiating to the half of the face. This point can be moxibusted.
[Indications]	Tinnitus, deviation of eye and mouth, trismus, toothache, and mumps.

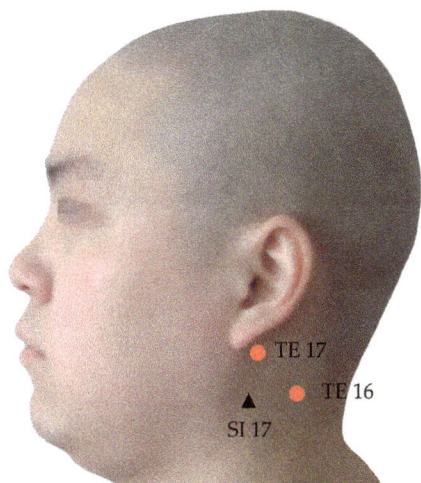

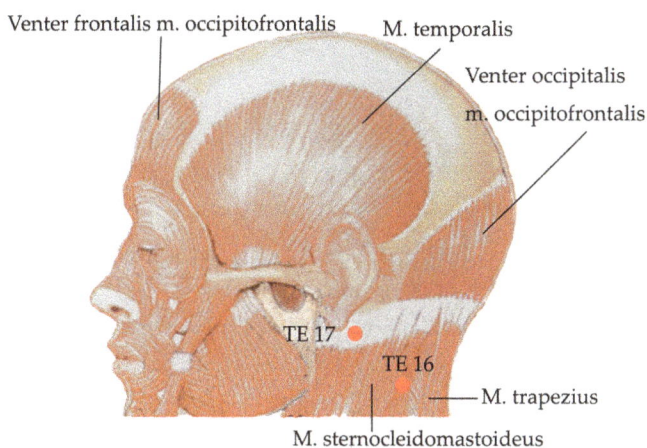

Venter frontalis m. occipitofrontalis   M. temporalis

Venter occipitalis
m. occipitofrontalis

TE 17

TE 16

M. trapezius

M. sternocleidomastoideus

TE 18 – Chì Mài

[Locating]	The point is located in the sitting position, anterior and inferior to the mastoid process, at lower third of the curved line connecting TE 20 (Jiǎo Sūn) to TE 17 (Yì Fēng) following the posterior line of the helix of the ear.
[Regional Anatomy]	The needle passes through the skin and subcutaneous fascia, and enters m. auricularis posterior.
[Acupuncture and Moxibustion]	Insert the needle subcutaneously 0.3~0.5 cun deep and stimulate until there is a sour and distending sensation in the local area. Or prick with a three-edged needle to bleed. This point can be moxibusted.
[Indications]	Tinnitus, and infantile convulsion.

TE 19 – Lú Xī

[Locating]	The point is located in the sitting position, at upper third of the curved line connecting TE 20 (Jiǎo Sūn) to TE 17 (Yì Fēng) following the posterior line of the helix of the ear.
[Regional Anatomy]	The needle passes through the skin and subcutaneous fascia, and penetrates the belly of m. occipitofrontalis.
[Acupuncture and Moxibustion]	Insert the needle subcutaneously 0.3~0.5 cun deep and stimulate until there is a sour and distending sensation in the local area. This point can be moxibusted.
[Indications]	Tinnitus, infantile convulsion and vomiting.

TE 20 – Jiǎo Sūn

[Locating]	The point is located in the sitting position, at the hairline above the apex of the ear when the ear is bent forward.
[Regional Anatomy]	The needle passes through the skin and subcutaneous fascia, penetrates m. auricularis superior and m. temporalis, and reaches the periost.
[Acupuncture and Moxibustion]	Insert the needle subcutaneously 0.3~0.5 cun deep and stimulate until there is a sour and distending sensation in the local area radiating to the ear.
[Indications]	Parotitis and redness, swelling and pain of the eye.

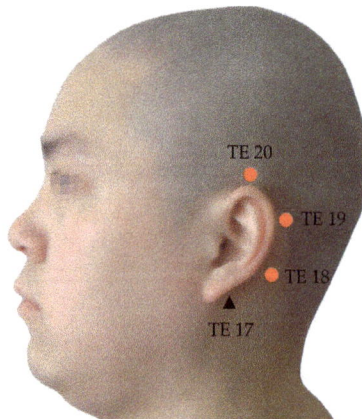

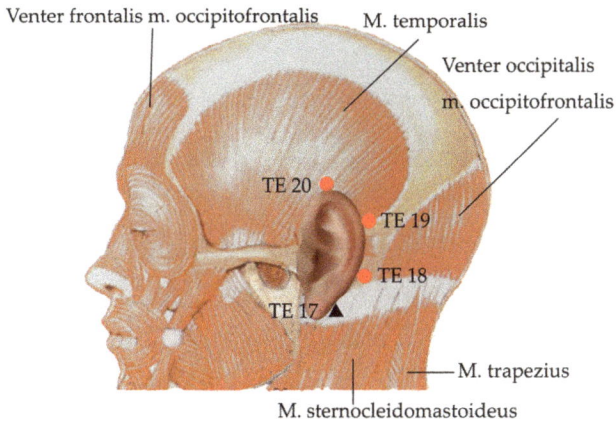

Venter frontalis m. occipitofrontalis M. temporalis

Venter occipitalis
m. occipitofrontalis

TE 20
TE 19
TE 18
TE 17

M. trapezius

M. sternocleidomastoideus

TE 21 – Ěr Mén

[Locating]	The point is located in the sitting position when the mouth is slightly open, in the depression anterior to the superior tragus notch.
[Regional Anatomy]	The needle passes through the skin and subcutaneous fascia, penetrates the upper portion of parotid gland.
[Acupuncture and Moxibustion]	Insert the needle perpendicularly 0.5~1.0 cun deep and stimulate until there is a sour and distending sensation in the local area radiating to the ear. This point can be moxibusted.
[Indications]	Tinnitus, deafness, ceruminal ear, and toothache.

TE 22 – ěr Hé Liáo

[Locating]	The point is located in the sitting position, on the posterior border of the hairline of the temple on the head, at the level with the root of the ear, posterior to the superficial temporal artery.
[Regional Anatomy]	The needle passes through the skin and subcutaneous fascia, and penetrates m. auricularis anterior and m. temporalis.
[Acupuncture and Moxibustion]	Avoid puncturing the artery, insert the needle obliquely 0.3~0.5 cun deep and stimulate until there is a sour and distending sensation in the local area. This point can be moxibusted.
[Indications]	Deviation of the eye and mouth, headache, and tinnitus.

TE 22

TE 21

SI 19

M. temporalis   Venter frontalis m. occipitofrontalis

Venter occipitalis
m. occipitofrontalis

TE 22
TE 21

Tuberositas os
occipitale

M. trapezius

M. sternocleidomastoideus

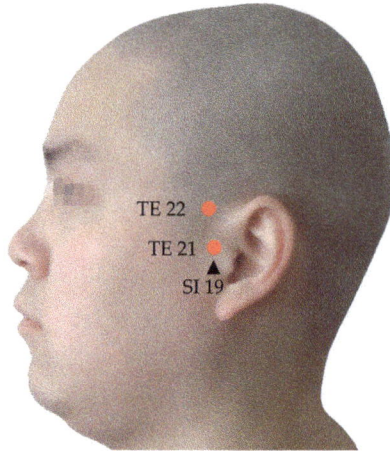

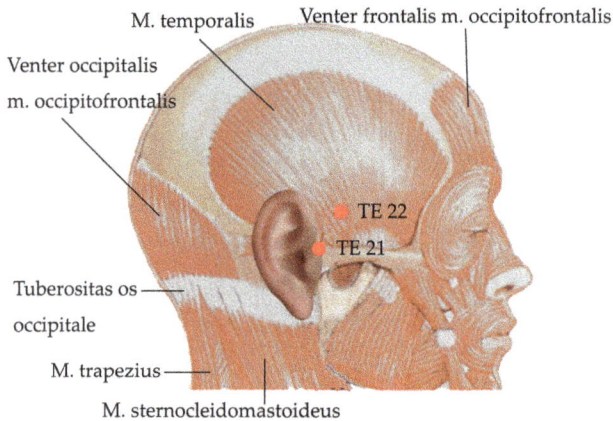

TE 23 – Sī Zhú Kōng

[Locating]	The point is located in the sitting position, on the lateral border of the frontal zygomatic process, in the depression at the lateral end of the eyebrow.
[Regional Anatomy]	The needle passes through the skin and subcutaneous tissue, penetrates m. orbicularis oculi, and reaches the periost of frontal bone.
[Acupuncture and Moxibustion]	Insert the needle subcutaneously 0.5~1.0 cun deep and stimulate until there is a sore and numbing sensation in the local area. Or prick with a three-edged needle to bleed. The point is contraindicated for moxibustion.
[Indications]	Headache, epilepsy, redness, swelling and pain of the eye and twitching of the eyelid.

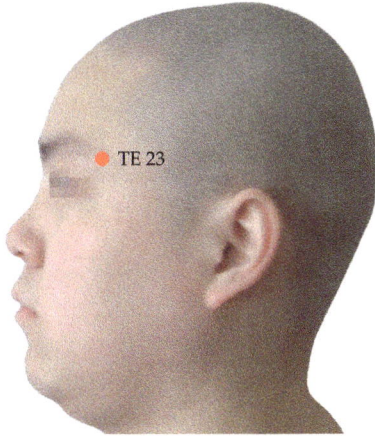

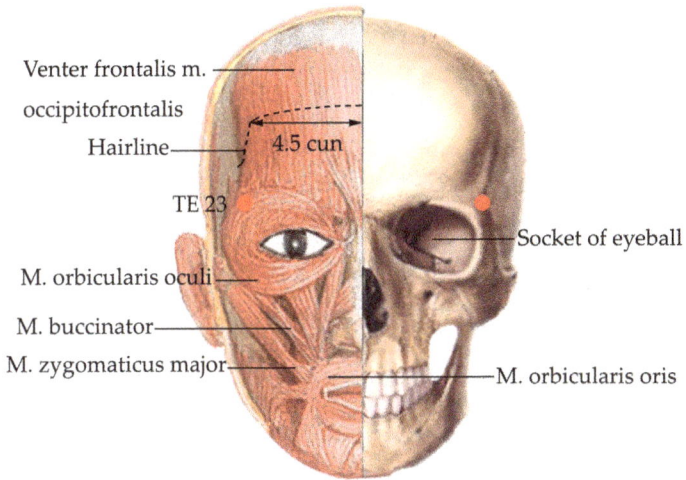

Venter frontalis m. occipitofrontalis

Hairline

4.5 cun

TE 23

M. orbicularis oculi

M. buccinator

M. zygomaticus major

Socket of eyeball

M. orbicularis oris

CHAPTER 12

Gallbladder Channel of Foot Shaoyang; GB

There are forty-four acupuncture points on the Gallbladder Channel of the Foot *Shaoyang* and eighty-eight points in total on both sides. There are twenty points on the face and head, one point on the shoulder, seven points on the lateral side of the chest, abdomen and waist, sixteen points on the lateral side of the lower extremities. The first point is GB 1 (Tóng Zǐ Liáo) and the last point is GB 44 (Zú Qiào Yīn). The indications of this channel are diseases of the head, ear, eye and throat, mental diseases, febrile diseases and the symptoms along the course of the channel.

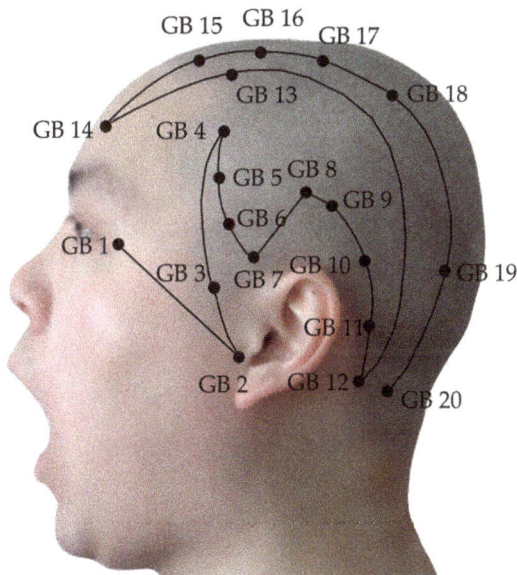

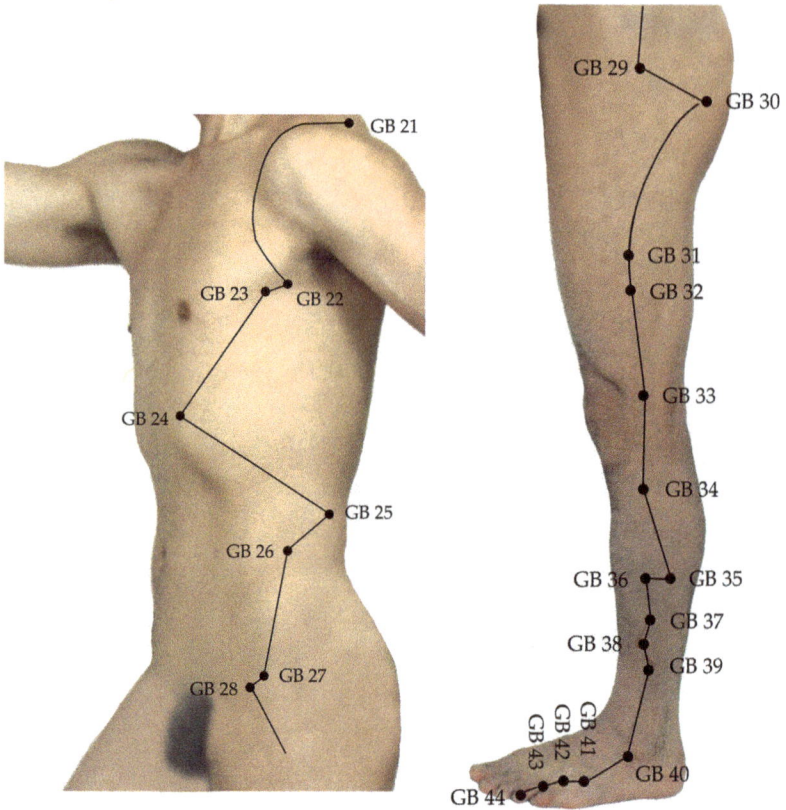

Points labeled: GB 21, GB 23, GB 22, GB 24, GB 25, GB 26, GB 28, GB 27, GB 29, GB 30, GB 31, GB 32, GB 33, GB 34, GB 36, GB 35, GB 37, GB 38, GB 39, GB 43, GB 42, GB 41, GB 40, GB 44

GB 1 – Tóng Zǐ Liáo

[Locating]	The point is located in the sitting position with eyes closed, on the face lateral to the outer canthus, 0.5 cun depression on the lateral aspect of the eye.
[Regional Anatomy]	The needle passes through the skin and the subcutaneous tissues and penetrates the M. orbicularis oculiand m. temporalis.
[Acupuncture and Moxibustion]	① Insert the needle obliquely backward 0.5~0.8 cun deep and stimulate until there is a sore and numbing sensation in the local area radiating to the ear. ② Prick with a three-edged needle to bleed. ③ Not suitable for moxibustion.
[Indications]	Headache and dizziness, deviation of the eye and mouth, pain of the eye, and excessive lacrimation.

GB 2 – Tīng Huì

[Locating]	The point is located in the sitting position with an open mouth, in the depression anterior to the intertragic notch, on the posterior border of the condyloid process of the mandible.
[Regional Anatomy]	The needle passes through the skin and the subcutaneous tissues and penetrates the tissue near the parotid gland.
[Acupuncture and Moxibustion]	Insert the needle perpendicularly 0.5~1.0 cun deep and stimulate until there is a sore and numbing sensation in the local area. This point can be moxibusted.
[Indications]	Headache, dizziness and tinnitus.

GB 3 – Shàng Guān

[Locating]	The point is located in the sitting or lateral position with an open mouth, superior 1 cun to ST 7 (Xià Guān), in the depression on the upper border of the zygomatic arch.
[Regional Anatomy]	The needle passes through the skin and the subcutaneous tissues and penetrates the temporal fascia and m. temporalis.
[Acupuncture and Moxibustion]	Insert the needle perpendicularly 0.5~0.8 cun deep and stimulate until there is a sore and numbing sensation in the local area. This point can be moxibusted.
[Indications]	Headache, facial pain, and tinnitus.

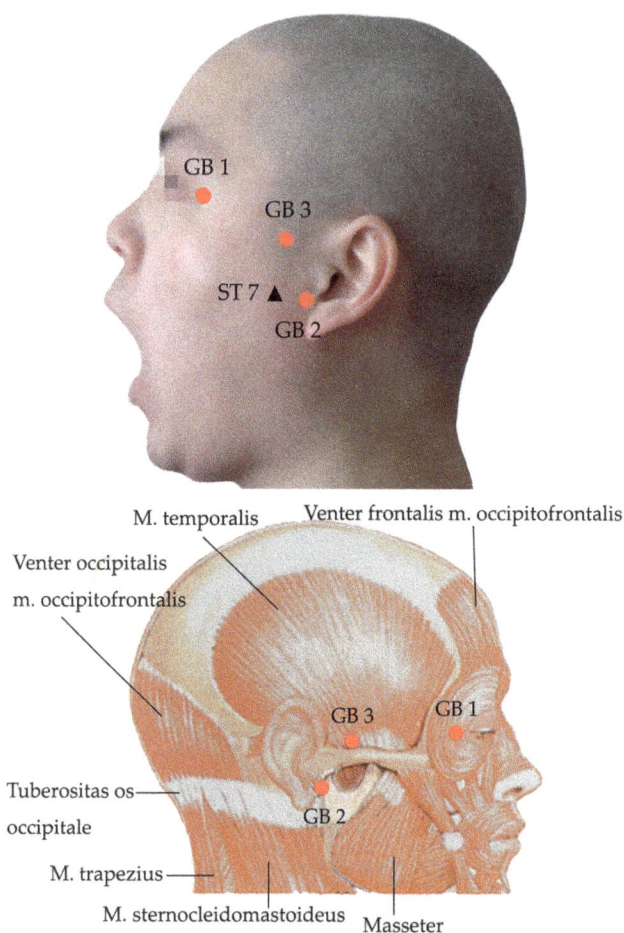

M. temporalis   Venter frontalis m. occipitofrontalis

Venter occipitalis
m. occipitofrontalis

Tuberositas os
occipitale

M. trapezius

M. sternocleidomastoideus   Masseter

GB 4 – Hàn Yàn

[Locating]	The point is located in the sitting or lateral position, in the upper 1/4 and the lower 3/4 of the arc connecting ST 8 (Tóu Wéi) and GB 7 (Qū Bìn).
[Regional Anatomy]	The needle passes through the skin and the subcutaneous tissues and penetrates the temporal fascia and m. temporalis.
[Acupuncture and Moxibustion]	Insert the needle subcutaneously 0.3~0.5 cun deep and stimulate until there is a sore and numbing sensation in the local area. This point can be moxibusted.
[Indications]	Headache and dizziness, tinnitus and deafness.

GB 5 – Xuán Lú

[Locating]	The point is located in the sitting or lateral position, in the middle of the arc connecting ST 8 (Tóu Wéi) and GB 7 (Qū Bìn).
[Regional Anatomy]	The same as GB 4 (Hàn Yàn).
[Acupuncture and Moxibustion]	Insert the needle subcutaneously 0.5~0.8 cun deep and stimulate until there is a sore and numbing sensation in the local area. This point can be moxibusted.
[Indications]	Migraine.

GB 6 – Xuán Lí

[Locating]	The point is located in the sitting or lateral position, in the upper 3/4 and the lower 1/4 of the arc connecting ST 8 (Tóu Wéi) and GB 7 (Qū Bìn).
[Regional Anatomy]	The same as GB 4 (Hàn Yàn).
[Acupuncture and Moxibustion]	Insert the needle subcutaneously 0.5~0.8 cun deep and stimulate until there is a sore and numbing sensation in the local area. This point can be moxibusted.
[Indications]	Headache and dizziness.

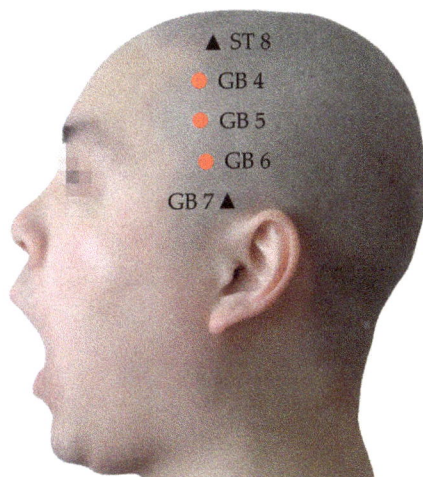

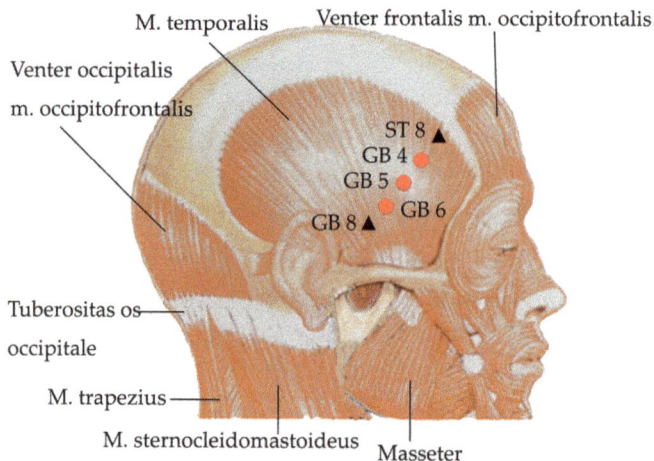

Labels on figure:
M. temporalis
Venter frontalis m. occipitofrontalis
Venter occipitalis
m. occipitofrontalis
ST 8 ▲
GB 4 ●
GB 5 ●
GB 8 ▲ ● GB 6
Tuberositas os
occipitale
M. trapezius
M. sternocleidomastoideus
Masseter

GB 7 – Qū Bìn

[Locating]	The point is located in the sitting or lateral position, on the temporal region of the head, within the hairline anterior to the ear, at the level with the apex of the ear, in front of the Jiǎosūn about 1 horizontal finger.
[Regional Anatomy]	The same as GB 4 (Hàn Yàn).
[Acupuncture and Moxibustion]	Insert the needle subcutaneously 0.5~0.8 cun deep and stimulate until there is a sore and numbing sensation in the local area. This point can be moxibusted.
[Indications]	Headache and dizziness.

GB 8 – Shuài Gǔ

[Locating]	The point is located in the sitting or lateral position, 1.5 cun superior to the tip of the ear.
[Regional Anatomy]	The needle passes through the skin and the subcutaneous tissues, penetrates the M. auricularis superior, temporal fascia and m. temporalis
[Acupuncture and Moxibustion]	Insert the needle subcutaneously 0.5~0.8 cun deep and stimulate until there is a sore and numbing sensation in the local area radiating to the temporal side of the head. This point can be moxibusted.
[Indications]	Headache, dizziness and infantile convulsion.

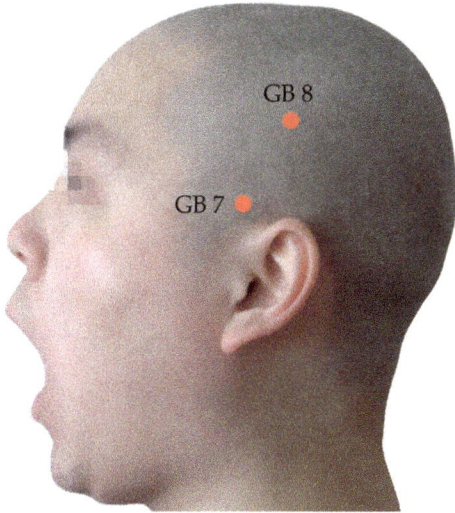

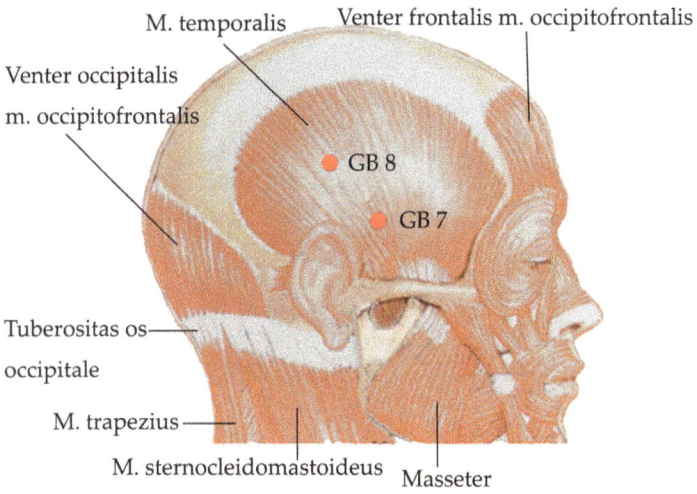

M. temporalis

Venter frontalis m. occipitofrontalis

Venter occipitalis
m. occipitofrontalis

GB 8

GB 7

Tuberositas os
occipitale

M. trapezius

M. sternocleidomastoideus   Masseter

GB 9 – Tiān Chōng

[Locating]	The point is located in the sitting or lateral position, superior to the posterior border of the ear, 2.0 cun within the hairline, 0.5 cun posterior to GB 8 (Shuài Gǔ).
[Regional Anatomy]	The needle passes through the skin and the subcutaneous tissues, penetrates the M. auricularis superior, temporal fascia and m. temporalis.
[Acupuncture and Moxibustion]	Insert the needle subcutaneously 0.5~0.8 cun deep and stimulate until there is a sore and numbing sensation in the local area. This point can be moxibusted.
[Indications]	Headache and dizziness.

GB 10 – Fú Bái

[Locating]	The point is located in the sitting or lateral position, posterior and superior to the mastoid process behind the ear, at the upper 1/3 and lower 2/3 of the distance along the arc connecting GB 9 (Tiān Chōng) to GB 12 (Wán Gǔ).
[Regional Anatomy]	The needle passes through the skin and the subcutaneous tissues, penetrates the M. auricularis superior, temporal fascia and m. temporalis.
[Acupuncture and Moxibustion]	Insert the needle subcutaneously 0.5~0.8 cun deep and stimulate until there is a sore and numbing sensation in the local area. This point can be moxibusted.
[Indications]	Headache and neck stiffness.

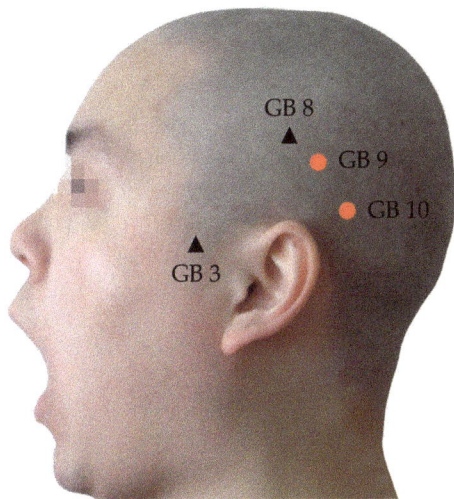

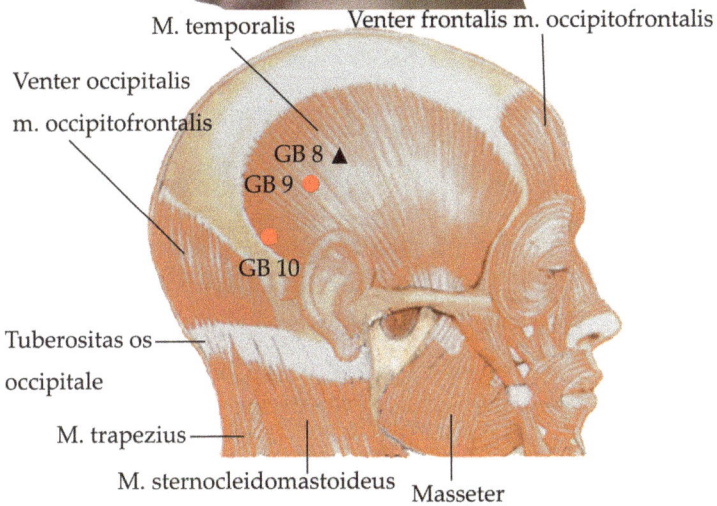

M. temporalis   Venter frontalis m. occipitofrontalis

Venter occipitalis
m. occipitofrontalis

GB 8 ▲
GB 9 ●

GB 10 ●

Tuberositas os
occipitale

M. trapezius

M. sternocleidomastoideus   Masseter

GB 11 – Tóu Qiào Yīn

[Locating]	The point is located in the sitting or lateral position, on the temporal part of the head, posterior and superior to the mastoid process behind the ear, or at the lower 1/3 and upper 2/3 of the distance along the arc connecting GB 9 (Tiān Chōng) to GB 12 (Wán Gǔ).
[Regional Anatomy]	The needle passes through the skin and the subcutaneous tissues, penetrates the auricularis posterior and occipital belly of m. occipitofrontalis.
[Acupuncture and Moxibustion]	Insert the needle subcutaneously 0.5~0.8 cun deep and stimulate until there is a sore and numbing sensation in the local area radiating to the posterior and lateral parts of the head. This point can be moxibusted.
[Indications]	Headache, tinnitus, chest pain, and bitter taste.

GB 12 – Wán Gǔ

[Locating]	The point is located in the sitting or lateral position, in the depression posterior and inferior to the mastoid process behind the ear.
[Regional Anatomy]	The needle passes through the skin and the subcutaneous tissues, penetrates the m. occipitofrontalis.
[Acupuncture and Moxibustion]	Insert the needle subcutaneously 0.5~0.8 cun deep and stimulate until there is a sore and numbing sensation in the local area radiating to the vertex of the head. This point can be moxibusted.
[Indications]	Headache and dizziness, tinnitus and deafness.

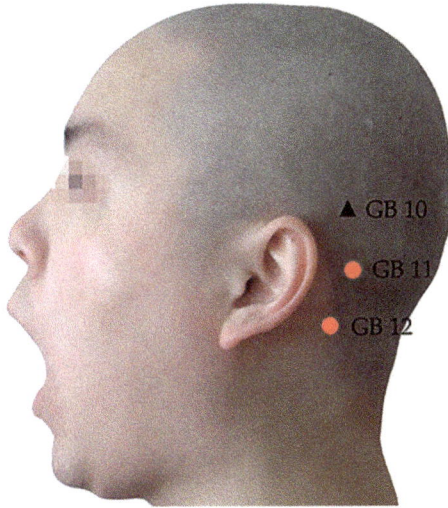

▲ GB 10
● GB 11
● GB 12

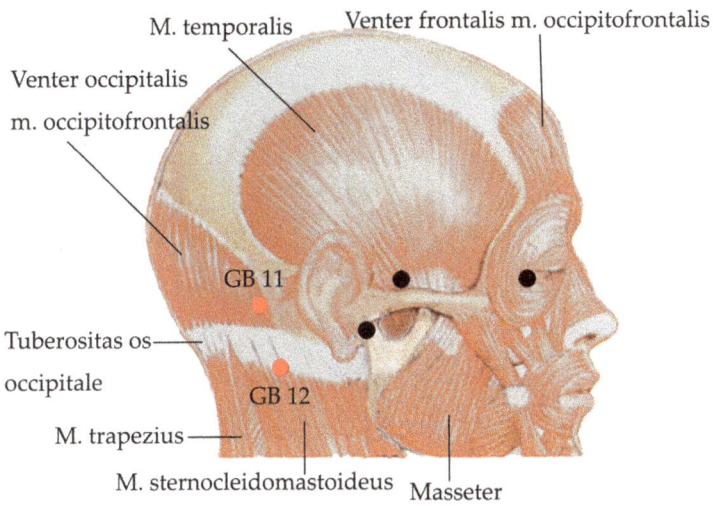

M. temporalis   Venter frontalis m. occipitofrontalis

Venter occipitalis
m. occipitofrontalis

GB 11

Tuberositas os—
occipitale

GB 12

M. trapezius—

M. sternocleidomastoideus   Masseter

GB 13 – Běn Shén

[Locating]	The point is located in the sitting or supine position, 0.5 cun within the anterior hairline of the forehead, 3 cun lateral to DU 24 (Shén Tíng).
[Regional Anatomy]	The needle passes through the skin and the subcutaneous tissues, penetrates the m. occipitofrontalis and the connective tissue beneath galea aponeurotica.
[Acupuncture and Moxibustion]	Insert the needle subcutaneously 0.5~0.8 cun deep and stimulate until there is a sore and numbing sensation in the local area.

This point can be moxibusted. |
| [Indications] | Headache, dizziness, neck stiffness and pain, and epilepsy. |

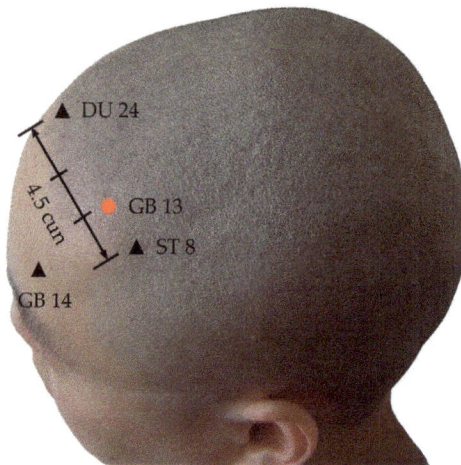

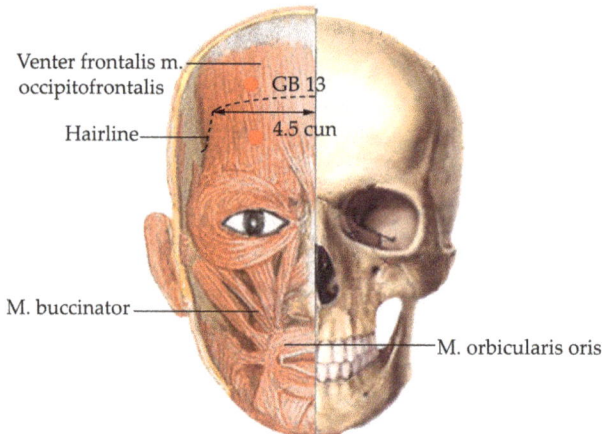

GB 14 – Yáng Bái

[Locating]	The point is located in the sitting or supine position, 1 cun superior to the eyebrow, directly above the pupil when looking forward.
[Regional Anatomy]	The needle passes through the skin and the subcutaneous tissues, penetrates the m. occipitofrontalis and the connective tissue beneath galea aponeurotica.
[Acupuncture and Moxibustion]	Insert the needle subcutaneously 0.5~0.8 cun deep and stimulate until there is a sore and numbing sensation in the local area. This point can be moxibusted.
[Indications]	Headache and dizziness, pain of the forehead and dry face, facial paralysis.

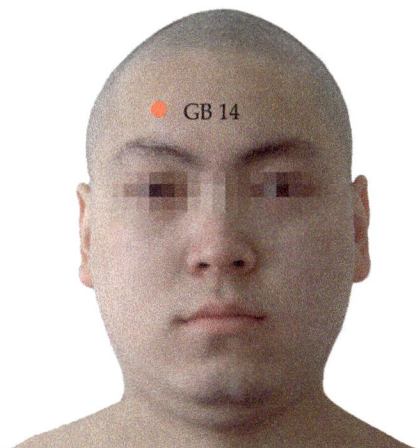

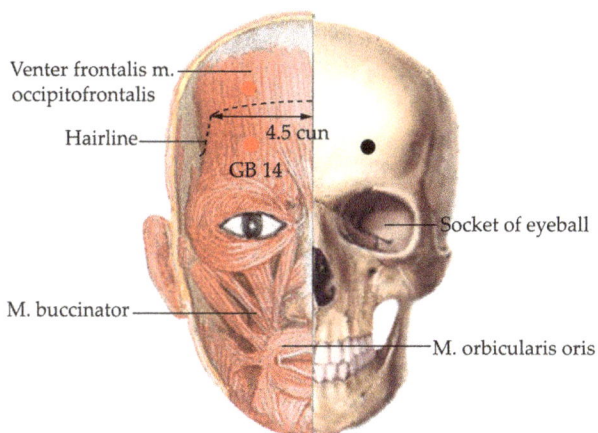

Venter frontalis m. occipitofrontalis
Hairline
4.5 cun
GB 14
Socket of eyeball
M. buccinator
M. orbicularis oris

GB 15 – Tóu Lín Qì

[Locating]	The point is located in the sitting or supine position, directly above GB 14 (Yáng Bái), 0.5 cun within the anterior hairline, at the midpoint of the line connecting DU 24 (Shén Tíng) to ST 8 (Tóu Wéi).
[Regional Anatomy]	The needle passes through the skin and the subcutaneous tissues, penetrates the m. occipitofrontalis and the connective tissue beneath galea aponeurotica.
[Acupuncture and Moxibustion]	Insert the needle subcutaneously 0.5~0.8 cun deep and stimulate until there is a sore and numbing sensation in the local area. This point can be moxibusted.
[Indications]	Headache and dizziness, redness, swelling and pain of the eye, tinnitus, and bitter taste.

GB 16 – Mù Chuāng

[Locating]	The point is located in the sitting or supine position, straight above the pupil when looking forward, 1 cun superior to GB 15 (Tóu Lín Qì), on the line connecting GB 14 (Tóu Lín Qì) to GB 20 (Fēng hí).
[Regional Anatomy]	The needle passes through the skin and the subcutaneous tissues, penetrates the galea aponeurotica and the connective tissue beneath galea aponeurotica.
[Acupuncture and Moxibustion]	Insert the needle subcutaneously 0.5~0.8 cun deep and stimulate until there is a sore and numbing sensation in the local area. This point can be moxibusted.
[Indications]	Headache and dizziness, redness, swelling and pain of the eye, myopia and hyperopia.

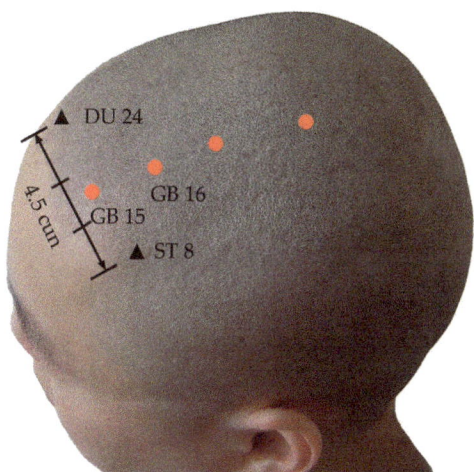

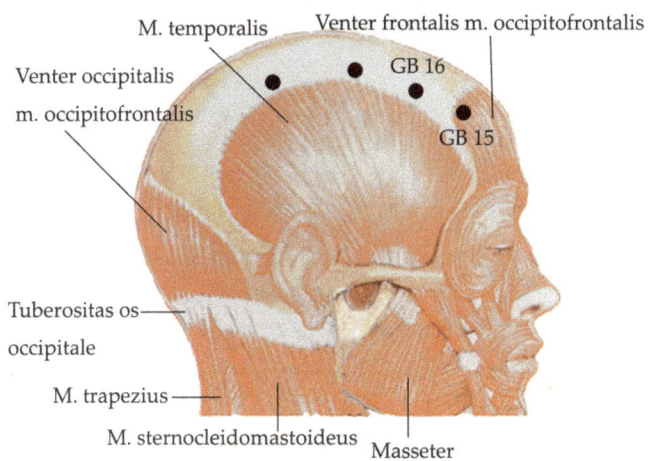

M. temporalis

Venter frontalis m. occipitofrontalis

GB 16

Venter occipitalis
m. occipitofrontalis

GB 15

Tuberositas os
occipitale

M. trapezius

M. sternocleidomastoideus   Masseter

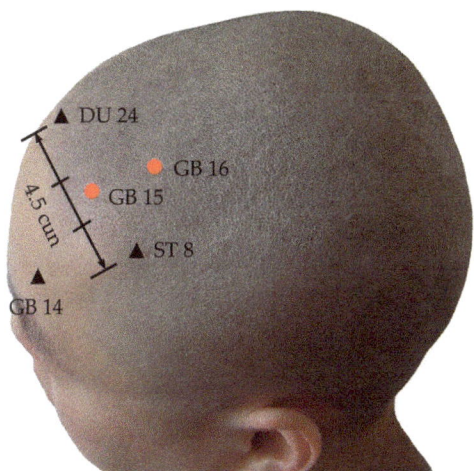

GB 17 – Zhèng Yíng

[Locating]	The point is located in the sitting or supine position, 2.5 cun posterior to the anterior hairline, 1 cun superior to GB 16 (Mùchuāng), on the line connecting GB 14 (Tóu Lín Qì) to GB 20 (Fēng Chí).
[Regional Anatomy]	The needle passes through the skin and the subcutaneous tissues, penetrates the galea aponeurotica and the connective tissue beneath galea aponeurotica.
[Acupuncture and Moxibustion]	Insert the needle subcutaneously 0.5~0.8 cun deep and stimulate until there is a sore and numbing sensation in the local area. This point can be moxibusted.
[Indications]	Headache and dizziness, swelling and redness of the face, and redness, swelling and pain of the eye.

GB 18 – Chéng Líng

[Locating]	The point is located in the sitting or supine position, 4 cun within the anterior hairline, on the line connecting GB 14 (Tóu Lín Qì) to GB 20 (Fēng Chí).
[Regional Anatomy]	The needle passes through the skin and the subcutaneous tissues, penetrates the galea aponeurotica and the connective tissue beneath galea aponeurotica.
[Acupuncture and Moxibustion]	Insert the needle subcutaneously 0.5~0.8 cun deep and stimulate until there is a sore and numbing sensation in the local area. This point can be moxibusted.
[Indications]	Headache, dizziness and nasal obstruction.

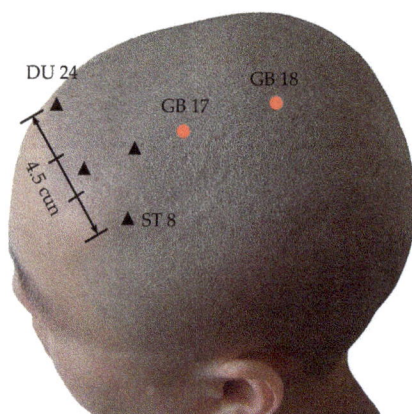

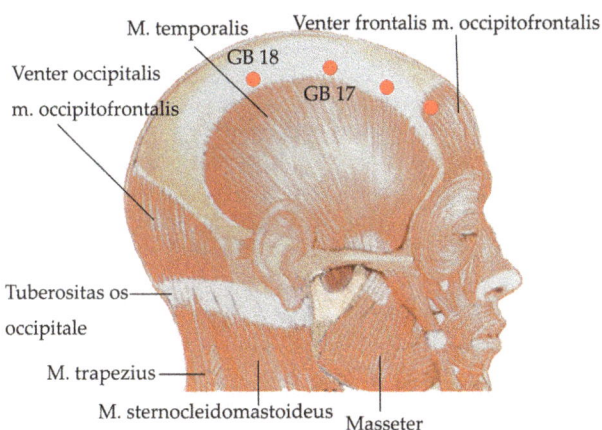

M. temporalis

Venter frontalis m. occipitofrontalis

GB 18

Venter occipitalis
m. occipitofrontalis

GB 17

Tuberositas os-
occipitale

M. trapezius

M. sternocleidomastoideus   Masseter

GB 19 – Năo Kōng

[Locating]	The point is located in the sitting or prone position, on the lateral aspect of the superior border of the external occipital protubearance, directly above GB 20 (Fēng Chí).
[Regional Anatomy]	The needle passes through the skin, subcutaneous tissues and penetrates the m. occipitofrontalis.
[Acupuncture and Moxibustion]	Insert the needle subcutaneously 0.5~0.8 cun deep and stimulate until there is a sore and numbing sensation in the local area, radiating to the posterior parts of the head. This point can be moxibusted.
[Indications]	Headache, epilepsy and fright, neck stiffness and pain.

GB 20 – Fēng Chí

[Locating]	The point is located in the sitting or prone position, on the nape, below the occipital bone, in the depression between m. sternocleidomastoideus and m. trapezius, at the level with DU 16 (Fēng Fǔ).
[Regional Anatomy]	The needle passes through the skin and the subcutaneous tissues, penetrates the fascia nuchalis, m. splenius capitis, m. semispinalis capitis and the m. rectus capitis posterior major.
[Acupuncture and Moxibustion]	Insert the needle obliquely towards the infraorbital internal ridge of the opposite side 0.5~0.8 cun deep and stimulate until there is a sore and numbing sensation in the local area radiating to the lateral parts of the head.
[Indications]	Headache and fever, stiff neck and pain, redness, swelling and pain of the eye, epistaxis, tinnitus, insomnia, and epilepsy.
[Note]	Avoid deep puncture to prevent injury to the medulla oblongata.

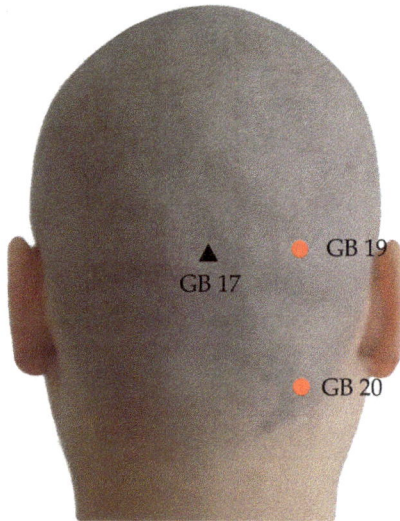

GB 17 GB 19 GB 20

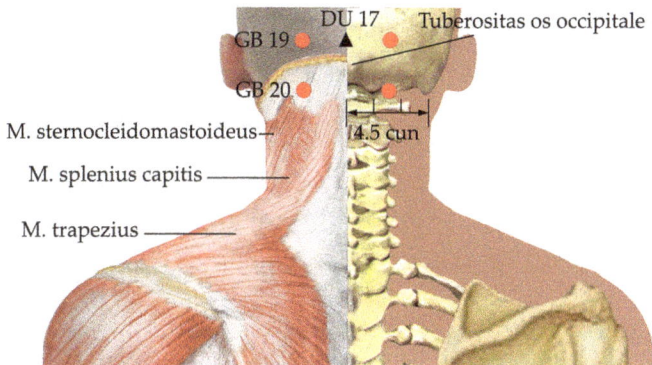

DU 17 Tuberositas os occipitale
GB 19
GB 20
M. sternocleidomastoideus
4.5 cun
M. splenius capitis
M. trapezius

GB 21 – Jiān Jǐng

[Locating]	The point is located in the sitting position, at the mid-point of the line connecting DU 14 (Dà Zhuī) and the acromion end of the clavicle.
[Regional Anatomy]	The needle passes through the skin and the subcutaneous tissues, penetrates the trapezius fascia, m. trapezius and the m. levator scapulae.
[Acupuncture and Moxibustion]	Insert the needle subcutaneously 0.5~0.8 cun deep and stimulate until there is a sore and numbing sensation in the local area radiating to the shoulder. This point can be moxibusted.
[Indications]	Mastitis and pain of the shoulder and arm.
[Note]	Avoid deep puncture to prevent injury to the top of pleura and apex of lung.

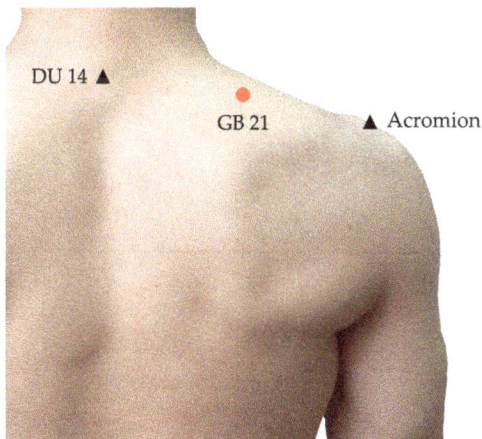

DU 14 ▲
GB 21
▲ Acromion

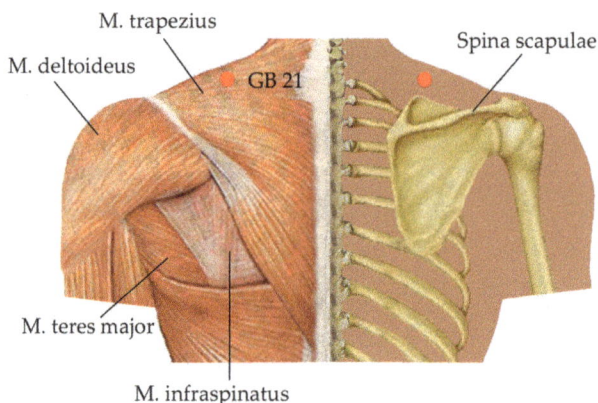

M. trapezius

M. deltoideus

GB 21

Spina scapulae

M. teres major

M. infraspinatus

GB 22 – Yuān Yè

[Locating]	The point is located in the sitting or lateral position, when the arm is raised, on the mid-axillary line, 3 cun directly below the axillary fossa, in the fourth intercostal space.
[Regional Anatomy]	The needle passes through the skin and the subcutaneous tissues, penetrates the deep thoracic fascia, m. serratus anterior and the fourth intercostal tissues.
[Acupuncture and Moxibustion]	Insert the needle subcutaneously 0.5~0.8 cun deep and stimulate until there is a sore and numbing sensation in the local area radiating to the chest and hypochondrium. This point can be moxibusted.
[Indications]	Chest congestion, pain and distention in the hypochondrium, swelling in the axillary fossa, pain of the shoulder and inability to raise the arm.
[Note]	Avoid puncture into thoracic cavity to prevent injury to the parietal pleura and lungs.

GB 23 - Zhé Jīn

[Locating]	The point is located in the sitting or lateral position, when the arm is raised, in the fourth intercostal space, 1 cun anterior to GB 22 (Yuān Yè).
[Regional Anatomy]	The needle passes through the skin and the subcutaneous tissues, penetrates the deep thoracic fascia, m. serratus anterior and the fourth intercostal tissues.
[Acupuncture and Moxibustion]	Insert the needle subcutaneously 0.5~0.8 cun deep and stimulate until there is a sore and numbing sensation in the local area radiating to the chest and hypochondrium. This point can be moxibusted.
[Indications]	Pain of the chest and hypochondrium, swelling in the axillary fossa, cough and asthma, and vomiting.
[Note]	The same as GB 22 (Yuān Yè).

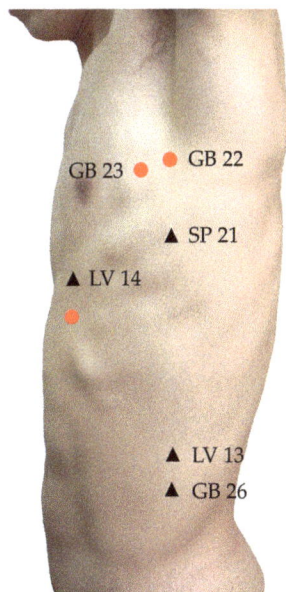

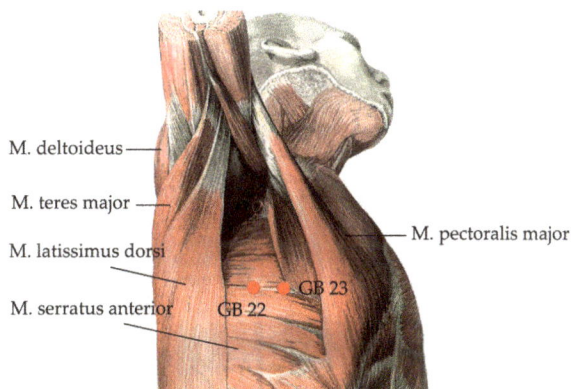

GB 24 – Rì Yuè

[Features]	Front-mu point of the Gallbladder Channel of Foot *Shaoyang*.
[Locating]	The point is located in the sitting or supine position, in the seventh intercostal space, 4 cun lateral to the anterior midline, directly below the nipple.
[Regional Anatomy]	The needle passes through the skin and the subcutaneous tissues, penetrates the m. obliquus externus abdominis aponeurosis, m. rectus abdominis and the intercostal tissues.
[Acupuncture and Moxibustion]	Insert the needle subcutaneously 0.5~0.8 cun deep and stimulate until there is a sore and numbing sensation in the local area radiating to the chest and hypochondrium. This point can be moxibusted.
[Indications]	Hiccup singultation, stomach ache, and acid regurgitation.
[Note]	The same as GB 22 (Yuān Yè).

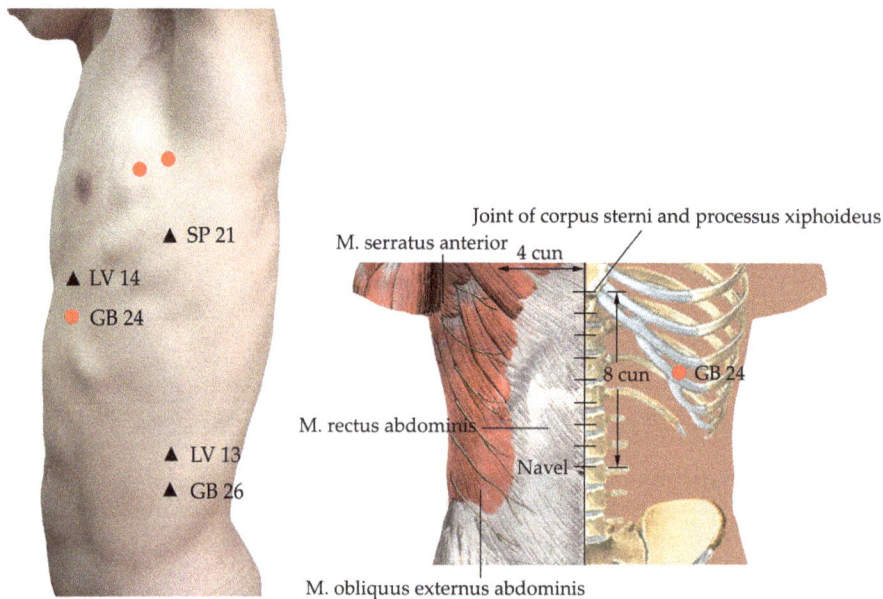

▲ SP 21
▲ LV 14
● GB 24
▲ LV 13
▲ GB 26

Joint of corpus sterni and processus xiphoideus
M. serratus anterior   4 cun
8 cun   ● GB 24
M. rectus abdominis
Navel
M. obliquus externus abdominis

GB 25 – Jīng Mén

[Features]	Front-mu point of the Kidney Channel of Foot *Shaoyin*.
[Locating]	The point is located in the lateral position, on the lower border of the end of the twelfth floating rib.
[Regional Anatomy]	The needle passes through the skin and the subcutaneous tissues, penetrates the abdominal fascia, m. obliquus externus abdominis and the m. obliquus internus abdominis.
[Acupuncture and Moxibustion]	Insert the needle subcutaneously 0.5~1.0 cun deep and stimulate until there is a sore and numbing sensation in the local area radiating to the lower back. This point can be moxibusted.
[Indications]	Chest distention and pain in the hypochondrium, abdominal distension, lumbago and backache.

GB 26 – Dài Mài

[Locating]	The point is located in the lateral or supine position, directly below the free end of the eleventh floating rib, at the level with the umbilicus.
[Regional Anatomy]	The needle passes through the skin and the subcutaneous tissues, penetrates the m. obliquus externus abdominis, m. obliquus internus abdominis and the transverse fascia.
[Acupuncture and Moxibustion]	Insert the needle obliquely 0.5~1.0 cun deep and stimulate until there is a sore and numbing sensation in the local area radiating to the lateral aspect of the abdomen. This point can be moxibusted.
[Indications]	Pain of the lower abdomen, irregular menstruation, red and white morbid leucorrhea, dysmenorrhea and infertility.

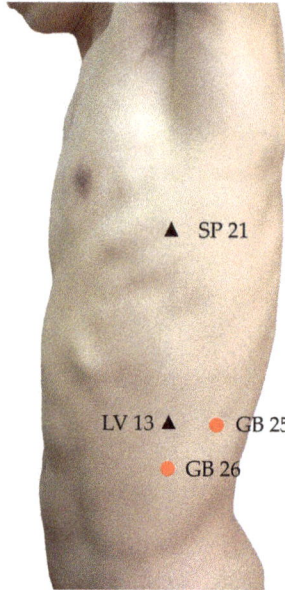

▲ SP 21

LV 13 ▲   ● GB 25

● GB 26

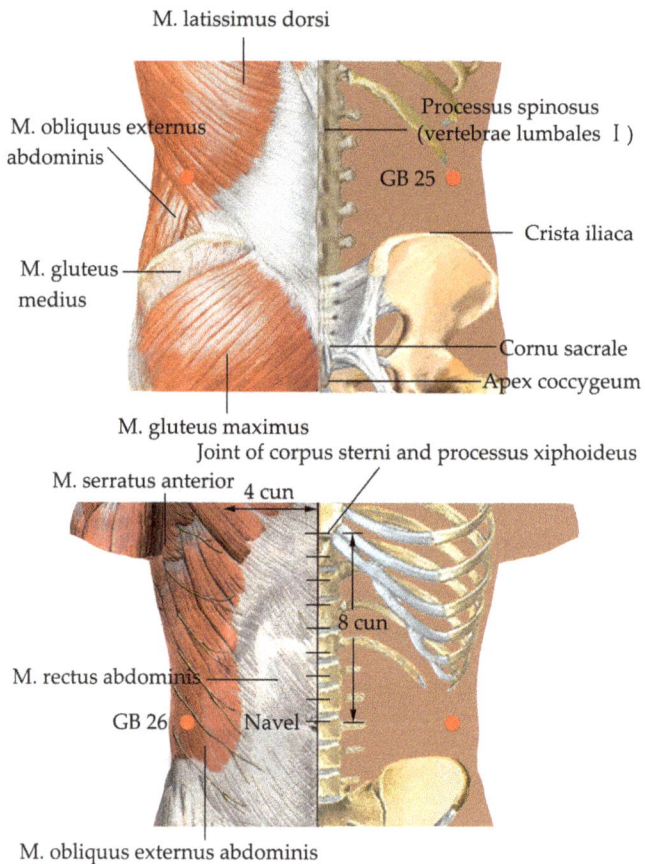

M. latissimus dorsi

M. obliquus externus
abdominis

M. gluteus
medius

Processus spinosus
(vertebrae lumbales Ⅰ)

GB 25 ●

Crista iliaca

Cornu sacrale

Apex coccygeum

M. gluteus maximus

Joint of corpus sterni and processus xiphoideus

M. serratus anterior   4 cun

8 cun

M. rectus abdominis

GB 26 ●   Navel

M. obliquus externus abdominis

GB 27 – Wǔ Shū

[Locating]	The point is located in the lateral position, in the depression on the internal border of the anterior superior iliac spine, 3 cun inferior to the level of the umbilicus, lateral to RN 4 (Guān Yuán).
[Regional Anatomy]	The needle passes through the skin and the subcutaneous tissues, penetrates the deep abdominal fascia, m. obliquus externus abdominis, m. obliquus internus abdominis and the transverse fascia.
[Acupuncture and Moxibustion]	Insert the needle perpendicularly 1.0~1.5 cun deep and stimulate until there is a sore and numbing sensation in the local area radiating to the groin. This point can be moxibusted.
[Indications]	Pain of the lower abdomen, irregular menstruation, and red and white morbid leucorrhea.

GB 28 – Wéi Dào

[Locating]	The point is located in the lateral position, 0.5 cun anterior and inferior to GB 27 (Wǔshū).
[Regional Anatomy]	The same as GB 27 (Wǔ Shū).
[Acupuncture and Moxibustion]	Insert the needle obliquely forwards and downward 1.0~1.5 cun deep and stimulate until there is a sore and numbing sensation in the local area radiating to the groin. This point can be moxibusted.
[Indications]	Irregular menstruation, red and white morbid leucorrhea.

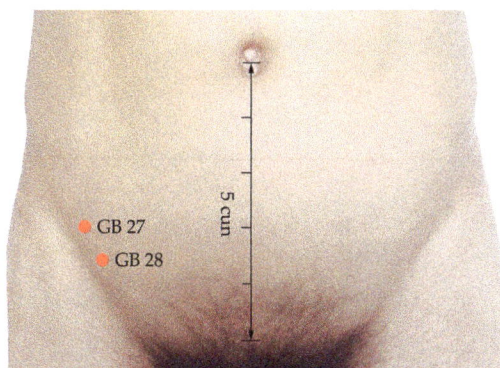

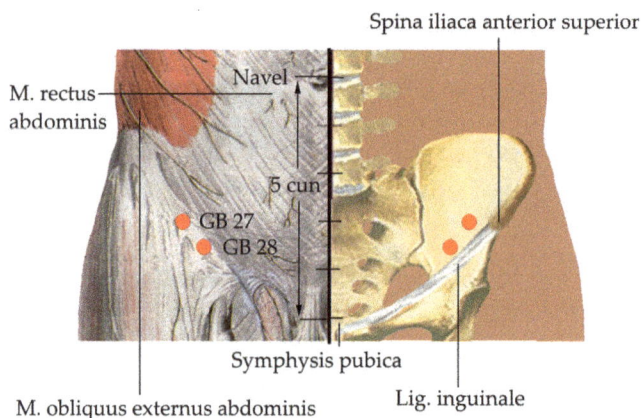

Spina iliaca anterior superior

M. rectus abdominis

Navel

5 cun

GB 27

GB 28

Symphysis pubica

M. obliquus externus abdominis

Lig. inguinale

GB 29 – Jū Liáo

[Locating]	The point is located in the lateral position, in the midpoint of the line connecting the anterior superior iliac spine and the highest point of the great trochanter of the femur.
[Regional Anatomy]	The needle passes through the skin and the subcutaneous tissues, penetrates the m. tensor fasciae latae and the m. gluteus medius
[Acupuncture and Moxibustion]	Insert the needle perpendicularly or obliquely 1.5~2.0 cun deep and stimulate until there is a sore and numbing sensation in the local area radiating to the hip, groin and hip joint. This point can be moxibusted.
[Indications]	Lumbar pain, weakness and numbness of the lower back and limbs, paralysis of the foot and hernia.

GB 30 – Huán Tiào

[Locating]	The point is located in the lateral position when the thigh is flexed and the leg is bent, at the junction of the lateral 1/3 and medial 2/3 of the line connecting the greater trochanter and the hiatus of the sacrum.
[Regional Anatomy]	The needle passes through the skin and the subcutaneous tissues, penetrates the fascia of gluteal muscles, m. gluteus maximus, sciatic nerve and the m. obturatorius internus.

[Acupuncture and Moxibustion]	Insert the needle perpendicularly 2.0~3.0 cun deep and stimulate until there is a sore and numbing sensation in the local area radiating to the lower limb. This point can be moxibusted.
[Indications]	Lumbar and hip pain, weakness and numbness of the lower back and limbs, rubella, and and hemiplegia.

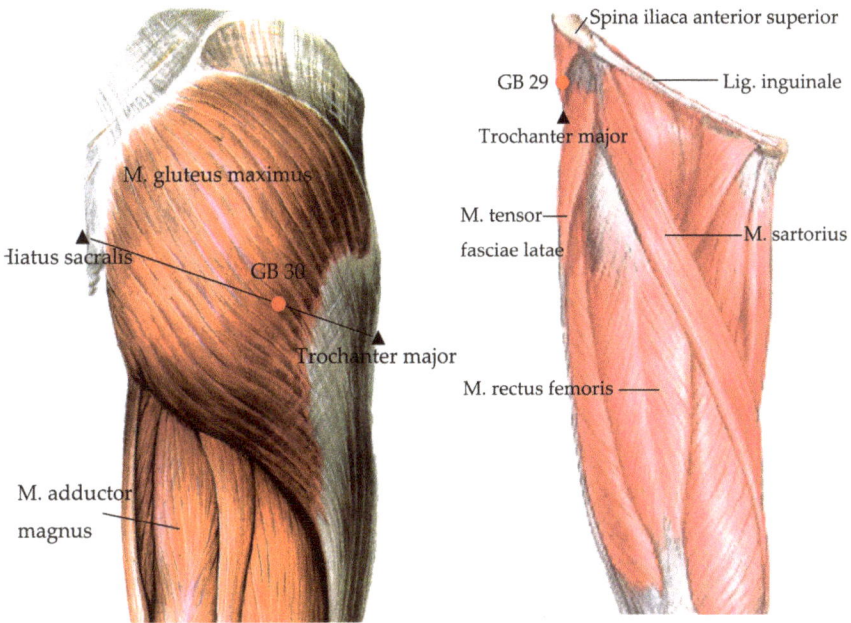

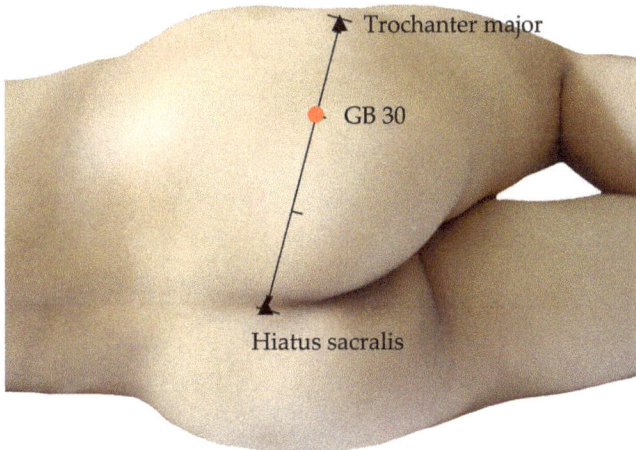

GB 31 – Fēng Shì

[Locating]	The point is located in the standing position with the hand resting on the side of the body, at the level with the tip of the middle finger placed naturally on the thigh. If the point is located in the lateral position, the point is 7 cun proximal to the transverse popliteal crease, on the midline of the lateral aspect of the thigh.
[Regional Anatomy]	The needle passes through the skin and the subcutaneous tissues, penetrates the fascia lata, iliotibial tract, m. vastus lateralis and the m. vastus intermedius.
[Acupuncture and Moxibustion]	Insert the needle perpendicularly 1.5~2.5 cun deep and stimulate until there is a sore and numbing sensation in the local area radiating downwards. This point can be moxibusted.
[Indications]	Hemiplegia, leg paralysis, and itching of the whole body.

GB 32 – Zhōng Dú

[Locating]	The point is located in the lateral position, on the midline of the lateral aspect of the thigh, 2 cun inferior to GB 31 (Fēng Shì), 5 cun proximal to the transverse popliteal crease.
[Regional Anatomy]	The needle passes through the skin and the subcutaneous tissues, penetrates the iliotibial tract, m. vastus lateralis and the m. vastus intermedius.
[Acupuncture and Moxibustion]	The same as GB 31 (Fēng Shì).
[Indications]	Pain, weakness and numbness of the lower limbs and hemiplegia.

GB 33 – Xī Yáng Guān

[Locating]	The point is located in the sitting position with the knee bent at 90° or in the supine position, in the posterior superior edge of lateral epicondyle of femur, the depression between the m. biceps femoris tendon and the iliotibial tract.

[Regional Anatomy]	The needle passes through the skin and the subcutaneous tissues, penetrates the iliotibial tract and the m. vastus lateralis.
[Acupuncture and Moxibustion]	Insert the needle perpendicularly 1.0~2.0 cun deep and stimulate until there is a sore and numbing sensation in the local area radiating to the hip or lateral aspect of the lower limb. This point can be moxibusted.
[Indications]	Swelling and pain of the knee, spasm of the muscle and numbness of the lower limbs.

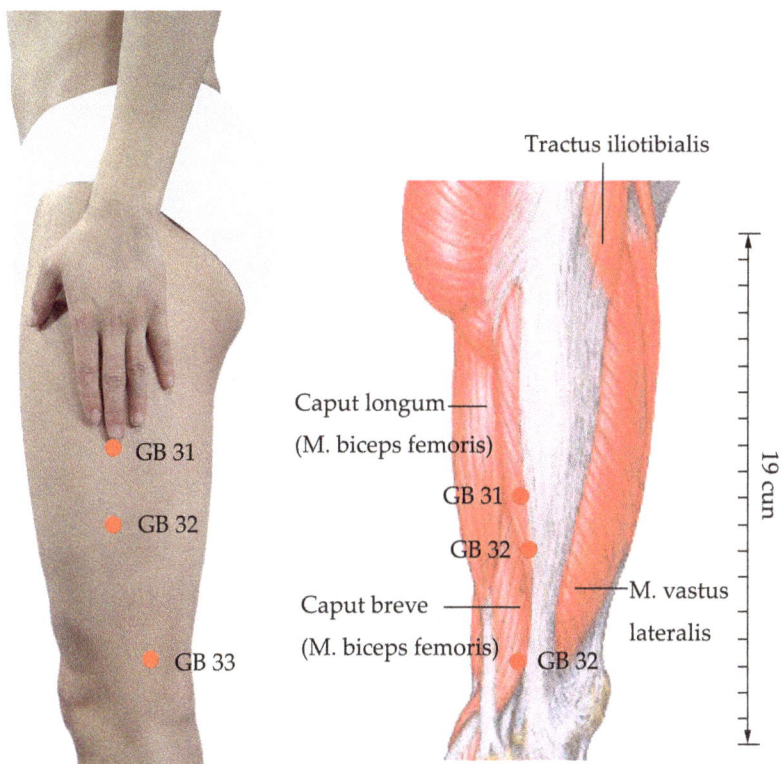

Tractus iliotibialis

GB 31

GB 32

GB 33

Caput longum (M. biceps femoris)

GB 31

GB 32

Caput breve (M. biceps femoris)

GB 32

M. vastus lateralis

19 cun

GB 34 – Yáng Líng Quán

[Features]	He-sea point of the Gallbladder Channel of the Foot *Shaoyang*; influential point of the sinews.
[Locating]	The point is located in the sitting position with the knee bent at 90°or in the supine position, in the depression anterior and inferior to the head of the fibula.
[Regional Anatomy]	The needle passes through the skin and the subcutaneous tissues, penetrates the deep crural fascia, m. peroneus longus and the m. peroneus brevis.
[Acupuncture and Moxibustion]	Insert the needle perpendicularly 1.0~3.0 cun deep and stimulate until there is a sore and numbing sensation in the local area radiating downwards. This point can be moxibusted.
[Indications]	Tinnitus, eye pain, pain of the chest, hypochondrium, asthma and cough, acid regurgitation, jaundice, swelling and pain of the knee, weakness and numbness of the lower extremities, and hemiplegia.

GB 35 – Yáng Jiāo

[Features]	Xi-cleft point of the Yang Linking Vessel.
[Locating]	The point is located in the sitting position with the feet resting on the ground or in the prone position, on the lateral aspect of the lower leg, 7 cun proximal to the tip of the external malleolus, on the posterior border of the fibula.
[Regional Anatomy]	The needle passes through the skin and the subcutaneous tissues, penetrates the m. peroneus longus, m. peroneus brevis, m. triceps surae and the m. flexor digitorum longus.
[Acupuncture and Moxibustion]	Insert the needle perpendicularly 1.0~1.5 cun deep and stimulate until there is a sore and numbing sensation in the local area radiating to the foot. This point can be moxibusted.
[Indications]	Pain of the knee, weakness and numbness of the lower limbs and foot.

GB 36 – Wài Qiū

[Features]	Xi-cleft point of the Gallbladder Channel of the Foot *Shaoyang*.
[Locating]	The point is located in the sitting position with the feet resting on the ground or in the prone position, 7 cun proximal to the tip of the external malleolus, on anterior border of the fibula.
[Regional Anatomy]	The needle passes through the skin and the subcutaneous tissues, penetrates the m. peroneus brevis, m. peroneus longus and the m. extensor digitorum longus.
[Acupuncture and Moxibustion]	Insert the needle perpendicularly 0.5~0.8 cun deep and stimulate until there is a sore and numbing sensation in the local area radiating to the foot. This point can be moxibusted.
[Indications]	Pain and numbness of the lower limbs, pain of the neck and epilepsy.

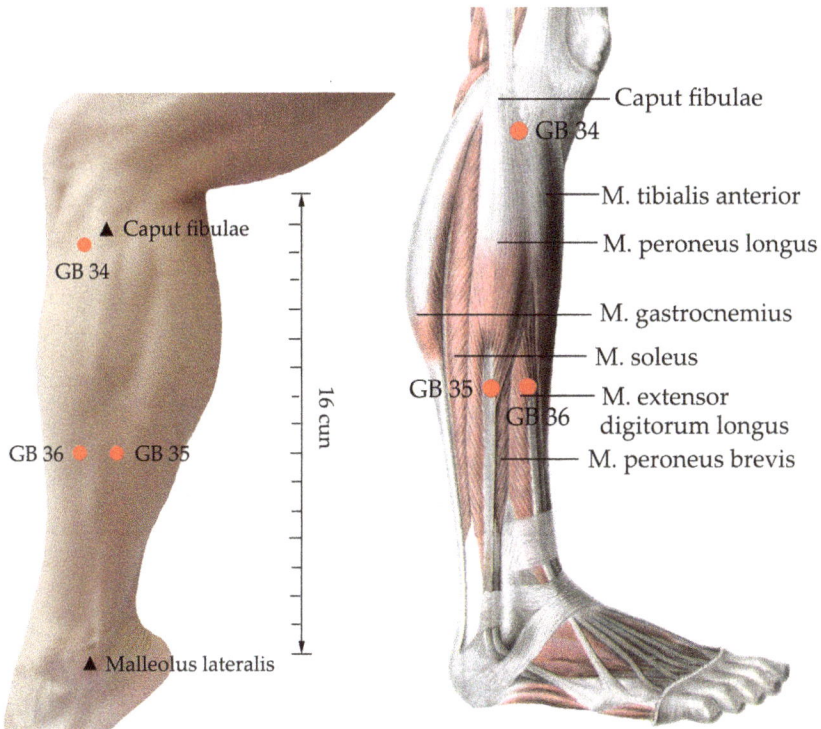

Caput fibulae
GB 34
▲ Caput fibulae
GB 34
M. tibialis anterior
M. peroneus longus
M. gastrocnemius
M. soleus
GB 35
GB 36
M. extensor digitorum longus
M. peroneus brevis
GB 36   GB 35
16 cun
▲ Malleolus lateralis

GB 37 – Guāng Míng

[Features]	Luo-connecting point the Gallbladder Channel of the Foot *Shaoyang*.
[Locating]	The point is located in the sitting position with the feet resting on the ground or in the prone position, 5 cun proximal to the tip of the external malleolus, on the anterior border of the fibula.
[Regional Anatomy]	The needle passes through the skin and the subcutaneous tissues, penetrates the m. peroneus longus, m. peroneus brevis, m. extensor digitorum longus and the m. flexor pollicis longus.
[Acupuncture and Moxibustion]	Insert the needle perpendicularly 0.8~1.2 cun deep and stimulate until there is a sore and numbing sensation in the local area. This point can be moxibusted.
[Indications]	Redness, swelling and pain of the eye and blurred vision.

GB 38 – Yáng Fǔ

[Features]	Jing-river point of the Gallbladder Channel of the Foot *Shaoyang*.
[Locating]	The point is located in the sitting position with the feet resting on the ground or in the prone position, 4 cun proximal to the tip of the external malleolus, slightly anterior to the anterior border of the fibula.
[Regional Anatomy]	The needle passes through the skin and the subcutaneous tissues, penetrates the m. peroneus longus, m. peroneus brevis, m. extensor digitorum longus and the m. flexor pollicis longus.
[Acupuncture and Moxibustion]	Insert the needle perpendicularly 0.8~1.2 cun deep and stimulate until there is a sore and numbing sensation in the local area. This point can be moxibusted.
[Indications]	Pain of the chest and hypochondrium, pain of the lower extremity lateral.

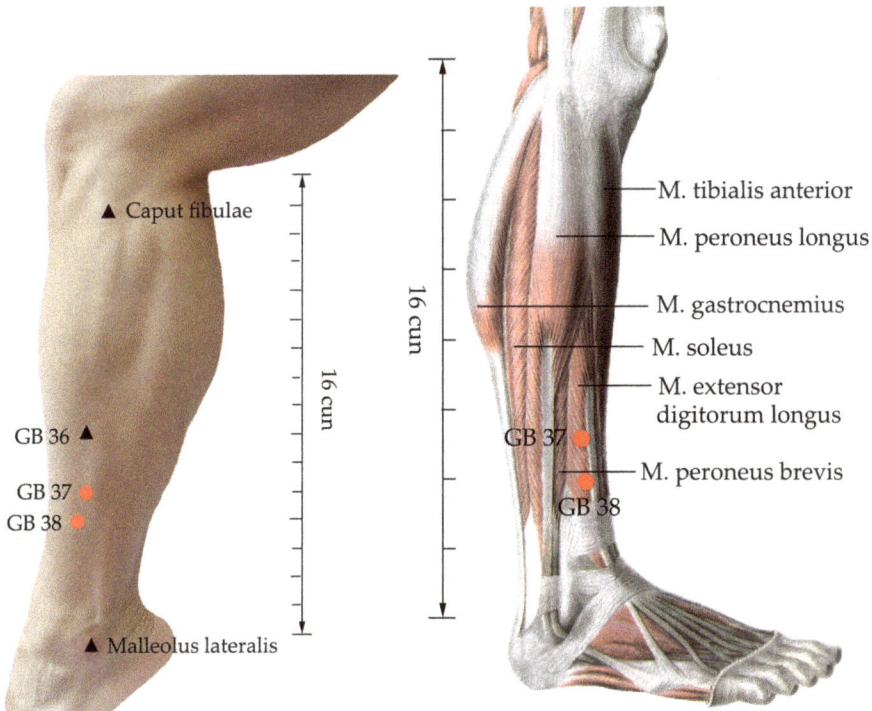

Labels on figure:
▲ Caput fibulae

16 cun
16 cun
16 cun

GB 36 ▲
GB 37 ●
GB 38 ●

▲ Malleolus lateralis

M. tibialis anterior
M. peroneus longus
M. gastrocnemius
M. soleus
M. extensor digitorum longus
M. peroneus brevis

GB 37 ●
GB 38 ●

GB 39 – Xuán Zhōng

[Features]	One of the Eight Strategic Nerve Points, influential point of the marrow.
[Locating]	The point is located in the sitting position with the feet resting on the ground or in the prone position, 3 cun proximal to the tip of the external malleolus, in the depression between the posterior order of fibula.
[Regional Anatomy]	The needle passes through the skin and the subcutaneous tissues, penetrates the m. peroneus longus, m. peroneus brevis and the m. extensor digitorum longus.
[Acupuncture and Moxibustion]	Insert the needle perpendicularly 0.5~0.8 cun deep and stimulate until there is a sore and numbing sensation in the local area. This point can be moxibusted.
[Indications]	Neck stiffness, arthralgia of extremities, hemiplegia, pain of the chest and hypochondrium, tinnitus.

GB 40 – Qiū Xū

[Features]	Yuan-source point of the Gallbladder Channel of the Foot *Shaoyang*.
[Locating]	The point is located in the sitting position with the feet resting on the ground or in the supine position, anterior and inferior to the external malleolus, in the depression on the lateral aspect of the tendon of m. extensor digitorum longus.
[Regional Anatomy]	The needle passes through the skin and the subcutaneous tissues, penetrates the dorsal fascia of foot and the m. extensor digitorum brevis.
[Acupuncture and Moxibustion]	Insert the needle perpendicularly 0.5~0.8 cun deep and stimulate until there is a sore and numbing sensation in the local area. This point can be moxibusted.
[Indications]	Pain of the chest, hypochondrium, and hernia.

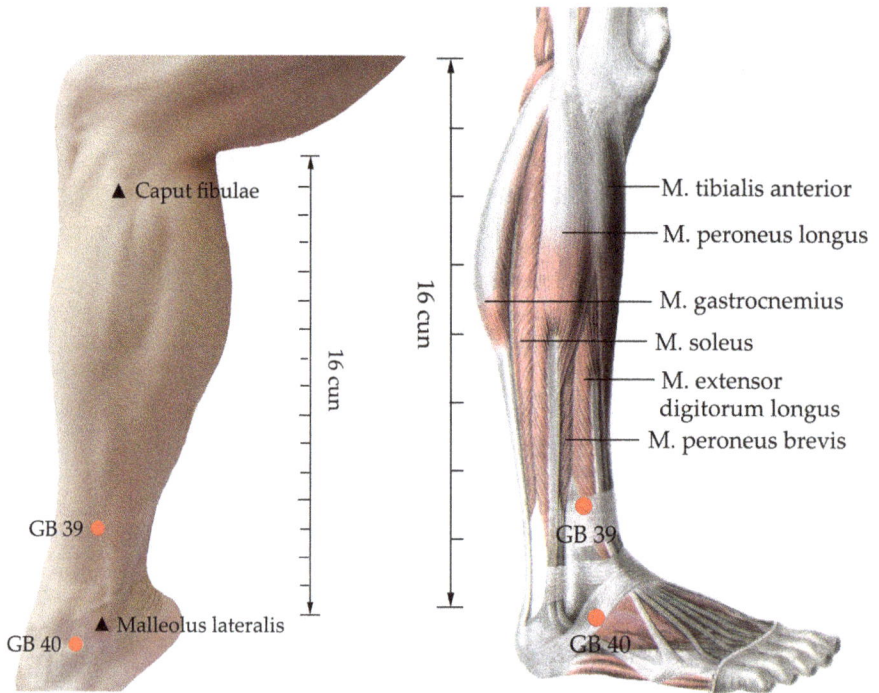

GB 41 – Zú Lín Qì

[Features]	Shu-stream points confluent point of the Girdling vessel, one of the eight confluent acupoints connecting the eight extra channels, confluent point of the girdling vessel.
[Locating]	The point is located in the sitting position with the feet resting on the ground or in the supine position, anterior to the fourth and the fifth basal metatarsal junction, in the depression on the lateral aspect of the tendon of m. extensor digit minimi of the foot.
[Regional Anatomy]	The needle passes through the skin and the subcutaneous tissues, penetrates the m. extensor digitorum brevis and the m. interossei dorsales.
[Acupuncture and Moxibustion]	Insert the needle perpendicularly 0.5~0.8 cun deep and stimulate until there is a sore and numbing sensation in the local area spreading to the toe. This point can be moxibusted.
[Indications]	Headache and dizziness, redness, swelling and pain of the eye, swelling of the throat, deafness, pain of the chest, and hypochondrium.

GB 42 – Dì Wǔ Huì

[Locating]	The point is located in the sitting position with the feet resting on the ground or in the supine position, between the fourth and fifth metatarsal bones, in the depression on the posterior to the fourth metatarsophalangeal joint.
[Regional Anatomy]	The needle passes through the skin and the subcutaneous tissues, penetrates the m. interossei dorsales.
[Acupuncture and Moxibustion]	Insert the needle perpendicularly or obliquely upwards 0.5~0.8 cun deep and stimulate until there is a sore and numbing sensation in the local area. Moxibustion is not allowed in ancient records.
[Indications]	Headache and dizziness, redness, swelling and pain of the eye, swelling of the throat, and deafness.

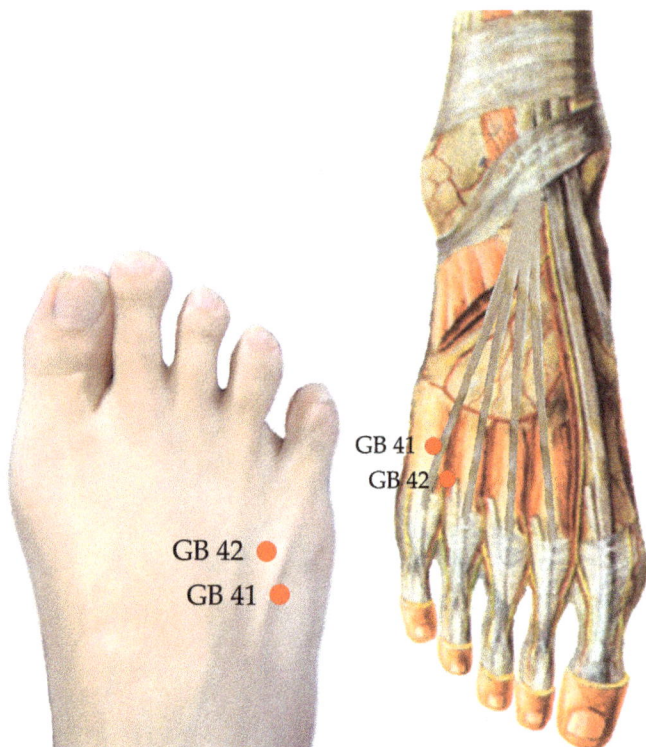

GB 43 – Xiá Xī

[Features]	Ying-spring point of the Gallbladder Channel of the Foot *Shaoyang*.
[Locating]	The point is located in the sitting position with the feet resting on the ground or in the supine position, proximal to the margin of the web between the fourth and fifth toes.
[Regional Anatomy]	The needle passes through the skin and the subcutaneous tissues, pierces deep dorsal fascia of foot, penetrates the m. extensor digitorum brevis and the m. interossei dorsales.
[Acupuncture and Moxibustion]	Insert the needle perpendicularly 0.5~0.8 cun deep and stimulate until there is a sore and numbing sensation in the local area. This point can be moxibusted.

[Indications]	Headache, tinnitus, deafness, pain of the eye, and cheek swelling.

GB 44 – Zú Qiào Yīn

[Features]	Jing-well point of the Gallbladder Channel of the Foot *Shaoyang*.
[Locating]	The point is located in the sitting position with the feet resting on the ground or in the supine position, at the junction of the line connecting the lateral border of the nail of the fourth toe and the base of the nail.
[Regional Anatomy]	The needle passes through the skin and the subcutaneous tissues, penetrates the dorsal digital aponeurosis.
[Acupuncture and Moxibustion]	① Insert the needle subcutaneously 0.1~0.2 cun deep and stimulate until there is a sore and numbing sensation in the local area. ② Prick with a three-edged needle to bleed. This point can be moxibusted.
[Indications]	Redness, swelling and pain of the eye, tinnitus and deafness, pain of the chest, and hypochondriumand.

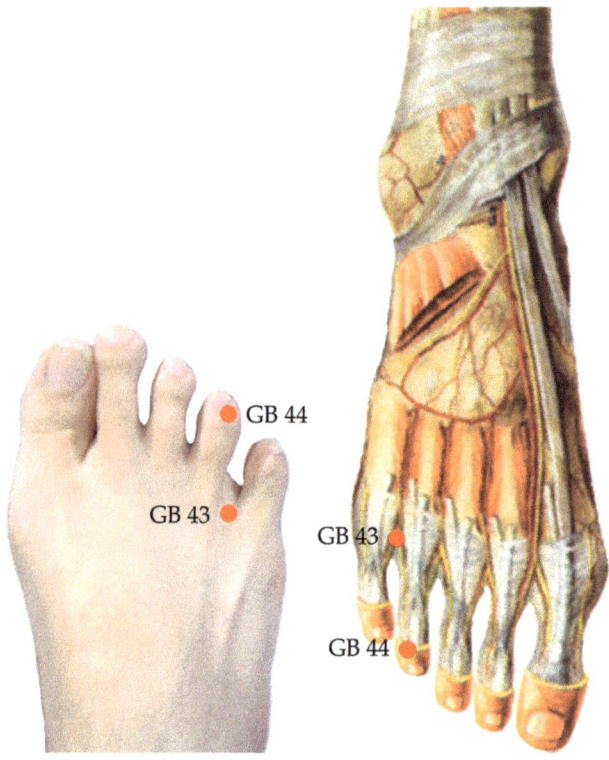

GB 44

GB 43

GB 43

GB 44

CHAPTER 13

Liver Channel of Foot Jueyin; LR

There are fourteen points on the Liver Channel of Foot *Jueyin* and twenty-eight in total on both sides. There are two points on the the chest and hypochondrium and twelve points are distributed on the medial aspect of the lower limb. The first point is LR 1 (Dà Dūn) and the last point is LR 14 (Qī Mén). The indications of the channel are diseases of the mind, head, ear, eye, throat and febrile diseases and symptoms along the course of the channel.

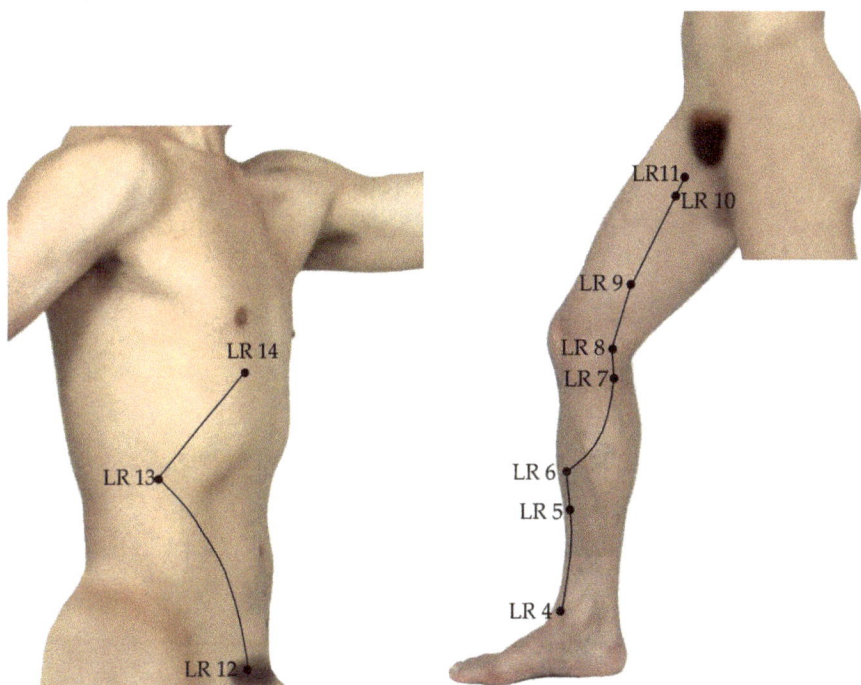

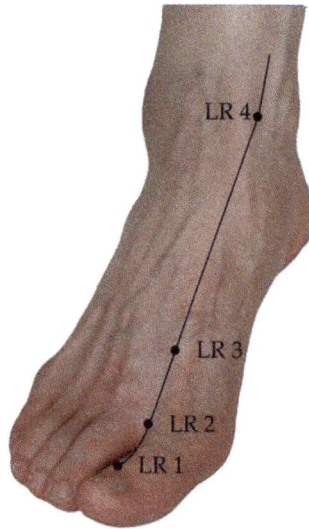

LR 1 – Dà Dūn

[Features]	Jing-well point of the Liver Channel of Foot *Jueyin*.
[Locating]	The point is located in the sitting position with the foot resting on the ground or in the supine position, at the junction of the line of the lateral border and base of the nail of the big toe, 0.1 cun lateral to the corner of the nail of the big toe.
[Regional Anatomy]	The needle passes through the skin and subcutaneous tissues, and penetrates the dorsal aponeurosis of phalanx.
[Acupuncture and Moxibustion]	① Insert the needle subcutaneously 0.1~0.2 cun deep and stimulate until there is a sour and distending sensation in the local area. ② Prick with a three-edged needle to bleed. This point can be moxibusted.
[Indications]	Amenorrhea, metrorrhagia, metrostaxis, prolapse of uterus, hernia, enuresis, and disuria.

LR 2 – Xíng Jiān

[Features]	Ying-spring point of the Liver Channel of Foot *Jueyin*.
[Locating]	The point is located in the sitting position with the foot resting on the ground or supine position, in the depression between the first and second toes, at the junction of the red and white skin.
[Regional Anatomy]	The needle passes through the skin and subcutaneous tissues,and penetrates the m. interossei dorsales.
[Acupuncture and Moxibustion]	Insert the needle subcutaneously 0.5~0.8 cun deep and stimulate until there is a sour and distending sensation in the local area radiating to the dorsum of the foot. This point can be moxibusted.
[Indications]	Headache, pain and redness of the eyes, coughing up blood, pain and distension in the chest and hypochondrium, dysphoria and dysmenorrhea.

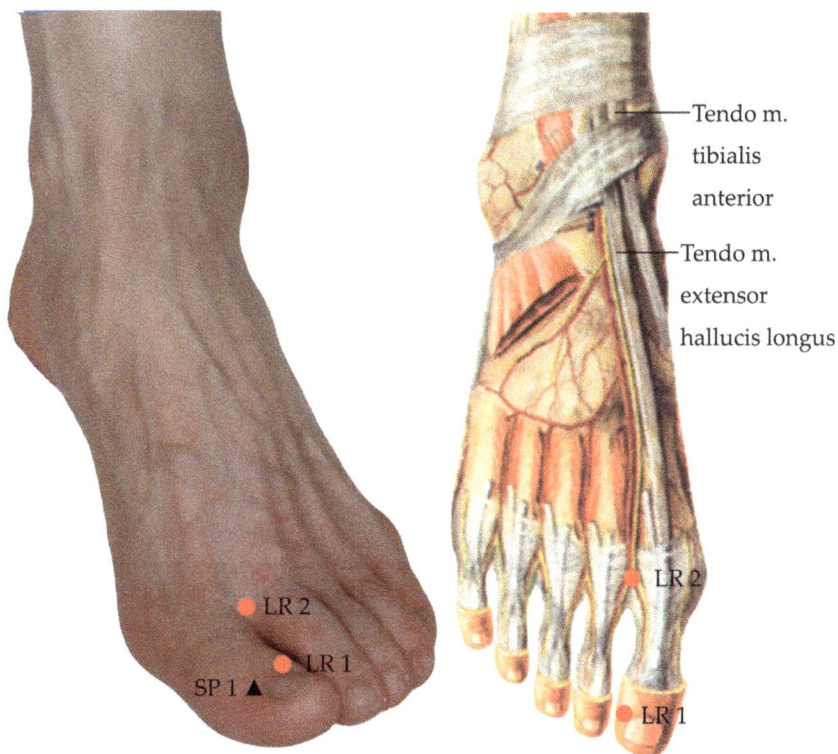

Tendo m. tibialis anterior

Tendo m. extensor hallucis longus

LR 2

LR 2

LR 1

SP 1 ▲

LR 1

LR 3 – Tài Chōng

[Features]	Shu-stream and yuan-source point of the Liver Channel of Foot *Jueyin*.
[Locating]	The point is located in the sitting position with the foot resting on the ground or supine position, on the dorsum of the foot, between the first and second metatarsal bone, in the depression lateral to the tendon of m. extensor pollicis longus.
[Regional Anatomy]	The needle passes through the skin and subcutaneous tissues, and penetrates the m. interossei dorsales.
[Acupuncture and Moxibustion]	Insert the needle perpendicularly upwards 0.5~1.0 cun deep and stimulate until there is a sore, distending or numbing sensation in the local area radiating to the sole of the foot. This point can be moxibusted.
[Indications]	Headache, pain of the throat, insomnia, hernia, enuresis, pain in the chest and hypochondrium, irregular menstruation, dysmenorrhea, weakness of the lower limbs, infantile convulsions and epilepsy.

LR 4 – Zhōng Fēng

[Features]	Jing-river point of the Liver Channel of Foot Jueyin.
[Locating]	The point is located when the foot is flexed, anterior and inferior to the medial malleolus, in the depression medial to the tendon of m. tibilis anterior.
[Regional Anatomy]	The needle passes through the skin and subcutaneous tissues and penetrates the m. interossei dorsales, between the tendon of m. tibialis anterior and tendon of m. extensor hallucis.
[Acupuncture and Moxibustion]	Insert the needle subcutaneously 0.5~0.8 cun deep and stimulate until there is a sour and distending sensation in the local area radiating to the dorsum of the foot. This point can be moxibusted.
[Indications]	Pain and swelling of the medial malleolus, lower abdominal pain, pharyngoxerosis and feet cold.

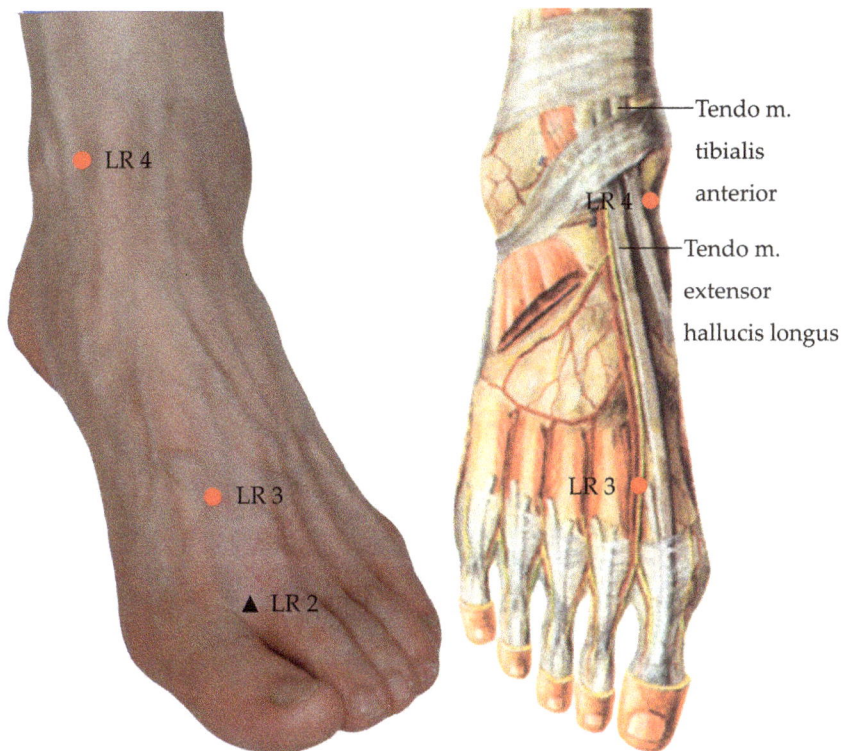

Tendo m. tibialis anterior

Tendo m. extensor hallucis longus

LR 5 – Lí Gōu

[Features]	Luo-connecting point of the Liver Channel of Foot *Jueyin*.
[Locating]	The point is located in the supine position, on the medial aspect of the lower limb, 5 cun superior l to the tip of the medial malleolus, in the center of the medial aspect of the tibia.
[Regional Anatomy]	The needle passes through the skin, subcutaneous tissues and penetrates the m. triceps surae (m. soleus), reaches the periost of the tibia.
[Acupuncture and Moxibustion]	Insert the needle subcutaneously 0.5~0.8 cun deep and stimulate until there is a sour and distending sensation in the local area. This point can be moxibusted.
[Indications]	Hernia, enuresis, irregular menstruation, morbid leucorrhea, pain of the uterus, metrorrhagia and metrostaxis.

LR 6 – Zhōng Dū

[Features]	Xi-cleft point of the Liver Channel of Foot *Jueyin*.
[Locating]	The point is located in the sitting or supine position, 7 cun above the tip of the medial marreolus, in the center of the medial aspect of the tibia.
[Regional Anatomy]	The needle passes through the skin, subcutaneous tissues and penetrates the m. triceps surae (m. soleus), reaches the periost of the tibia
[Acupuncture and Moxibustion]	Insert the needle subcutaneously 0.5~0.8 cun deep and stimulate until there is a sour and distending sensation in the local area. This point can be moxibusted.
[Indications]	Hernia, spermatorrhea, metrorrhagia, metrostaxis and retention of lochia.

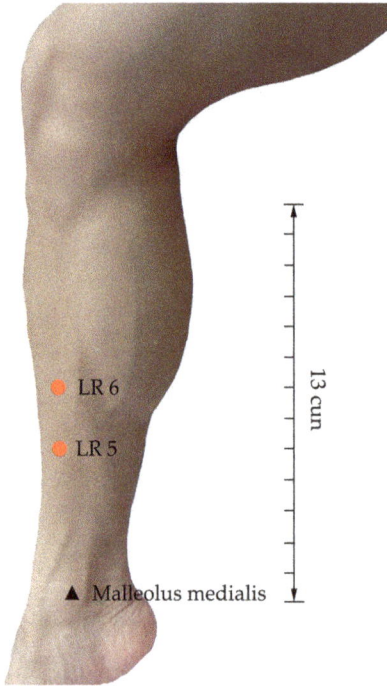

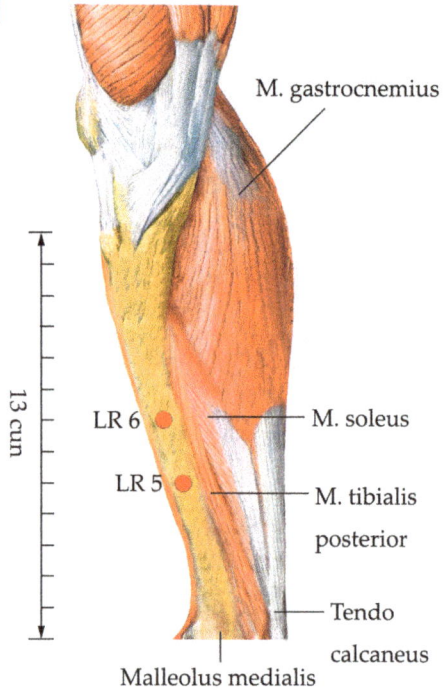

LR 7 – Xī Guān

[Locating]	The point is located in the sitting or supine position, on the medial aspect of the lower leg, posterior and inferior to the medial condyle of the tibia, 1 cun posterior SP 9 (Yīn Líng Quán).
[Regional Anatomy]	The needle passes through the skin and subcutaneous tissues and penetrates the m.sartorius,m. semimembranosus and m. semitendinosus.
[Acupuncture and Moxibustion]	Insert the needle perpendicularly 0.8~1.0 cun deep and stimulate until there is a sour and distending sensation in the local area with a numbing and electric sensation radiating to the sole of the foot. This point can be moxibusted.
[Indications]	Swelling and pain of the knee, atrophy and paralysis of the lower extremities and gout.

LR 8 – Qū Quán

[Features]	He-sea point of the Liver Channel of Foot *Jueyin*.
[Locating]	The point is located in the sitting or supine position when the knee is flexed, in the depression above the medial end of the transverse popliteal.
[Regional Anatomy]	The needle passes through the skin and subcutaneous tissues, and penetrates the m. vastus medialis.
[Acupuncture and Moxibustion]	Insert the needle perpendicularly 1.0~1.5 cun deep and stimulate until there is a sour and distending sensation in the local area spreading in the knee joint, and a numbing and electric sensation radiating to the lower. This point can be moxibusted.
[Indications]	Irregular menstruation, impotence, spermatorrhea, and dysuria.

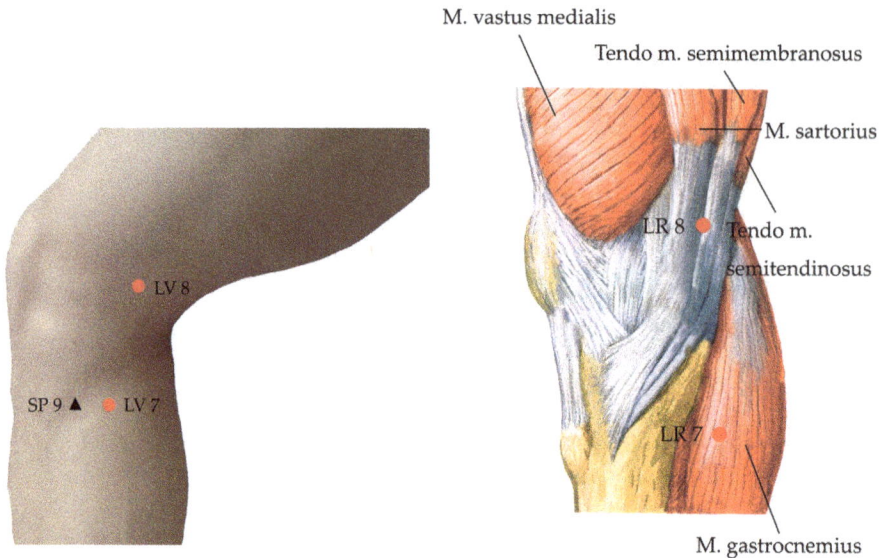

M. vastus medialis
Tendo m. semimembranosus
M. sartorius
LR 8
Tendo m. semitendinosus
LV 8
SP 9 ▲ LV 7
LR 7
M. gastrocnemius

LR 9 – Yīn Bāo

[Locating]	The point is located in the supine position, on the medial aspect of the thigh, 4 cun superior to the medial epicondyle of the femur, between m. vastus medialis and m. sartorius.
[Regional Anatomy]	The needle passes through the skin and subcutaneous tissues, and penetrates the m. adductor magnus.
[Acupuncture and Moxibustion]	Insert the needle perpendicularly 0.8~1.0 cun deep and stimulate until there is a sour and distending sensation in the local area. This point can be moxibusted.
[Indications]	Irregular menstruation and lower abdominal pain.

LR 10 – Zú Wǔ Lǐ

[Locating]	The point is located in the supine position when the lower limb is extended, 3 cun directly inferior to ST 30 (Qì Chōng).
[Regional Anatomy]	The needle passes through the subcutaneous tissues and penetrates the m. adductor brevis and m. adductor longus, m. adductor brevis.
[Acupuncture and Moxibustion]	Insert the needle perpendicularly 0.8~1.0 cun deep and stimulate until there is a sour and distending sensation in the local area. This point can be moxibusted.
[Indications]	Dysuria.

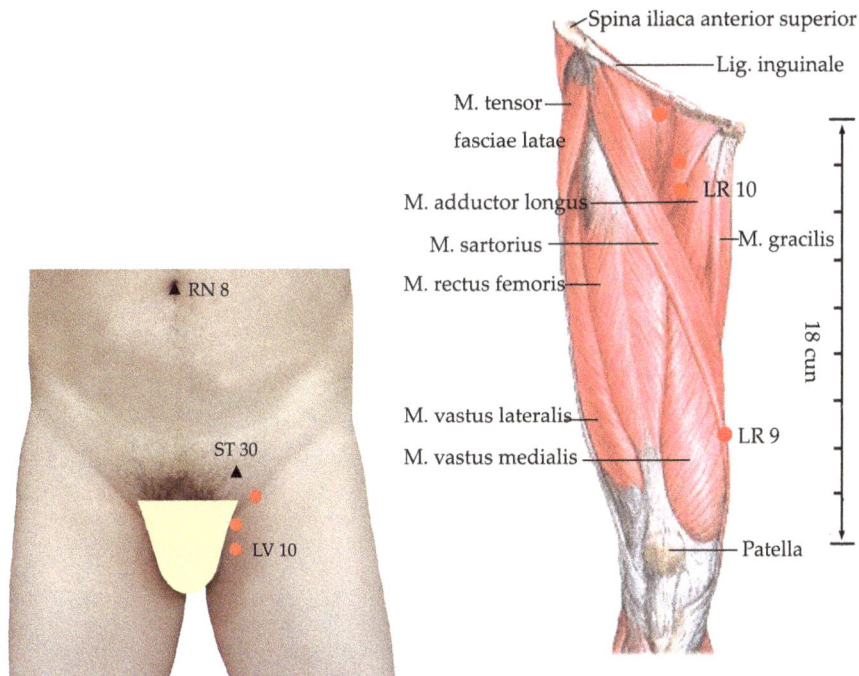

Spina iliaca anterior superior
Lig. inguinale
M. tensor fasciae latae
M. adductor longus
M. sartorius
M. rectus femoris
M. gracilis
LR 10
M. vastus lateralis
M. vastus medialis
LR 9
Patella
18 cun
RN 8
ST 30
LV 10

LR 11 – Yīn Lián

[Locating]	The point is located in the supine position when the lower limb is extended, 2 cun directly inferior ST 30 (Qì Chōng).
[Regional Anatomy]	The needle passes through the subcutaneous tissues and penetrates the m. adductor brevis and m. adductor longus.
[Acupuncture and Moxibustion]	Insert the needle perpendicularly 0.5~0.8 cun deep and stimulate until there is a sour and distending sensation in the local area. This point can be moxibusted.
[Indications]	Irregular menstruation, bloody and morbid leucorrhea, and lowers abdominal pain.

LR 12 - Jí Mài

[Locating]	The point is located in the supine position when the lower limb is extended, at the level with the lower border of the pubis, at the inguinal groove where the fermoral artery pulsates, 2.5 cun lateral to the anterior midline.
[Regional Anatomy]	The needle passes through the subcutaneous tissues and penetrates the m. pectineus and m. adductor brevis.
[Acupuncture and Moxibustion]	Insert the needle perpendicularly 0.8~1.0 cun deep and stimulate until there is a sour and distending sensation in the local area radiating to the external genitalia. This point can be moxibusted.
[Indications]	Lower abdominal pain, hernia, and pain in the external genitalia.

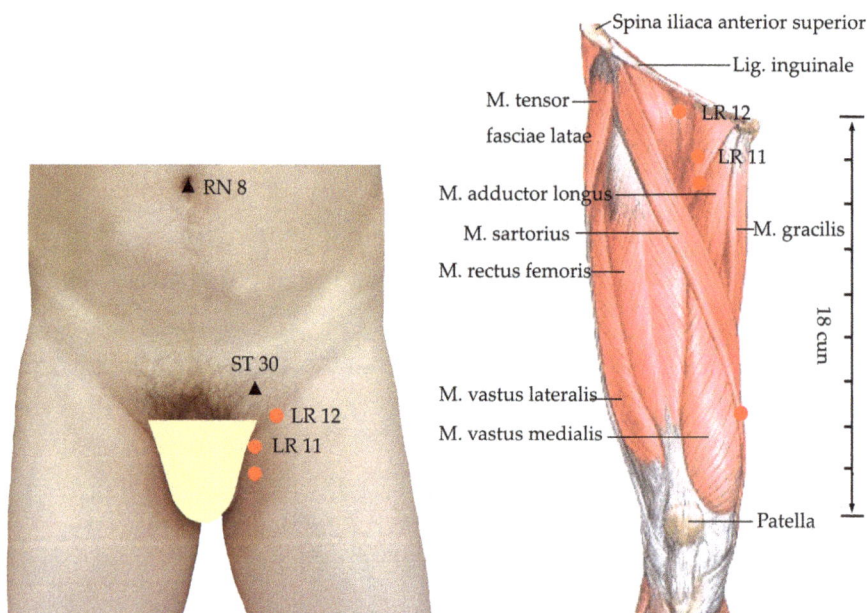

LR 13 – Zhāng Mén

[Features]	Front-mu Point of the Spleen and influential point of the Zang organs, below the free end of the eleventh floating rib.
[Locating]	The point is located in the supine or lateral position, on the mid-axillary line when the elbow is adducted and flexed, below the free end of the eleventh floating rib.
[Regional Anatomy]	The needle passes through the skin and subcutaneous tissues and penetrates the m. obliquus externus abdominis and m. transversus abdominis.
[Acupuncture and Moxibustion]	Insert the needle obliquely 0.5~0.8 cun deep and stimulate until there is a sour and distending sensation in the local area radiating to the external genitalia. This point can be moxibusted.
[Indications]	Abdominal congestion, pain in the chest and hypochondrium, and apocleisis.

LR 14 – Qī Mén

[Features]	Front-mu point of the Liver Channel of Foot *Jueyin*.
[Locating]	The point is located in the supine position, directly inferior to the nipple, in the sixth intercostal space, 4 cun lateral to the anterior midline.
[Regional Anatomy]	The needle passes through the skin, subcutaneous tissues and penetrates m. obliquus externus abdominis, m. intercostales externi and m. intercostales interni.
[Acupuncture and Moxibustion]	Insert the needle obliquely 0.5~0.8 cun deep and stimulate until there is a sour and distending sensation in the local area. This point can be moxibusted.
[Indications]	Distention of the chest and hypochondrium, vomiting and hiccups.
[Note]	Avoid deep insertion to prevent puncturing the lung.

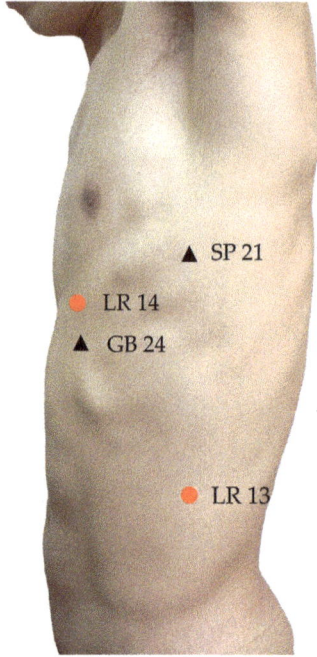

▲ SP 21

● LR 14

▲ GB 24

● LR 13

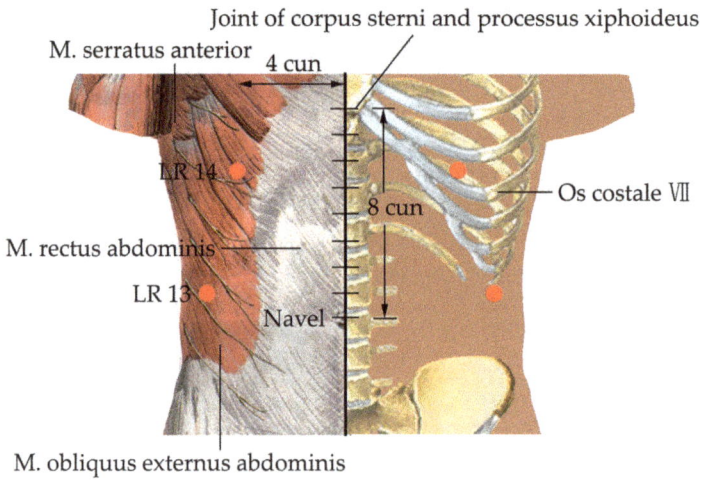

Joint of corpus sterni and processus xiphoideus

M. serratus anterior

4 cun

LR 14

Os costale VII

8 cun

M. rectus abdominis

LR 13

Navel

M. obliquus externus abdominis

CHAPTER 14

Du Vessel; DU

There are twenty-eight points on the Du Vessel. They are distributed along the midline of the head, face, neck, back, waist and sacrum. The first point is DU 1 (Cháng Qiáng) and the last one is DU 28 (Yín Jiāo). The indications of this channel are diseases of the respiratory, digestive, urogenital systems and the mind and the symptoms along the course of the channel.

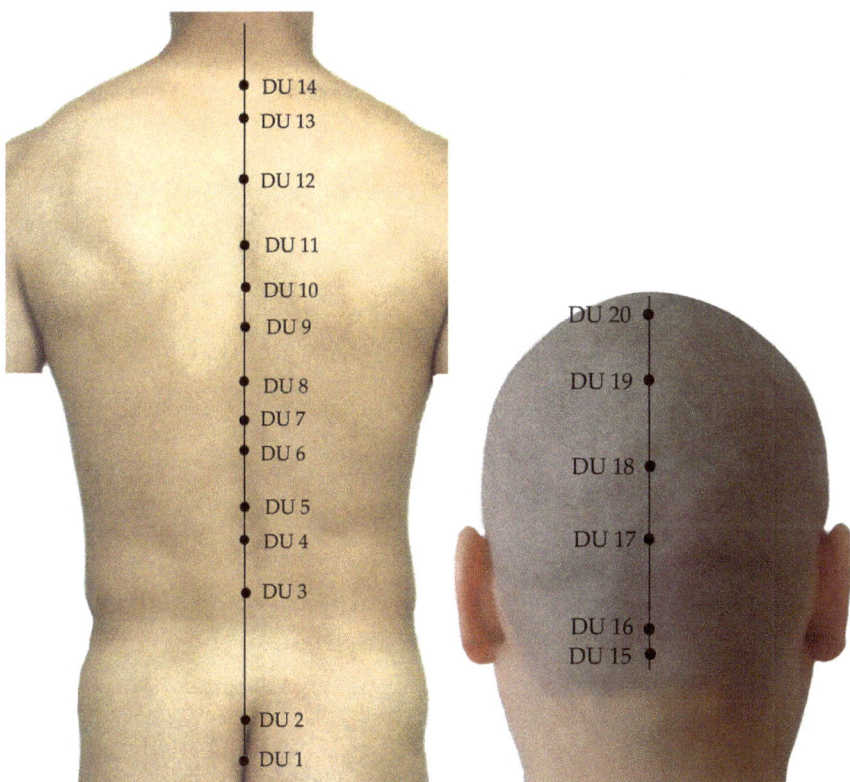

DU 14
DU 13
DU 12
DU 11
DU 10
DU 9
DU 8
DU 7
DU 6
DU 5
DU 4
DU 3
DU 2
DU 1

DU 20
DU 19
DU 18
DU 17
DU 16
DU 15

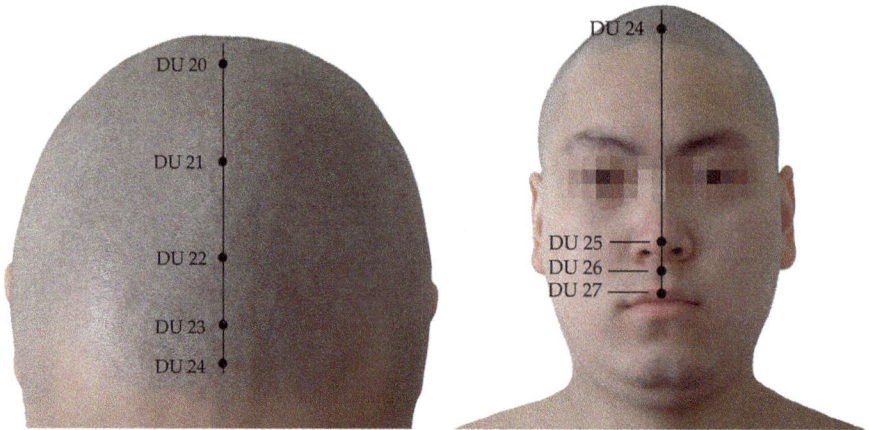

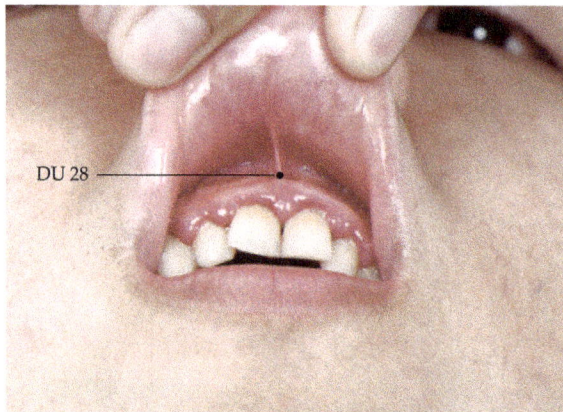

DU 1 – Cháng Qiáng

[Features]	Luo-connecting point of the Du Vessel.
[Locating]	The point is located in the prone position, below the tip of the coccyx, in the depression between the tip of the coccyx and the anus.
[Regional Anatomy]	The needle passes through the skin, subcutaneous tissues and the anococcygeal ligament, penetrates the m. coccygeus and m. levator ani.
[Acupuncture and Moxibustion]	Insert the needle obliquely upwards 0.5~1.0 cun deep proximally to the anterior border of the coccyx and penetrate between the coccyx and the rectum, stimulate until there is a sore and numbing sensation in the local area radiating to the coccyx and the anus. Moxibustion is prohibited.
[Indications]	Constipation, hemorrhoids, and prolapsus of the rectum.

DU 2 – Yāo Shū

[Locating]	The point is located in the prone position, on the posterior midline in the hiatus of the sacrum.
[Regional Anatomy]	The needle passes through the skin and the subcutaneous tissues, penetrates the dorsal sacrococcygeal ligament and the sacral canal.
[Acupuncture and Moxibustion]	Insert the needle obliquely 0.5~1.0 cun deep and stimulate until there is a sore and numbing sensation in the local area radiating to the lumbosacral region. This point can be moxibusted.
[Indications]	Diarrhea, constipation, hemorrhoids, uroschesis, and pain in the coccyx and scacral region.

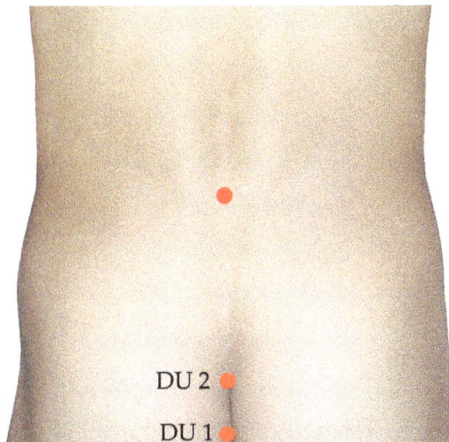

DU 2
DU 1
M. latissimus dorsi

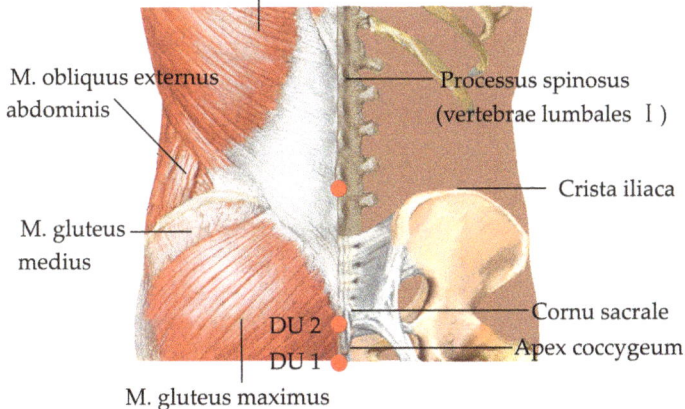

M. obliquus externus abdominis
Processus spinosus (vertebrae lumbales I)

Crista iliaca

M. gluteus medius

Cornu sacrale
Apex coccygeum

DU 2
DU 1
M. gluteus maximus

DU 3 – Yāo Yáng Guān

[Locating]	The point is located in the prone position, in the depression inferior to the spinous process of the fourth lumbar vertebra, on the posterior midline, at the level with the crista iliaca.
[Regional Anatomy]	The needle passes through the skin and the subcutaneous tissues, penetrates the supraspinal ligament and the interarcuate ligament.
[Acupuncture and Moxibustion]	Insert the needle perpendicularly 0.5~1.0 cun deep and stimulate until there is a sore and numbing sensation in the local area radiating to the lower limbs. This point can be moxibusted.
[Indications]	Lumbosacral pain and weakness, pain and numbness of the lower limbs, spermatorrhea, impotence, and irregular menstruation.

DU 4 – Mìng Mén

[Locating]	The point is located in the prone position, in the depression inferior to the spinous process of the second lumbar vertebra, on the posterior midline.
[Regional Anatomy]	The needle passes through the skin and the subcutaneous tissues, penetrates the supraspinal ligament, interspinal ligament and the interarcuate ligament.
[Acupuncture and Moxibustion]	Insert the needle perpendicularly 0.5~1.0 cun deep and stimulate until there is a sore and numbing sensation in the local area with an electric sensation radiating to the hip and lower limbs. This point can be moxibusted.
[Indications]	Spermatorrhea, impotence, infertility, lumbago due to consumptive disease, and stiffness and pain of the lumbar and lower limbs.

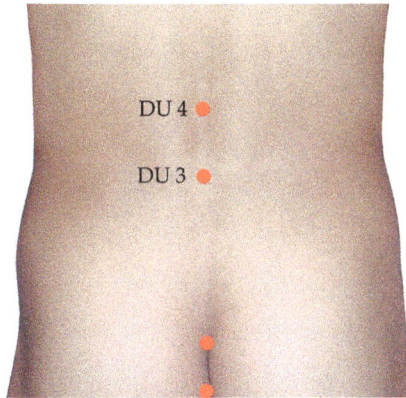

M. latissimus dorsi

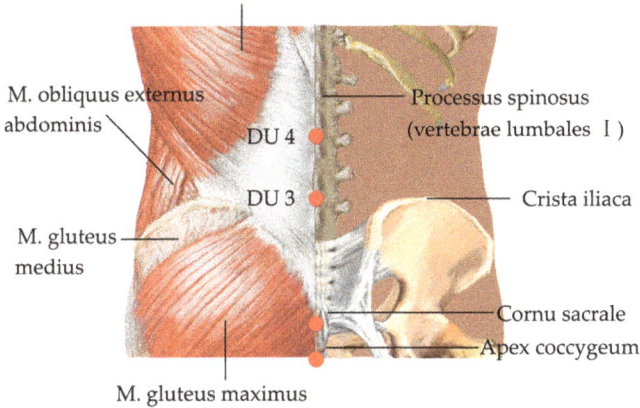

M. obliquus externus abdominis

M. gluteus medius

M. gluteus maximus

Processus spinosus (vertebrae lumbales Ⅰ)

Crista iliaca

Cornu sacrale

Apex coccygeum

DU 4

DU 3

DU 5 – Xuán Shū

[Locating]	The point is located in the sitting or prone position, in the depression inferior to the spinous process of the first lumbar vertebra, on the posterior midline.
[Regional Anatomy]	The needle passes through the skin and the subcutaneous tissues, penetrates the supraspinal ligament, interspinal ligament and the interarcuate ligament.
[Acupuncture and Moxibustion]	Insert the needle perpendicularly 0.5~1.0 cun deep with the twirling or rotating needling technique and stimulate until there is a sore and numbing sensation in the local area. This point can be moxibusted.
[Indications]	Abdominal pain, abdominal distention, undigested food and diarrhea, stiffness, and pain of the lumbar.

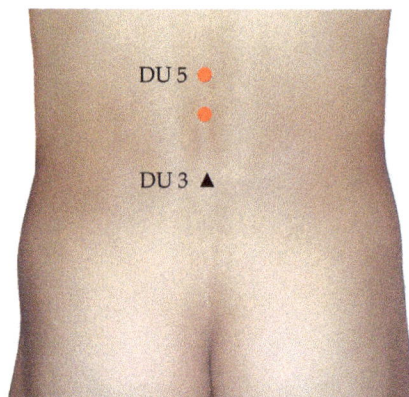

M. latissimus dorsi

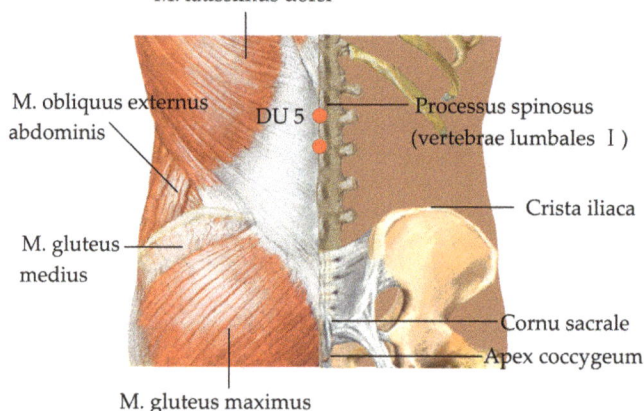

M. obliquus externus
abdominis

DU 5

Processus spinosus
(vertebrae lumbales I)

Crista iliaca

M. gluteus
medius

Cornu sacrale

Apex coccygeum

M. gluteus maximus

DU 6 – Jǐ Zhōng

[Locating]	The point is located in the prone position, in the depression inferior to the spinous process of the eleventh thoracic vertebra, on the posterior midline of the back.
[Regional Anatomy]	The needle passes through the skin and the subcutaneous tissues, penetrates the supraspinal ligament, interspinal ligament and the interarcuate ligament.
[Acupuncture and Moxibustion]	Insert the needle perpendicularly 0.5~1.0 cun deep with the twirling or rotating needling technique and stimulate until there is a sore and numbing sensation in the local area radiating to the lower limbs. This point can be moxibusted.
[Indications]	Diarrhea, dysentery and hemorrhoids.

DU 7 – Zhōng Shū

[Locating]	The point is located in the prone position, in the depression inferior to the spinous process of the tenth thoracic vertebra, on the posterior midline of the back.
[Regional Anatomy]	The needle passes through the skin and the subcutaneous tissues, penetrates the supraspinal ligament, interspinal ligament and the interarcuate ligament.
[Acupuncture and Moxibustion]	Insert the needle obliquely 0.5~1.0 cun deep with the twirling or rotating needling technique and stimulate until there is a sore and numbing sensation in the local area radiating to the lower limbs. This point can be moxibusted.
[Indications]	Vomiting, abdominal distention, poor appetite, pain of the lumbar, and lower back.

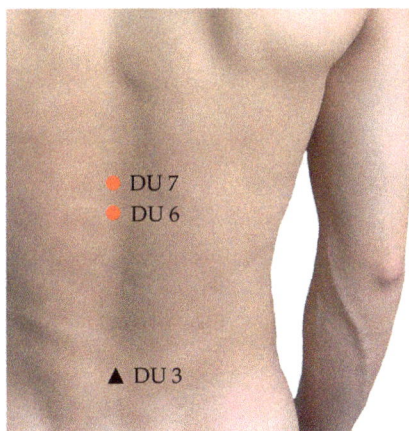

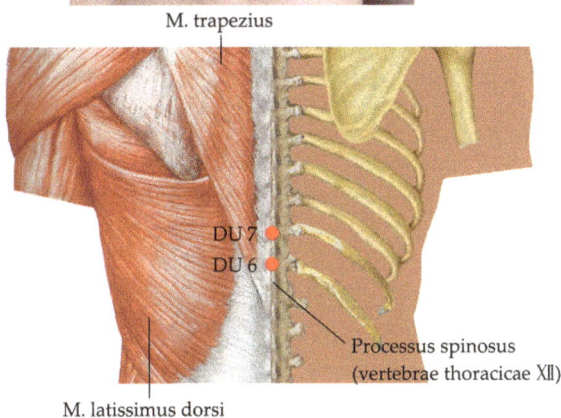

M. trapezius

DU 7
DU 6

Processus spinosus
(vertebrae thoracicae XII)

M. latissimus dorsi

DU 8 – Jīn Suō

[Locating]	The point is located in the prone position, in the depression inferior to the spinous process of the ninth thoracic vertebra, on the posterior midline of the back.
[Regional Anatomy]	The needle passes through the skin and the subcutaneous tissues, penetrates the supraspinal ligament, interspinal ligament and the interarcuate ligament.
[Acupuncture and Moxibustion]	Insert the needle obliquely 0.5~1.0 cun deep and stimulate with the twirling or rotating needling technique until there is a sore and numbing sensation in the local area. This point can be moxibusted.
[Indications]	Spasms and stiffness of the back, and epilepsy.

DU 9 – Zhì Yáng

[Locating]	The point is located in the prone position with arm adducted, in the depression inferior to the spinous process of the seventh thoracic vertebra, on the posterior midline of the back.
[Regional Anatomy]	The needle passes through the skin and the subcutaneous tissues, penetrates the supraspinal ligament, interspinal ligament and the interarcuate ligament.
[Acupuncture and Moxibustion]	Insert the needle obliquely 0.5~1.0 cun deep and stimulate until there is a sore and numbing sensation in the local area spreading to the back and chest. This point can be moxibusted.
[Indications]	Swelling and pain of the chest and hypochondrium, jaundice, lumbago, and stiffness of the spine.

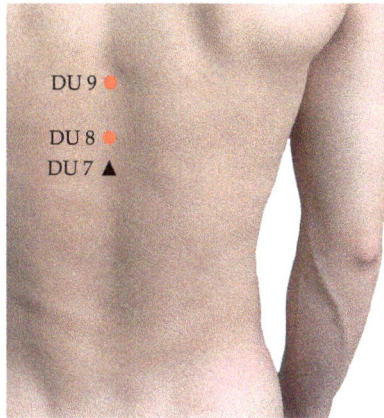

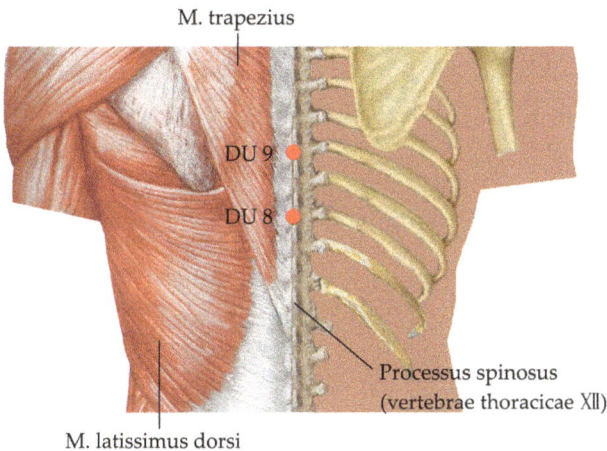

DU 9
DU 8
DU 7

M. trapezius

DU 9
DU 8

Processus spinosus
(vertebrae thoracicae XⅡ)

M. latissimus dorsi

DU 10 – Líng Tái

[Locating]	The point is located in the prone position, in the depression inferior to the spinous process of the sixth thoracic vertebra, on the posterior midline of the back.
[Regional Anatomy]	The needle passes through the skin and the subcutaneous tissues, penetrates the supraspinal ligament, interspinal ligament and the interarcuate ligament.
[Acupuncture and Moxibustion]	Insert the needle obliquely 0.5~1.0 cun deep and stimulate until there is a sore and numbing sensation in the local area spreading to the back and chest. This point can be moxibusted.
[Indications]	Furuncles, cough and asthma, and neck stiffness and back pain.

DU 11 – Shén Dào

[Locating]	The point is located in the prone position, in the depression inferior to the spinous process of the fifth thoracic vertebra, on the posterior midline of the back.
[Regional Anatomy]	The needle passes through the skin and the subcutaneous tissues, penetrates the supraspinal ligament, interspinal ligament and the interarcuate ligament.
[Acupuncture and Moxibustion]	Insert the needle obliquely 0.5~1.0 cun deep with the twirling or rotating needling technique and stimulate until there is a sore and numbing sensation in the local area spreading to the back and chest. This point can be moxibusted.
[Indications]	Insomnia and amnesia, and shoulder and back pain.

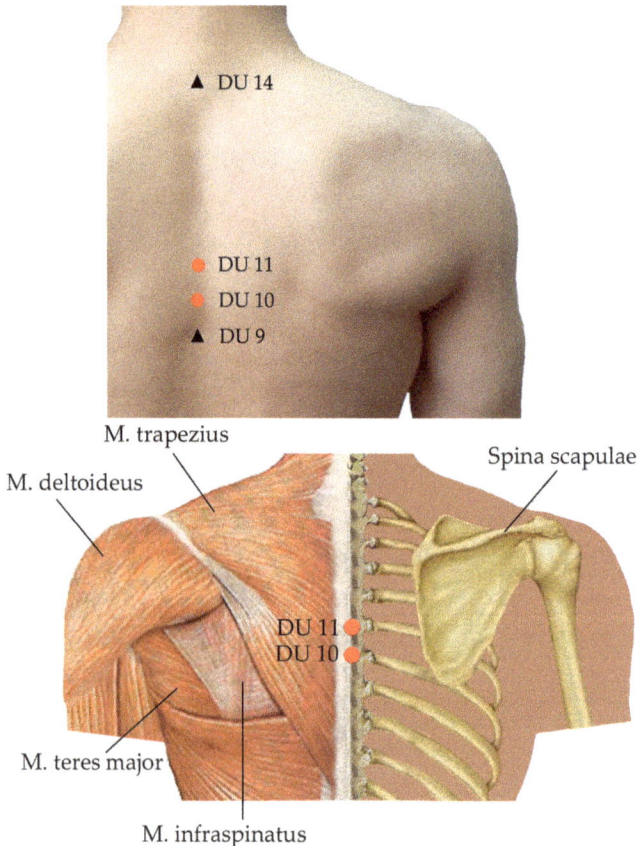

▲ DU 14

● DU 11
● DU 10
▲ DU 9

M. trapezius

M. deltoideus

Spina scapulae

DU 11 ●
DU 10 ●

M. teres major

M. infraspinatus

DU 12 – Shēn Zhù

[Locating]	The point is located in the prone position, in the depression inferior to the spinous process of the third thoracic vertebra, on the posterior midline of the back.
[Regional Anatomy]	The needle passes through the skin and the subcutaneous tissues, penetrates the supraspinal ligament, interspinal ligament and the interarcuate ligament.
[Acupuncture and Moxibustion]	Insert the needle obliquely 0.5~1.0 cun deep with the twirling or rotating needling technique and stimulate until there is a sore and numbing sensation in the local area. This point can be moxibusted.
[Indications]	Cough and asthma, and furuncles.

DU 13 – Táo Dào

[Locating]	The point is located in the prone position, in the depression inferior to the spinous process of the first thoracic vertebra, on the posterior midline of the back.
[Regional Anatomy]	The needle passes through the skin and the subcutaneous tissues, penetrates the supraspinal ligament, interspinal ligament and the interarcuate ligament.
[Acupuncture and Moxibustion]	Insert the needle obliquely 0.5~1.0 cun deep with the twirling or rotating needling technique and stimulate until there is a sore and numbing sensation in the local area radiating to the shoulder and upper limbs. This point can be moxibusted.
[Indications]	Aversion to cold and fever.

DU 14 – Dà Zhuī

[Locating]	The point is located in the sitting or prone position when the neck is flexed, in the depression inferior to the spinous process of the seventh cervical vertebra, on the posterior midline of the neck.
[Regional Anatomy]	The needle passes through the skin and the subcutaneous tissues, penetrates the supraspinal ligament, interspinal ligament and the interarcuate ligament.
[Acupuncture and Moxibustion]	① Insert the needle obliquely 0.5~1.0 cun deep and stimulate until there is a sore and numbing sensation in the local area. ② Prick with a three-edged needle to bleed. This point can be moxibusted.
[Indications]	Aversion to cold and fever, pain and stiffness of the neck and pain of the shoulder and back, rubella, cough and asthma, epilepsy, and manic psychosis.

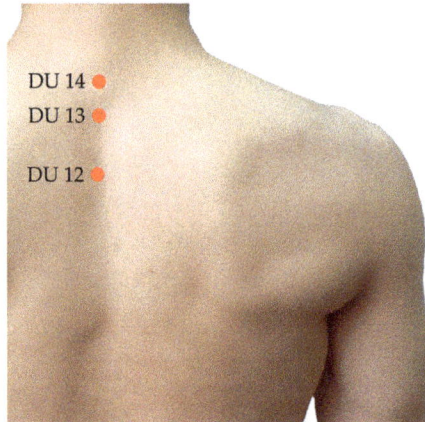

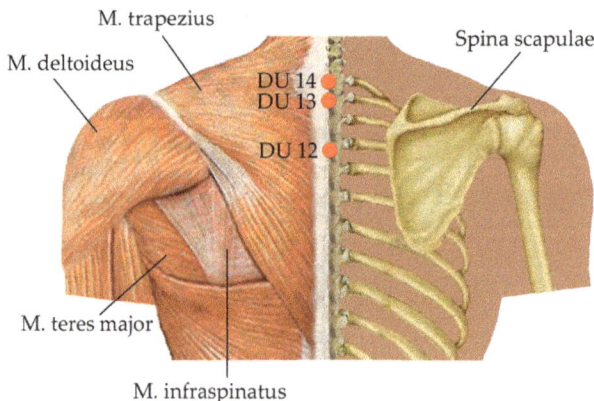

DU 14
DU 13
DU 12

M. trapezius
M. deltoideus
Spina scapulae
DU 14
DU 13
DU 12
M. teres major
M. infraspinatus

DU 15 – Yǎ Mén

[Locating]	The point is located in the sitting position when the head bends forwards slightly, on the back of the neck, 0.5 cun superior to the posterior hairline.
[Regional Anatomy]	The needle passes through the skin and the subcutaneous tissues, penetrates the region between left and right m. trapezius, nuchal ligament, interspinal ligament and interarcuate ligament.
[Acupuncture and Moxibustion]	With the sitting position when the head bends forwards slightly, relax neck muscles, insert the needle obliquely towards the mandible 0.5~1.0 cun deep and stimulate until there is a sore and numbing sensation in the local area. Moxibustion is prohibited.
[Indications]	Deaf and mute syndrome, and headache.
[Note]	Needle insertion is absolutely not directed toward the nose, avoid deep insertion to prevent injury to the medulla oblongata.

DU 16 – Fēng Fǔ

[Locating]	The point is located in the sitting position when the head is bent forward, on the back of the neck, 0.5 cun superior to the midpoint of the posterior hairline.
[Regional Anatomy]	The needle passes through the skin and the subcutaneous tissues, penetrates the region between left and right m. trapezius, nuchal ligament and posterior altantoccipital membrane.
[Acupuncture and Moxibustion]	With the sitting position when the head bends forwards slightly, relax neck muscles, insert the needle obliquely towards the mandible 0.5~1.0 cun deep and stimulate until there is a sore and numbing sensation in the local area. Moxibustion is prohibited.
[Indications]	Stroke, stiffness and pain of the head and neck, dizziness, nasal obstruction, and epilepsy.
[Note]	The same as DU 15 (Yǎ Mén).

DU 17 – Năo Hù

[Locating]	On the head, in the depression superior to the external occipital protuberance.
[Regional Anatomy]	The needle passes through the skin and the subcutaneous tissues, penetrates the m. occipitofrontalis and the connective tissue beneath aponeurosis.
[Acupuncture and Moxibustion]	Insert the needle subcutaneously 0.5~0.8 cun deep and stimulate until there is a sore and distending sensation in the local area.
[Indications]	Dizziness, headache, and neck stiffness.

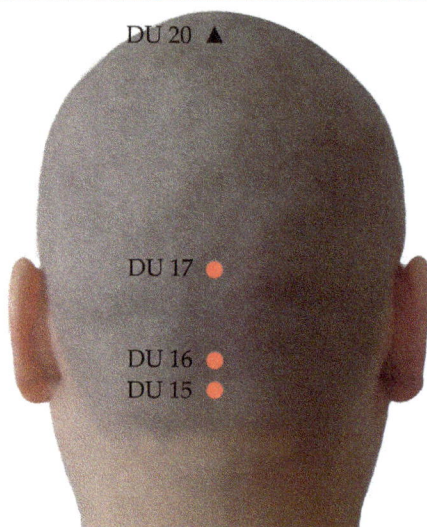

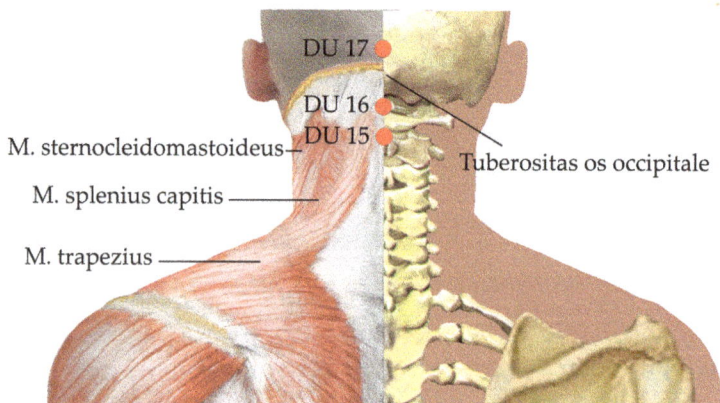

DU 18 – Qiáng Jiān

[Locating]	On the head, 4 cun superior to the midpoint of the posterior hairline, 1.5 cun superior to DU 17 (Nǎo Hù).
[Regional Anatomy]	The needle passes through the skin and the subcutaneous tissues, penetrates the galea aponeurotica and the connective tissue beneath aponeurosis.
[Acupuncture and Moxibustion]	Insert the needle subcutaneously 0.5~0.8 cun deep and stimulate until there is a sore and distending sensation in the local area. This point can be moxibusted.
[Indications]	Headache, dizziness, and epilepsy.

DU 19 – Hòu Dǐng

[Locating]	The point is located in the sitting or supine position, on the posterior midline of the neck, 1.5 cun superior to DU 18 (Qiáng Jiān), 5.5 cun superior to the posterior hairline.
[Regional Anatomy]	The needle passes through the skin and the subcutaneous tissues, penetrates the galea aponeurotica and the connective tissue beneath aponeurosis.
[Acupuncture and Moxibustion]	Insert the needle subcutaneously 0.5~0.8 cun deep and stimulate until there is a sore and distending sensation in the local area. This point can be moxibusted.
[Indications]	Neck stiffness, headache, dizziness, and insomnia.

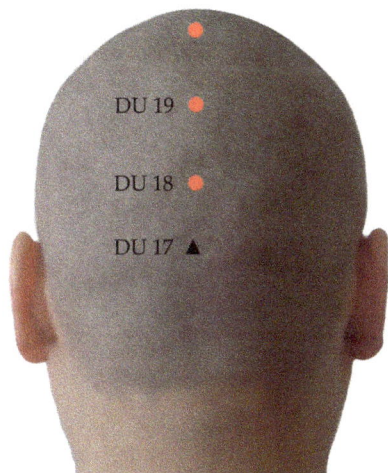

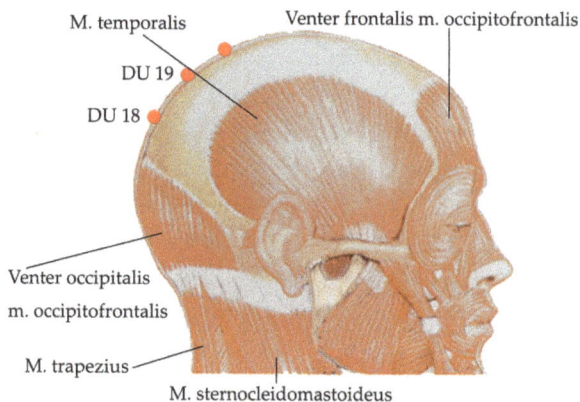

M. temporalis

Venter frontalis m. occipitofrontalis

DU 19

DU 18

Venter occipitalis
m. occipitofrontalis

M. trapezius

M. sternocleidomastoideus

DU 20 – Bǎi Huì

[Locating]	The point is located in the sitting or supine position, on the midline, 1.5 cun superior to DU 19 (Hòu Dǐng), 7 cun posterior to the posterior hairline, and at the midpoint of the line between the two ears.
[Regional Anatomy]	The needle passes through the skin and the subcutaneous tissues, penetrates the galea aponeurotica and the connective tissue beneath aponeurosis.
[Acupuncture and Moxibustion]	Insert the needle subcutaneously 0.5~0.8 cun deep and stimulate until there is a sore and distending sensation in the local area.
	This point can be moxibusted.
[Indications]	Stroke, loss of the consciousness, epilepsy, dizziness, headache, prolapsed rectum and hemorrhoids, prolapsed uterus.

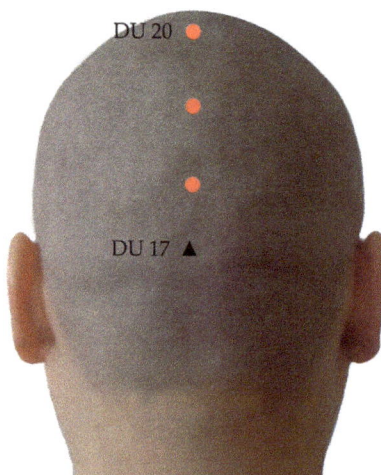

DU 20

DU 17 ▲

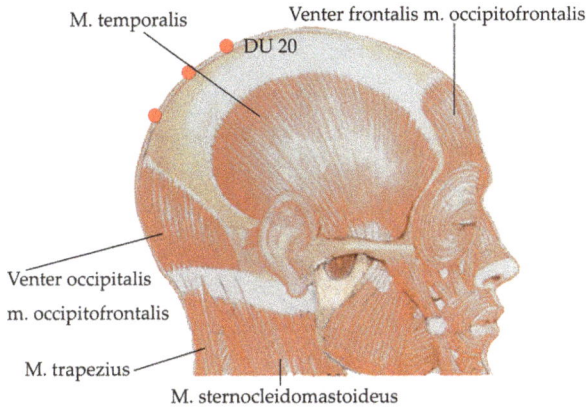

M. temporalis

Venter frontalis m. occipitofrontalis

DU 20

Venter occipitalis
m. occipitofrontalis

M. trapezius

M. sternocleidomastoideus

DU 21 – Qián Dǐng

[Locating]	The point is located in the sitting or supine position, on the midline, 1.5 cun superior to DU 20 (Bǎi Huì), 3.5 cun superior to the anterior hairline.
[Regional Anatomy]	The needle passes through the skin and the subcutaneous tissues, penetrates the galea aponeurotica and the connective tissue beneath aponeurosis.
[Acupuncture and Moxibustion]	Insert the needle subcutaneously 0.3~0.5 cun deep and stimulate until there is a heavy and distending sensation in the local area. This point can be moxibusted.
[Indications]	Febrile Convulsion, headache, dizziness, and epilepsy.

DU 22 – Xìn Huì

[Locating]	The point is located in the sitting or supine position, on the midline, 1.5 cun superior to DU 19 (Qián Dǐng), 2 cun superior to the anterior hairline.
[Regional Anatomy]	The needle passes through the skin and the subcutaneous tissues, penetrates the galea aponeurotica and the connective tissue beneath aponeurosis.
[Acupuncture and Moxibustion]	Insert the needle subcutaneously 0.3~0.5 cun deep and stimulate until there is a heavy and distending sensation in the local area. This point can be moxibusted.
[Indications]	The same as DU 19 (Qiándǐng).

DU 20 ▲
1.5 cun
DU 21 ●
1.5 cun
DU 22 ●
1 cun
1 cun

M. temporalis
Venter frontalis m. occipitofrontalis
DU 21   DU 22

Venter occipitalis
m. occipitofrontalis
M. trapezius
M. sternocleidomastoideus

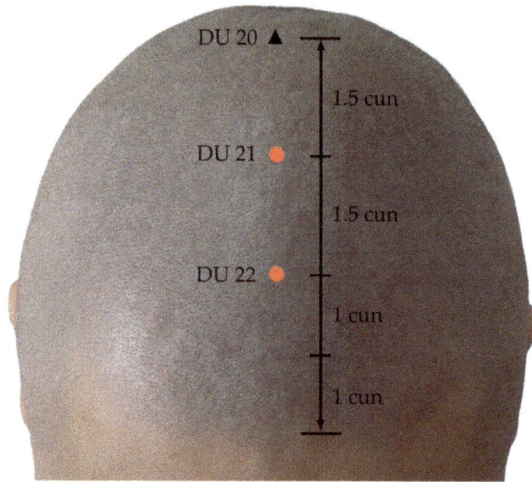

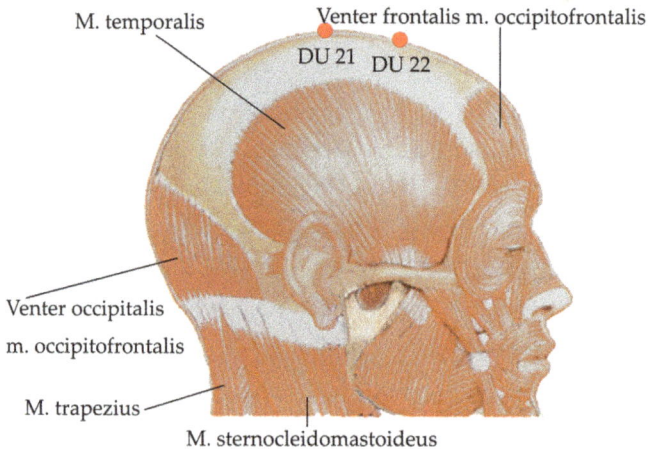

DU 23 – Shàng Xīng

[Locating]	The point is located in the sitting or supine position, on the midline, 1 cun superior to the anterior hairline.
[Regional Anatomy]	The needle passes through the skin and the subcutaneous tissues, penetrates the galea aponeurotica and the connective tissue beneath aponeurosis.
[Acupuncture and Moxibustion]	Insert the needle subcutaneously 0.3~0.5 cun deep and stimulate until there is a heavy and distending sensation in the local area. This point can be moxibusted.
[Indications]	Headache, dizziness, and epistaxis.

DU 24 – Shén Tíng

[Locating]	The point is located in the sitting or supine position, on the midline, 0.5 cun superior to anterior hairline.
[Regional Anatomy]	The needle passes through the skin and the subcutaneous tissues, penetrates the m. frontalis occipitalis.
[Acupuncture and Moxibustion]	Insert the needle subcutaneously 0.3~0.5 cun deep and stimulate until there is a heavy and distending sensation in the local area. This point can be moxibusted.
[Indications]	Epilepsy, palpitations and easily frightened, insomnia, headache, dizziness, nasosinusitis and rhinorrhea.

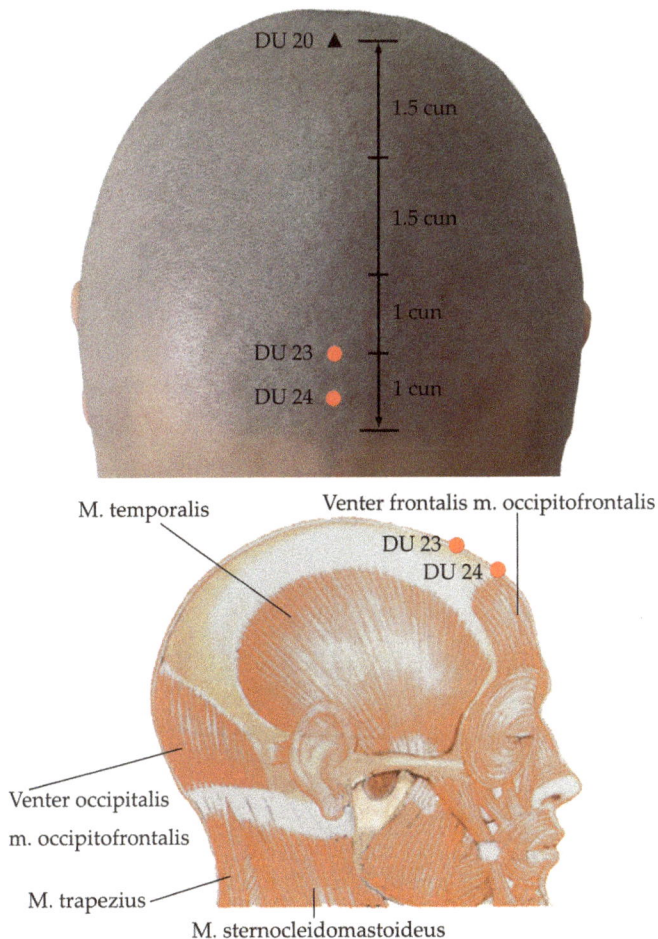

DU 20 ▲
1.5 cun
1.5 cun
1 cun
DU 23 ●
DU 24 ●
1 cun

M. temporalis
Venter frontalis m. occipitofrontalis
DU 23 ●
DU 24 ●
Venter occipitalis m. occipitofrontalis
M. trapezius
M. sternocleidomastoideus

DU 25 – Sù Liáo

[Locating]	The point is located in the sitting or supine position, on the face, on the tip of the nose.
[Regional Anatomy]	The needle passes through the skin and subcutis and penetrates the nasal perichondrium.
[Acupuncture and Moxibustion]	① Insert the needle obliquely upwards 0.3~0.5 cun deep and stimulate until there is a sore and distending sensation in the local area spreading in the nose. ② Prick with a three-edged needle to bleed. Moxibustion is prohibited.
[Indications]	Easily frightened, and loss of the consciousness, neonatal asphyxia, nasal congestion, and rhinorrhea.

DU 26 – Shuǐ Gōu

[Locating]	The point is located in the sitting or supine position, at the superior 1/3 and inferior 2/3 of the philtrum.
[Regional Anatomy]	The needle passes through the skin and subcutis and penetrates the m. orbicularis oris.
[Acupuncture and Moxibustion]	Insert the needle obliquely towards the center of the nose 0.2~0.3 cun deep and stimulate until there is a pain sensation in the local area, or nail pinching. Moxibustion is prohibited.
[Indications]	Loss of consciousness, syncope, epilepsy, lumbago, febrile convulsion, deviation of the eye and mouth.

DU 27 – Duì Duān

[Locating]	The point is located in the sitting or supine position, at the border of the upper lip, at the juncture of the skin of the philtrum and the upper lip.
[Regional Anatomy]	The needle passes through the skin and subcutis and penetrates the m. orbicularis oris.
[Acupuncture and Moxibustion]	Insert the needle obliquely 0.5~0.8 cun deep and stimulate until there is a sore and distending sensation in the local area. Moxibustion is prohibited.
[Indications]	Loss of consciousness and syncope, and nasal obstruction.

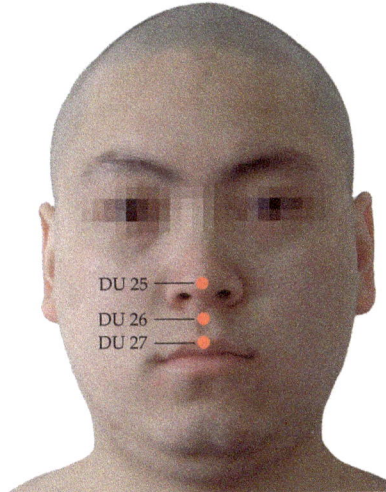

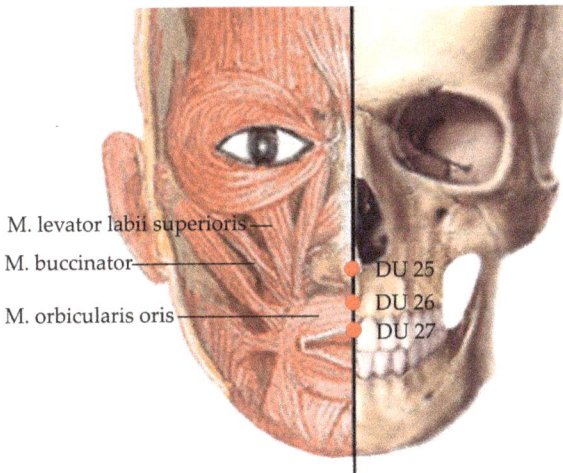

DU 25
DU 26
DU 27

M. levator labii superioris
M. buccinator
M. orbicularis oris

DU 25
DU 26
DU 27

DU 28 – Yín Jiāo

[Locating]	The point is located in the sitting or supine position by pulling up the upper lip, inside the upper lip, at the junction of the frenulum of the upper lip and the gum.
[Regional Anatomy]	The needle passes through the mucosa and penetrates the deep layer of mucosa.
[Acupuncture and Moxibustion]	① Insert the needle obliquely upwards 0.2~0.3 cun deep and stimulate until there is a sore and distending sensation in the local area. ② Prick with a three-edged needle to bleed. Moxibustion is prohibited.
[Indications]	Manic psychosis, hysteria, and hemorrhoids.

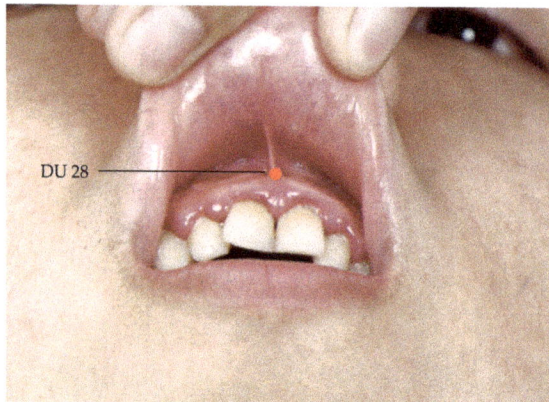

DU 28

Ren Vessel; RN

There are twenty-four points on the Ren vessel. They are distributed on the midline of the face, neck, chest and abdomen. The first point is RN 1 (Huì Yīn) and the last one is RN 24 (Chéng Jiāng). The indications for this vessel are the diseases of the mental, respiratory, digestive and urogenital system and the symptoms along the course of the channel.

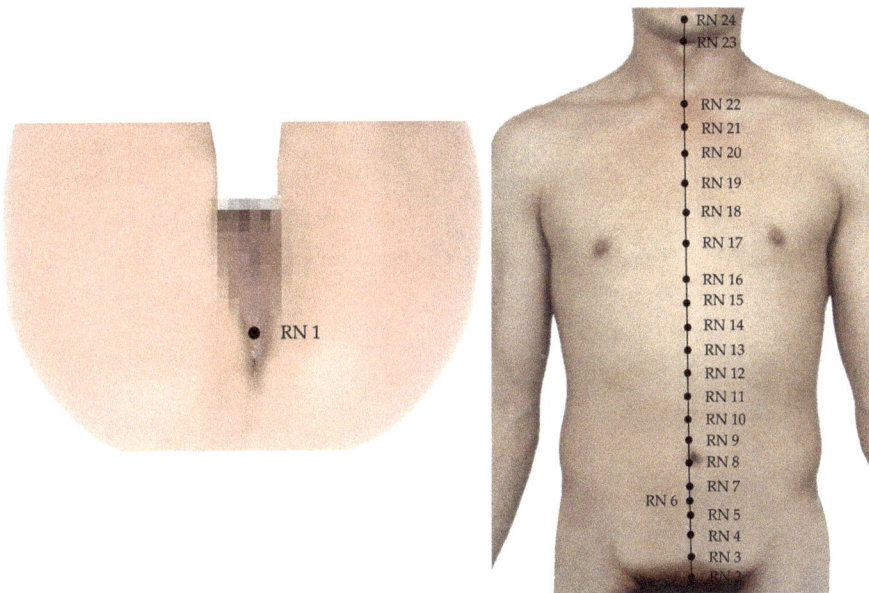

RN 1 – Huì Yīn

[Locating]	On the perineum, at the midpoint between the anus and the root of the scrotum in males and between the anus and the posterior labial commissure in females.
[Regional Anatomy]	The needle passes through the skin and subcutaneous tissues and penetrates the central tendon of perineum.

[Acupuncture and Moxibustion]	Insert the needle perpendicularly 0.5~1.0 cun deep and stimulate until there is a sore and distending sensation in the local area radiating to the anterior and posterior of the genetalia. This point can be moxibusted.
[Indications]	Pain and itching of the genitalia, pudendal swelling, and drowning suffocation.
[Note]	The point is prohibited during pregnancy.

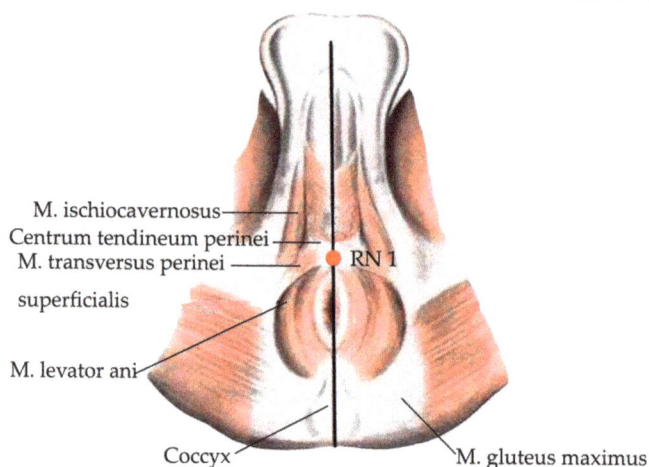

M. ischiocavernosus
Centrum tendineum perinei
M. transversus perinei
superficialis

M. levator ani

RN 1

Coccyx

M. gluteus maximus

RN 2 – Qū Gǔ

[Locating]	The point is located in the supine position, on the anterior midline, in the depression of the midpoint of the upper border of the symphysis pubis.
[Regional Anatomy]	The needle passes through the skin and the subcutaneous tissues, penetrates the median umbilical fold.
[Acupuncture and Moxibustion]	Insert the needle perpendicularly 0.5~1.0 cun deep and stimulate until there is a sore and distending sensation in the local area radiating to the genitalia. This point can be moxibusted.
[Indications]	Spermatorrhea, impotence and enuresis, and irregular menstruation.
[Note]	Acupuncture is prohibited during pregnancy. Request the patient empty their bladder before the puncturing this point.

RN 3 – Zhōng Jí

[Features]	Front-mu point of the Bladder Channel of Foot *Tai-yang*.
[Locating]	The point is located in the supine position, on the anterior midline, 4 cun inferior to the umbilicus.
[Regional Anatomy]	The same as RN 2 (Qū Gǔ).
[Acupuncture and Moxibustion]	The same as RN 2 (Qū Gǔ).
[Indications]	Hernia, spermatorrhea, and dysuria.
[Note]	The same as RN 2 (Qū Gǔ).

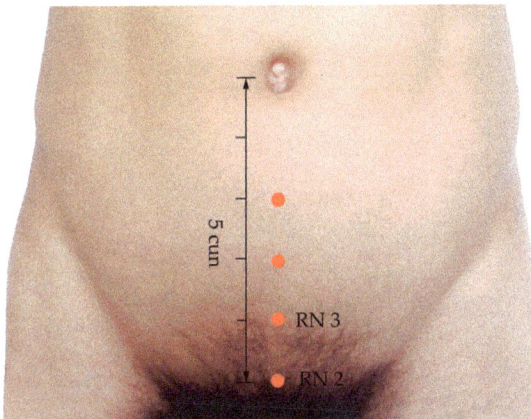

5 cun

RN 3

RN 2

Spina iliaca anterior superior

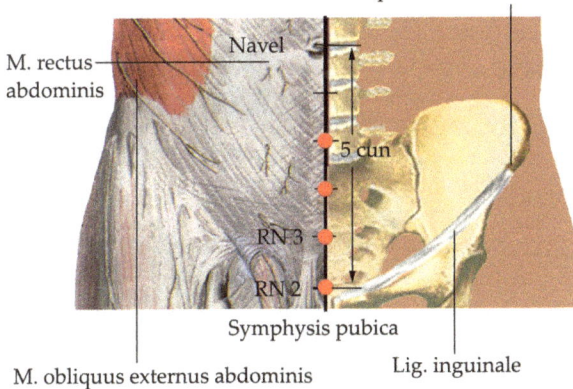

Navel

M. rectus abdominis

5 cun

RN 3

RN 2

M. obliquus externus abdominis

Symphysis pubica

Lig. inguinale

RN 4 – Guān Yuán

[Features]	Front-mu point of the Small intestine of Hand *Taiyang*.
[Locating]	The point is located in the supine position, on the anterior midline, 3 cun inferior to the umbilicus.
[Regional Anatomy]	The same as RN 2 (Qū Gǔ).
[Acupuncture and Moxibustion]	The same as RN 2 (Qū Gǔ).
[Indications]	Abdominal pain, impotence, amenorrhea, infertility and general weakness.
[Note]	The same as RN 2 (Qū Gǔ).

RN 5 – Shí Mén

[Features]	Front-mu point of the Sanjiao Channel of Hand *Shaoyang*.
[Locating]	The point is located in the supine position, on the anterior midline, 2 cun inferior to the umbilicus.
[Regional Anatomy]	The same as RN 2 (Qū Gǔ).
[Acupuncture and Moxibustion]	The same as RN 2 (Qū Gǔ).
[Indications]	Amenorrhea and morbid leucorrhea.

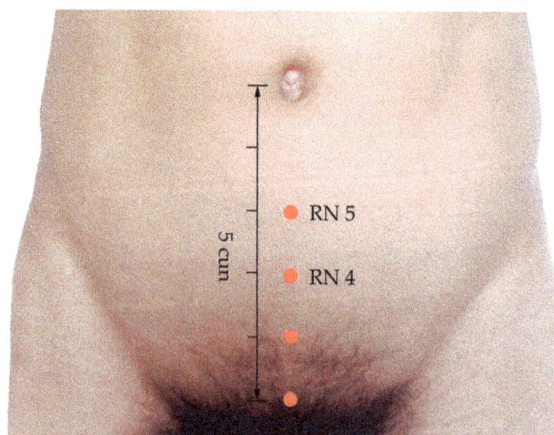

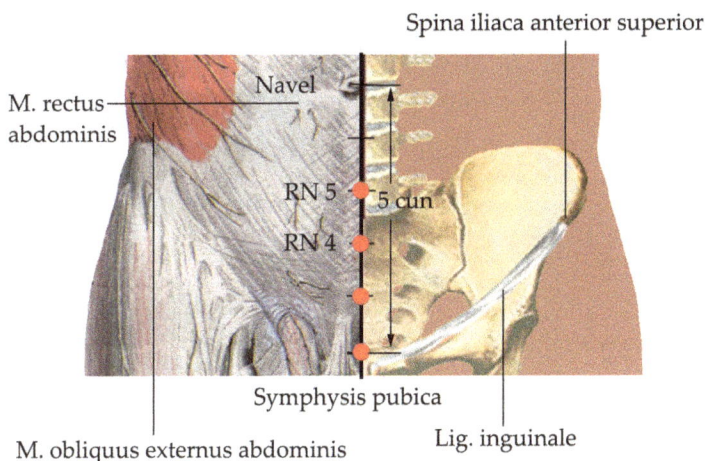

Spina iliaca anterior superior

M. rectus abdominis

Navel

RN 5 — 5 cun

RN 4

Symphysis pubica

M. obliquus externus abdominis

Lig. inguinale

RN 6 – Qì Hǎi

[Features]	Yuan-source point of Huang.
[Locating]	The point is located in the supine position, on the anterior midline, 1.5 cun inferior to the umbilicus.
[Regional Anatomy]	The same as RN 2 (Qū Gǔ).
[Acupuncture and Moxibustion]	The same as RN 2 (Qū Gǔ).
[Indications]	Lower abdomen diseases, women's diseases, gastrointestinal disease, and general weakness.

RN 7 – Yīn Jiāo

[Locating]	The point is located in the supine position, on the anterior midline, 1 cun below the umbilicus.
[Regional Anatomy]	The same as RN 2 (Qū Gǔ).
[Acupuncture and Moxibustion]	The same as RN 2 (Qū Gǔ).
[Indications]	metrorrhagia and morbid leucorrhea.

RN 8 – Shén Què

[Locating]	On the abdomen, in the center of the umbilicus.
[Regional Anatomy]	The needle passes through the skin, subcutaneous tissues and fibrous ring of umbilicus
[Acupuncture and Moxibustion]	Acupuncture is prohibited, moxibustion is allowed.
[Indications]	Syncope and chills in limbs caused by weakness and cold, borborygums and abdominal pain, irregular menstruation, metrorrhagia, spermatorrhea, enuresis, and infertility.

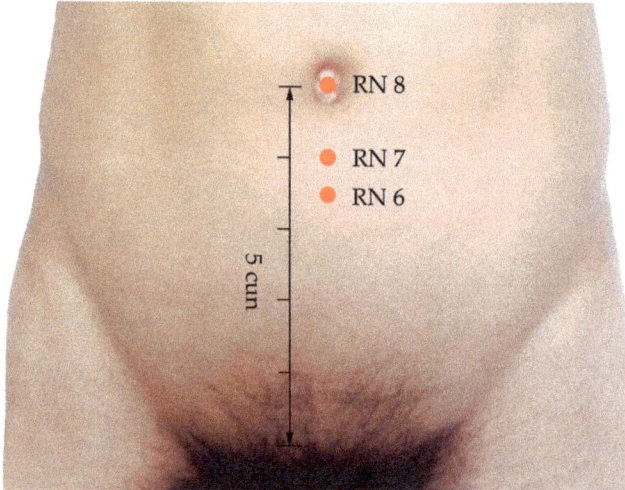

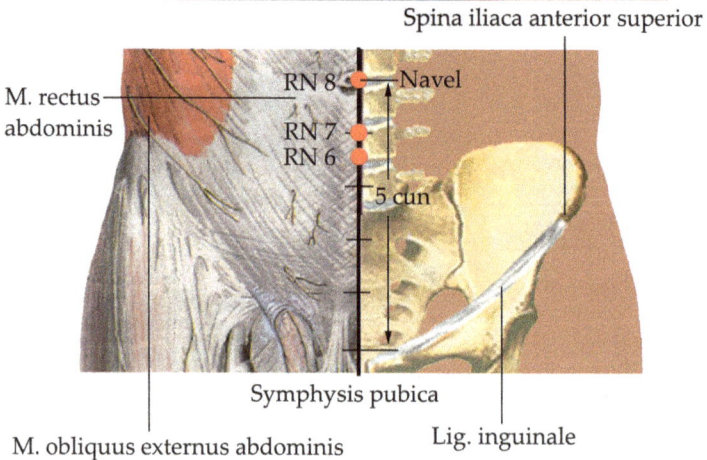

RN 9 – Shuǐ Fēn

[Locating]	The point is located in the supine position, on the anterior midline, 1 cun superior to the umbilicus.
[Regional Anatomy]	The needle passes through the skin and the subcutaneous tissues, penetrates the median umbilical fold.
[Acupuncture and Moxibustion]	Insert the needle perpendicularly 0.5~1.0 cun deep and stimulate until there is a sore and distending sensation in the local area. This point can be moxibusted.
[Indications]	Spermatorrhea, impotence, irregular menstruation, and enuresis.

RN 10 – Xià Wǎn

[Locating]	The point is located in the supine position, on the anterior midline, 2 cun above the umbilicus.
[Regional Anatomy]	The same as RN 9 (Shuǐ Fēn).
[Acupuncture and Moxibustion]	The same as RN 9 (Shuǐ Fēn).
[Indications]	Borborygums and abdominal pain, abdominal distention, vomiting and hiccup singultation.

RN 11 – Jiàn Lǐ

[Locating]	The point is located in the supine position, on the anterior midline, 3 cun superior to the umbilicus.
[Regional Anatomy]	The same as RN 9 (Shuǐ Fēn).
[Acupuncture and Moxibustion]	The same as RN 9 (Shuǐ Fēn).
[Indications]	Borborygums and abdominal pain and vomiting.

RN 12 – Zhōng Wǎn

[Features]	Front-mu point of the Stomach Channel of the Foot *Yangming*, influential point of the fu organs.
[Locating]	The point is located in the supine position, on the anterior midline, 4 cun superior to the umbilicus.
[Regional Anatomy]	The same as RN 9 (Shuǐ Fēn).
[Acupuncture and Moxibustion]	The same as RN 9 (Shuǐ Fēn).
[Indications]	The diseases of the digestive system, manic psychosis, and irregular menstruation.

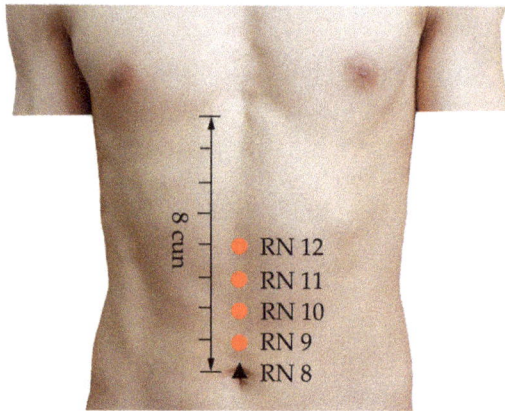

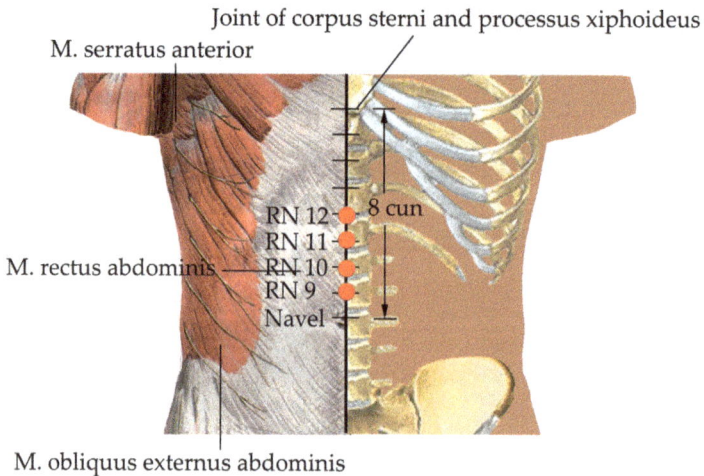

8 cun

RN 12
RN 11
RN 10
RN 9
RN 8

Joint of corpus sterni and processus xiphoideus

M. serratus anterior

8 cun

RN 12
RN 11
M. rectus abdominis — RN 10
RN 9
Navel

M. obliquus externus abdominis

RN 13 – Shàng Wǎn

[Locating]	The point is located in the supine position, on the anterior midline, 5 cun superior to the umbilicus.
[Regional Anatomy]	The same as RN 9 (Shuǐ Fēn).
[Acupuncture and Moxibustion]	The same as RN 9 (Shuǐ Fēn).
[Indications]	Stomach ache, vomiting, hiccup singultation, indigestion, and loss of appetite.
[Note]	Avoid deep puncture to prevent injury to the internal organs.

RN 14 – Jù Què

[Features]	Front-mu point of the Heart Channel of Hand *Shaoyin*.
[Locating]	The point is located in the supine position, on the anterior midline, 6 cun superior to the umbilicus.
[Regional Anatomy]	The same as RN 9 (Shuǐ Fēn).
[Acupuncture and Moxibustion]	The same as RN 9 (Shuǐ Fēn).
[Indications]	Stomach ache, vomiting, hiccup singultation, indigestion, and loss of appetite.
[Note]	The same as RN 13 (Shàng Wǎn).

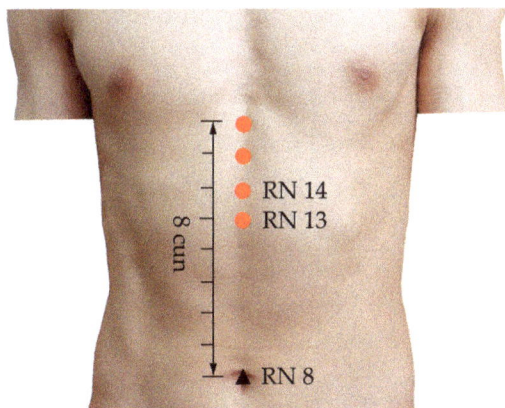

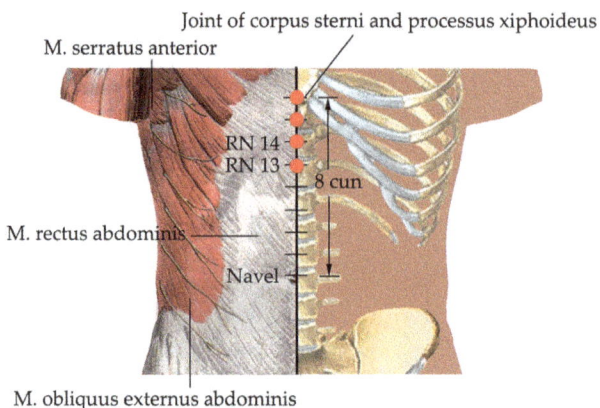

Joint of corpus sterni and processus xiphoideus
M. serratus anterior
RN 14
RN 13
8 cun
M. rectus abdominis
Navel
M. obliquus externus abdominis

RN 15 – Jiū Wěi

[Features]	Yuan-source point of Huang, Luo-connecting point of the Ren vessel.
[Locating]	The point is located in the supine position, on the anterior midline, 1 cun inferior to the sternocostal angle.
[Regional Anatomy]	The same as RN 9 (Shuǐ Fēn).
[Acupuncture and Moxibustion]	Insert the needle obliquely downwards 0.5~1.0 cun deep and stimulate until there is a sore and distending sensation in the local area. This point can be moxibusted.
[Indications]	Stomach ache, vomiting, hiccup singultation, indigestion and loss of appetite.
[Note]	The same as RN 13 (Shàngwǎn).

RN 16 – Zhōng Tíng

[Locating]	The point is located in the supine position, on the anterior midline, at the sternocostal angle.
[Regional Anatomy]	The needle passes through the skin and the subcutaneous tissues, penetrates the sternal body.
[Acupuncture and Moxibustion]	Insert the needle subcutaneously 0.3~0.5 cun deep and stimulate until there is a sore and distending sensation in the local area. This point can be moxibusted.
[Indications]	Pain of the chest, cancer of the esophagus, and vomiting.

Joint of corpus sterni and processus xiphoideus

M. serratus anterior

RN 16
RN 15

8 cun

M. rectus abdominis

Navel

M. obliquus externus abdominis

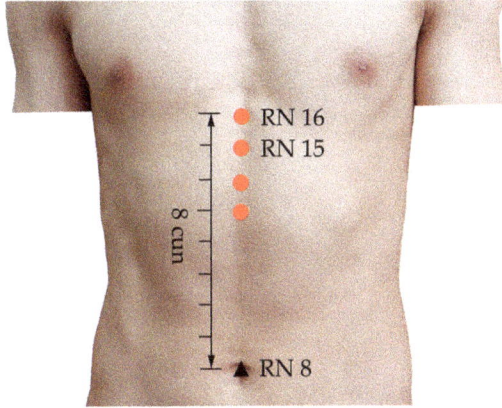

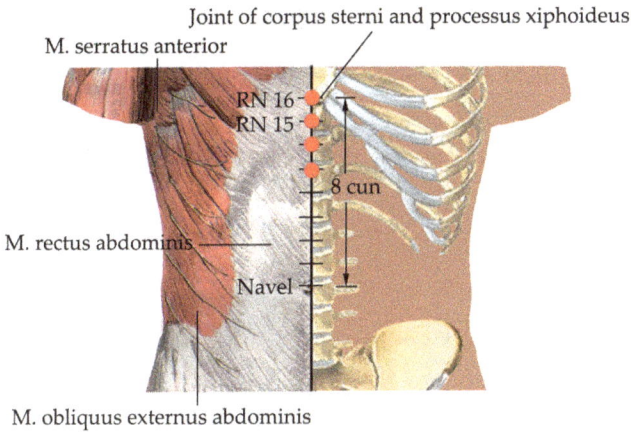

RN 17 – Dàn Zhōng

[Regional Anatomy]	Front-mu point of the Pericardium Channel of Hand *Jueyin*; influential point of Qi.
[Locating]	The point is located in the supine position, on the anterior midline, at the level with the fourth intercostal space.
[Regional Anatomy]	The needle passes through the skin and the subcutaneous tissues, penetrates the sterna body.
[Acupuncture and Moxibustion]	Insert the needle subcutaneously 0.3~0.5 cun deep and stimulate until there is a sore and distending sensation in the local area radiating to the chest. This point can be moxibusted.
[Indications]	Chest distention, heart palpitation, cough and asthma, insufficient lactation.

RN 18 – Yù Táng

[Locating]	On the chest, on the anterior midline, at the level of the third intercostal space.
[Regional Anatomy]	The same as RN 17 (Dàn Zhōng).
[Acupuncture and Moxibustion]	The same as RN 17 (Dàn Zhōng).
[Indications]	Cough, and shortness of breath.

RN 19 – Zǐ Gōng

[Locating]	On the chest, on the anterior midline, at the level of the second intercostal space.
[Regional Anatomy]	The same as RN 17 (Dàn Zhōng).
[Acupuncture and Moxibustion]	The same as RN 17 (Dàn Zhōng).
[Indications]	Cough and asthma, and chest pain.

RN 20 – Huá Gài

[Locating]	On the chest, on the anterior midline, at the level of the first intercostal space.
[Regional Anatomy]	The same as RN 17 (Dàn Zhōng).
[Acupuncture and Moxibustion]	The same as RN 17 (Dàn Zhōng).
[Indications]	Cough and asthma, and chest pain.

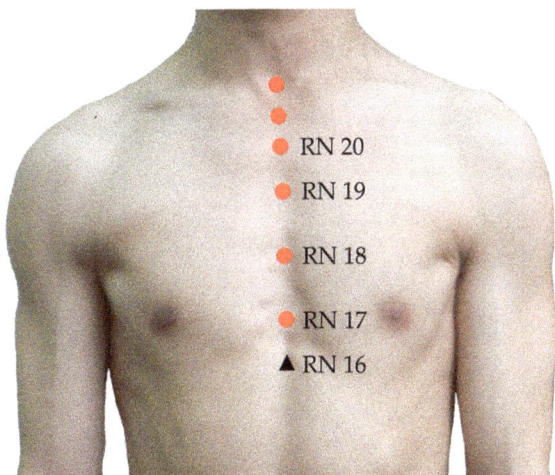

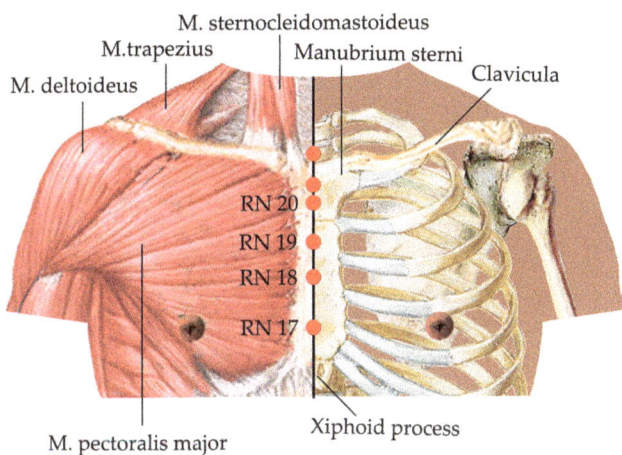

M. sternocleidomastoideus
M.trapezius
Manubrium sterni
M. deltoideus
Clavicula

RN 20
RN 19
RN 18
RN 17

M. pectoralis major
Xiphoid process

RN 21 – Xuán Jī

[Locating]	On the chest, on the anterior midline, 1 cun inferior to RN 22 (Tiān Tū).
[Regional Anatomy]	The same as RN 17 (Dàn Zhōng).
[Acupuncture and Moxibustion]	The same as RN 17 (Dàn Zhōng).
[Indications]	Cough and asthma, and sore throat.

RN 22 – Tiān Tū

[Locating]	The point is located in the sitting or supine position, on the anterior midline, in the center of the suprasternal fossa.
[Regional Anatomy]	The needle passes through the skin and the subcutaneous tissues, penetrates the space anterior to trachea.
[Acupuncture and Moxibustion]	Insert the needle perpendicularly 0.2~0.3 cun deep and insert the needle between the posterior border of the sternum and the anterior border of the trachea 0.5~1.0 cun deep and stimulate until there is a sore and distending sensation in the local area. This point can be moxibusted.
[Indications]	Cough and asthma, and sore throat.

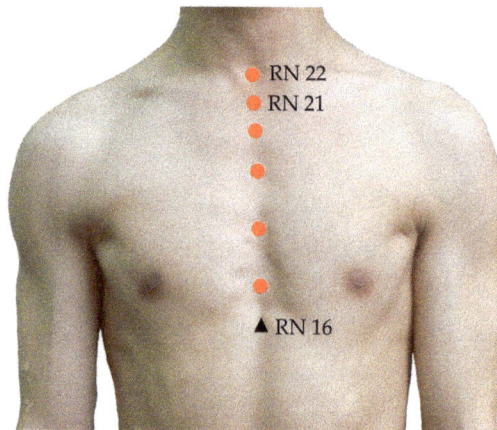

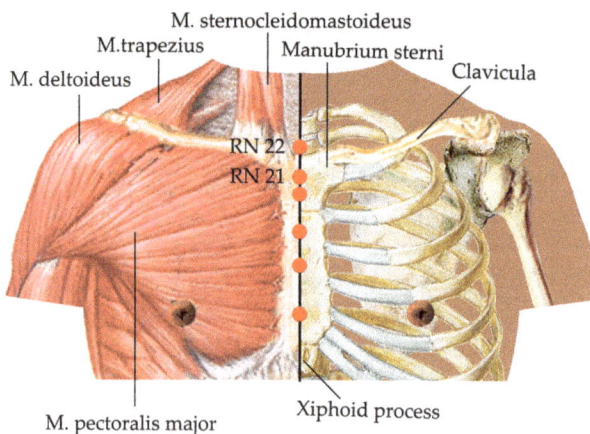

RN 23 – Lián Quán

[Locating]	The point is located in the sitting or supine position, between the Adam's Apple and the lower jaw, in the depression above the upper border of the hyoid bone.
[Regional Anatomy]	The needle passes through the skin and the subcutaneous tissues, penetrates the thyroid gland, hyoid bone and median ligament.
[Acupuncture and Moxibustion]	Insert the needle perpendicularly 0.5~0.8 cun deep and stimulate until there is a sore and distending sensation in the local area. This point can be moxibusted.
[Indications]	Tongue swelling and pain, sudden loss of the voice, and aphtha of the mouth and tongue.

RN 24 – Chéng Jiāng

[Locating]	The point is located in the sitting or supine position, on the anterior midline, below the lower lip, in the depression in the center of the mentolabial groove.
[Regional Anatomy]	The needle passes through the skin and the subcutaneous tissues, penetrates the m. orbicularis oris, m. depressor labii inferioris and m. mentalis.
[Acupuncture and Moxibustion]	Insert the needle obliquely 0.3~0.5 cun deep and stimulate until there is a sore and distending sensation in the local area spreading to the lips. This point can be moxibusted.
[Indications]	Stroke, loss of conciseness, epilepsy, deviation of the eye and mouth, and salivation.

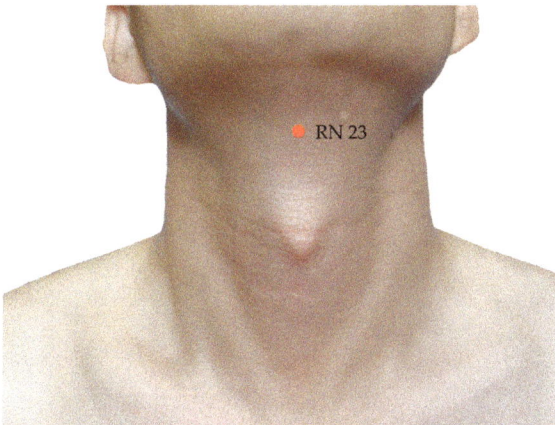

RN 23

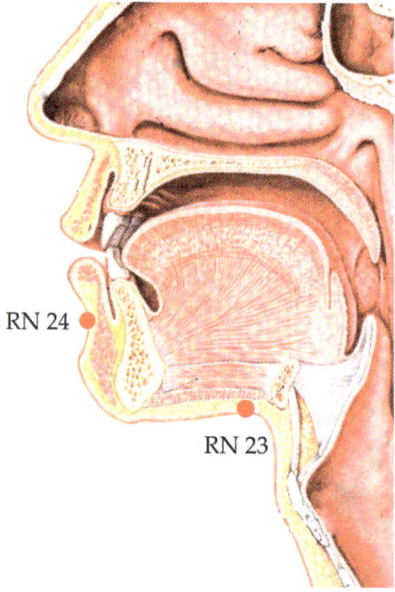

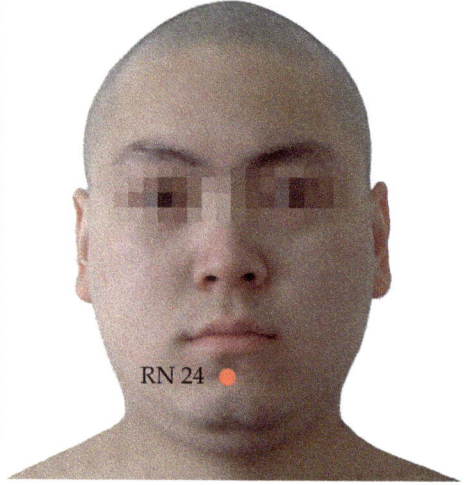

CHAPTER 15

Extrapoints; EX

EX 1 – Sì Shén Cōng

[Locating]	The point is located in the sitting or supine position, at the vertex, 1 cun posterior, anterior and lateral to DU 20 (Bǎi Huì), a group of 4 points.
[Regional Anatomy]	The needle passes through the skin and the subcutaneous tissues, penetrates the galea aponeurotica and the loose connective tissue beneath aponeurosis and periost.
[Acupuncture and Moxibustion]	Insert the needle subcutaneously 0.5~0.8 cun deep and stimulate until there is a sore and distending sensation in the local area. This point can be moxibusted.
[Indications]	Neck stiffness, headache, vertigo, and insomnia.

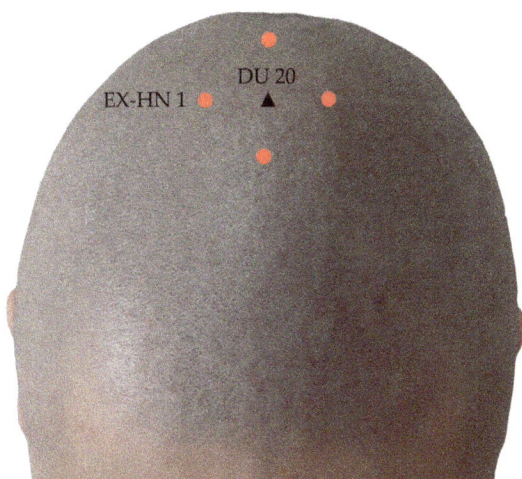

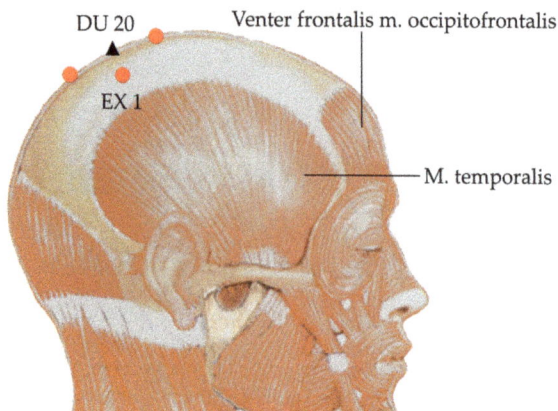

DU 20

Venter frontalis m. occipitofrontalis

EX 1

M. temporalis

EX 2 – Yìn Táng

[Locating]	The point is located in the sitting or supine position, in the depression of the midpoint of the medial ends of the two eyebrows.
[Regional Anatomy]	The needle passes through the skin and the subcutaneous tissues, penetrates the m. procerus and m. corrugator supercilii.
[Acupuncture and Moxibustion]	Lift and squeeze the skin, insert the needle subcutaneously downwards 0.3~0.5 cun deep and stimulate until there is a sore and distending sensation in the local area. This point can be moxibusted.
[Indications]	Insomnia, epistaxis, and epilepsy.

EX 3 – Yú Yāo

[Locating]	The point is located in the sitting or supine position, at the midpoint of the eyebrows, directly above the pupil.
[Regional Anatomy]	The needle passes through the skin and the subcutaneous tissues, penetrates the m. orbicularis oculi.
[Acupuncture and Moxibustion]	Insert the needle subcutaneously towards the left and right 0.3~0.5 cun deep and stimulate until there is a sore and distending sensation in the local area. Moxibustion is prohibited.
[Indications]	Blepharoptosis, pain in the supraorbital region, and trigeminal neuralgia.

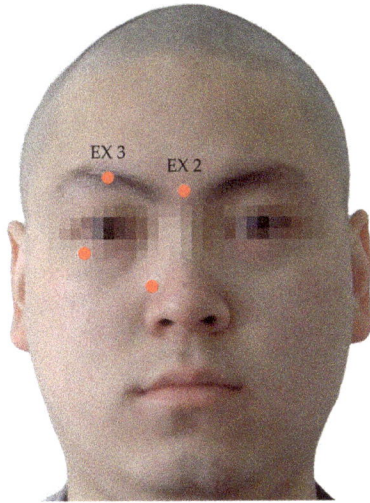

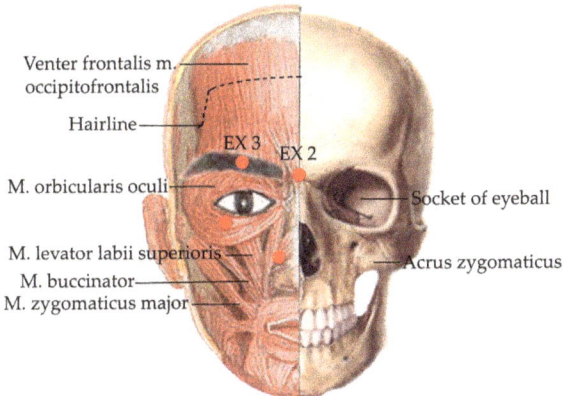

Venter frontalis m. occipitofrontalis
Hairline
EX 3
EX 2
M. orbicularis oculi
Socket of eyeball
M. levator labii superioris
Acrus zygomaticus
M. buccinator
M. zygomaticus major

EX 4 - Qiú Hòu

[Locating]	The point is located in the sitting or supine position when the eyes are closed, at the junction of the lateral 1/4 and the medial 3/4 of the infraorbital margin.
[Regional Anatomy]	The needle passes through the skin and the subcutaneous tissues, penetrates the m. orbicularis oculi, m. tarsalis inferior and m. oblique inferior.
[Acupuncture and Moxibustion]	Push the eyeball upwards gently and insert the needle perpendicularly 0.5-1.2 cun deep slowly along the lower orbital margin towards the optic nerve. Moxibustion is prohibited.
[Indications]	Optic neuritis, and glaucoma and myopia.

EX 5 – Shàng Yíng Xiāng

[Locating]	The point is located in the sitting or supine position, at the junction of the nasal alar cartilage and the turbinate, at the highest point of the nasolabial groove.
[Regional Anatomy]	The needle passes through the skin, subcutaneous tissues and reaches the m. levator labii superioris alaeque nasi.
[Acupuncture and Moxibustion]	Insert the needle subcutaneously upwards and inwards 0.5-0.8 cun deep and stimulate until there is a sore and distending sensation in the local area. This point can be moxibusted.
[Indications]	Rhinitis.

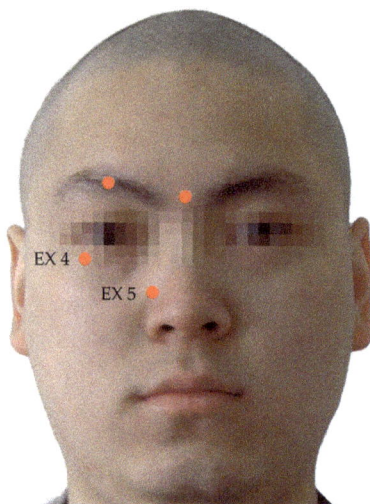

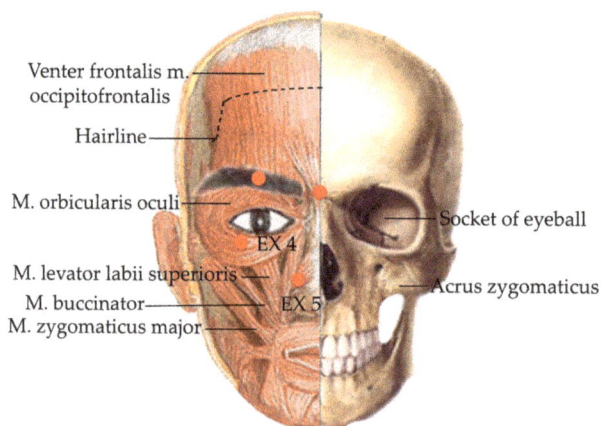

EX 6 – Tài Yáng

[Locating]	The point is located in the sitting or supine position, in the depression about one finger breadth posterior to the midpoint between the lateral end of the eyebrow and the outer canthus.
[Regional Anatomy]	The needle passes through the skin and the subcutaneous tissues, penetrates the m. orbicularis oculi, temopral fascia and m. temporalis.
[Acupuncture and Moxibustion]	① Insert the needle obliquely 0.3~0.5 cun deep and stimulate until there is a sore and distending sensation in the local area. ② Prick with a three-edged needle to bleed. This point can be moxibusted.
[Indications]	Headache, insomnia, and vertigo.

EX 7 – Qiān Zhèng

[Locating]	The point is located in the sitting or lateral position, 0.5-1.0 cun anterior to the auricular lobe, at the level with the midpoint of the auricular lobe.
[Regional Anatomy]	The needle passes through the skin and the subcutaneous tissues, penetrates the parotid gland and the masseter.
[Acupuncture and Moxibustion]	Insert the needle perpendicularly 0.5-1.0 cun deep and stimulate until there is a sore and distending sensation in the local area spreading to the face.
[Indications]	Deviation of the eyes and mouth.

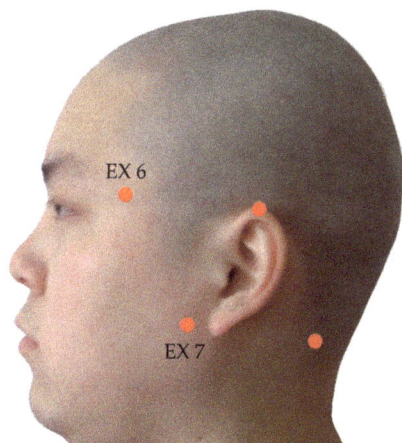

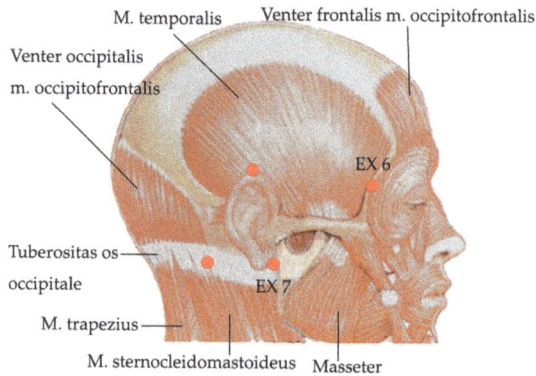

M. temporalis   Venter frontalis m. occipitofrontalis

Venter occipitalis
m. occipitofrontalis

EX 6

Tuberositas os
occipitale   EX 7

M. trapezius

M. sternocleidomastoideus   Masseter

EX 8 – Ěr Jiān

[Locating]	The point is located in the sitting or lateral position, fold the ear, the point is at the apex of the ear when it is folded forward.
[Regional Anatomy]	The needle passes through the skin and the subcutaneous tissues, penetrates the auricular cartilage.
[Acupuncture and Moxibustion]	① Insert the needle perpendicularly 0.1-0.2 deep and stimulate until there is a sore sensation in the local area. ② Prick with a three-edged needle to bleed. This point can be moxibusted.
[Indications]	Febrile disease, acute conjunctivitis, and sore throat.

EX 9 – Ān Mián

[Locating]	The point is located in the sitting or lateral position, at the midpoint between SJ 17 (Yì Fēng) and GB 20 (Fēng Chí).
[Regional Anatomy]	The needle passes through the skin and the subcutaneous tissues, penetrates the platysma and the m. splenius capitis.
[Acupuncture and Moxibustion]	Insert the needle perpendicularly 0.5-1.0 cun deep and stimulate until there is a sore and distending sensation in the local area. This point can be moxibusted.
[Indications]	Insomnia.

M. temporalis Venter frontalis m. occipitofrontalis

Venter occipitalis
m. occipitofrontalis

EX 8

Tuberositas os— EX 9
occipitale

M. trapezius —

M. sternocleidomastoideus Masseter

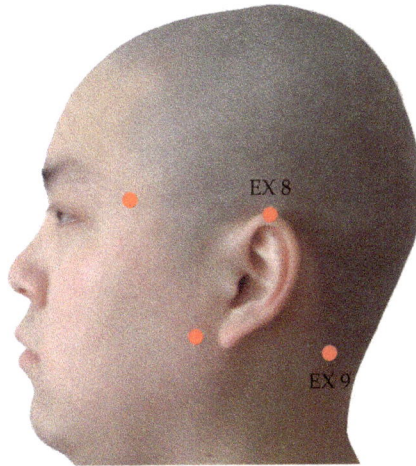

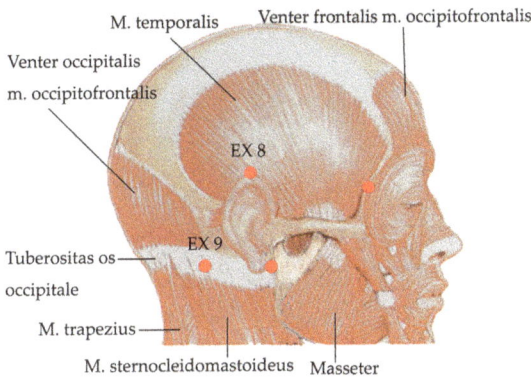

EX 10 – Jǐng Bǎi Láo

[Locating]	The point is located in the sitting or prone position when the neck is flexed, 2 cun superior to the spinous process of the seventh cervical vertebra, 1 cun lateral to the posterior midline.
[Regional Anatomy]	The needle passes through the skin and the subcutaneous tissues, penetrates the m. trapezius, m. splenius cervicis and the m. semispinalis capitis.
[Acupuncture and Moxibustion]	Insert the needle perpendicularly 0.3-0.5 cun deep and stimulate until there is a sore and distending sensation in the local area. This point can be moxibusted.
[Indications]	Cough and asthma, pulmonary tuberculosis, crvical spondylopathy.

EX 11 – Xuè Yā Diǎn

[Locating]	The point is located in the sitting or prone position when the neck is flexed, at the level of the intravertebral space between the sixth and the seventh cervical vertebra, 2 cun lateral to the posterior midline.
[Regional Anatomy]	The needle passes through the skin and the subcutaneous tissues, penetrates the m. trapezius, m. levator scapulae and the m. splenius capitis.
[Acupuncture and Moxibustion]	Insert the needle perpendicularly 0.5-1.0 cun deep and stimulate until there is a sore and distending sensation in the local area spreading to the scapular region. This point can be moxibusted.
[Indications]	Hypertension and hypotension, crvical spondylopathy, and neck stiffness.

EX 12 – Dìng Chuǎn

[Locating]	The point is located in the sitting or prone position when the neck is flexed, 0.5 cun lateral to DU 14 (Dà Zhuī).
[Regional Anatomy]	The needle passes through the skin and the subcutaneous tissues, penetrates the m. trapezius and the m. rhomboideus.
[Acupuncture and Moxibustion]	Insert the needle perpendicularly or obliquely inwards 0.5-0.8 cun deep and stimulate until there is a sore and heavy sensation in the local area. This point can be moxibusted.
[Indications]	Asthma and cough.

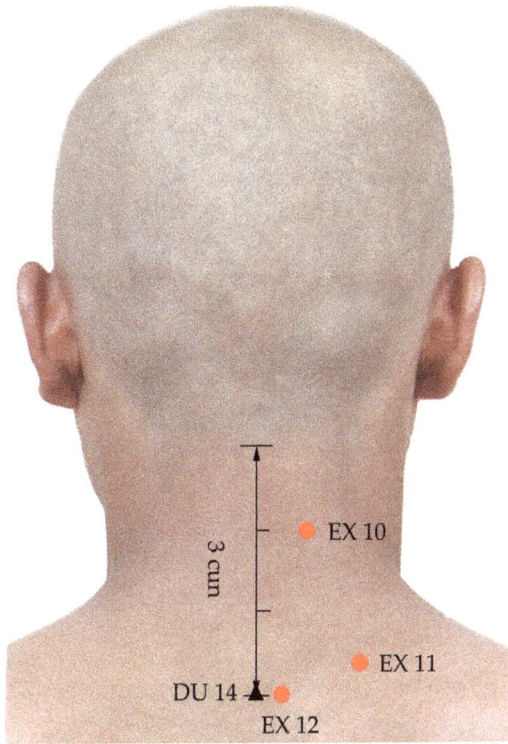

3 cun

EX 10

EX 11

DU 14

EX 12

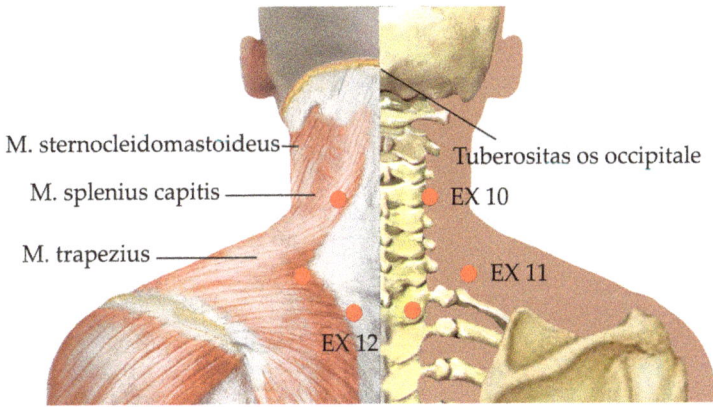

M. sternocleidomastoideus

M. splenius capitis

M. trapezius

Tuberositas os occipitale

EX 10

EX 11

EX 12

EX 13 – Shí Qī Zhuī

[Locating]	The point is located in the prone position, along the posterior midline, in the depression inferior to the spinous process of the fifth lumbar vertebra.
[Regional Anatomy]	The needle passes through the skin and the subcutaneous tissues, penetrates the supraspinal ligament, interspinal ligament and the interarcuate ligament.
[Acupuncture and Moxibustion]	Insert the needle perpendicularly 0.5-1.0 cun deep and stimulate until there is a sore and heavy sensation in the local area. This point can be moxibusted.
[Indications]	Lumbosacral pain, thigh pain, and enuresis.

EX 14 – Yāo Qí

[Locating]	The point is located in the prone position, on the lower back, 2 cun superior to the tip of the coccyx.
[Regional Anatomy]	The needle passes through the skin and the subcutaneous tissues, penetrates the sacrococcygeal ligament.
[Acupuncture and Moxibustion]	Insert the needle subcutaneously upwards 1.0-2.0 deep and stimulate until there is a sore and heavy sensation in the local area. This point can be moxibusted.
[Indications]	Lumbago, frequent micturition, general weakness, and gynecological diseases.

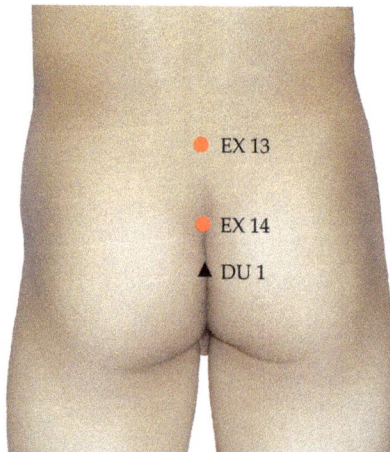

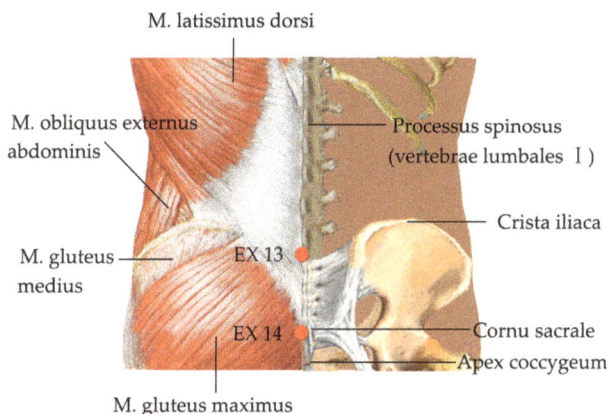

M. latissimus dorsi

M. obliquus externus abdominis

M. gluteus medius

EX 13

M. gluteus maximus

Processus spinosus (vertebrae lumbales I)

Crista iliaca

EX 14

Cornu sacrale

Apex coccygeum

EX 15 – Pǐ Gēn

[Locating]	The point is located in the prone position, at the level inferior to the spinous process of the first lumbar vertebra, 3.5 cun lateral to the posterior midline.
[Regional Anatomy]	Muscular: M. latissimus dorsi, m. sacrospinalis and m. quadratus lumborum.
	Innervations: The posterior rami of the 12th thoracic nerve and the 1st and 2nd lumbar nerves. The needle passes through the subcutaneous tissues and penetrates the m. latissimus dorsi and m. sacrospinalis and then reaches m. quadratus lumborum.
[Acupuncture and Moxibustion]	Insert the needle perpendicularly 0.5-0.8 cun deep and stimulate until there is a sore and heavy sensation in the local area.
[Indications]	Hepatosplenomegaly, and lumbar muscle strain.

EX 16 – Jiē Jǐ

[Locating]	The point is located in the prone position, in the depression below the spinous process of the twelfth thoracic vertebra.
[Regional Anatomy]	The needle passes through the skin and the subcutaneous tissues, penetrates the supraspinal ligament, interspinal ligament and the interarcuate ligament.
[Acupuncture and Moxibustion]	Insert the needle obliquely 0.5~1.0 cun deep and stimulate until there is a sore and heavy sensation in the local area.
	This point can be moxibusted.
[Indications]	Abdominal pain, prolapsus of the rectum, epilepsy.

EX 17 – Jiá Jǐ

[Locating]	The point is located in the prone position, 0.5 cun lateral to the lower border of each spinous process from the first thoracic vertebra to the fifth lumbar vertebra, a group of 17 points on one side of the spinal column.
[Regional Anatomy]	The muscles, blood vessels and nerves involved are different because of the different positions of the acupoints. Generally the needle passes through the skin and the subcutaneous tissues, penetrates the superficial muscles: m. trapezius, latissimus dorsi, m. serratus posterior superior, m. serratus posterior inferior, and the deep muscle: m.sacrospinalis, intertransversarii.
[Acupuncture and Moxibustion]	① Insert the needle perpendicularly 0.3-0.5 cun deep and stimulate until there is a sore and heavy sensation in the local area. ② Prick with plum-blossom needle. This point can be moxibusted.
[Indications]	Pain of the back and lumbar, pain and numbness of the limb.

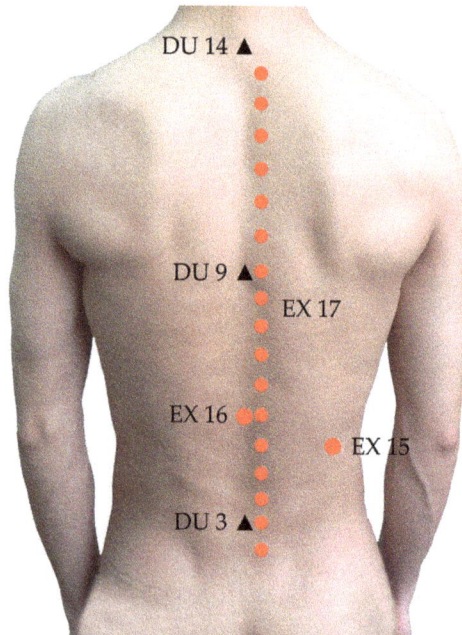

DU 14 ▲
DU 9 ▲
EX 17
EX 16
EX 15
DU 3 ▲

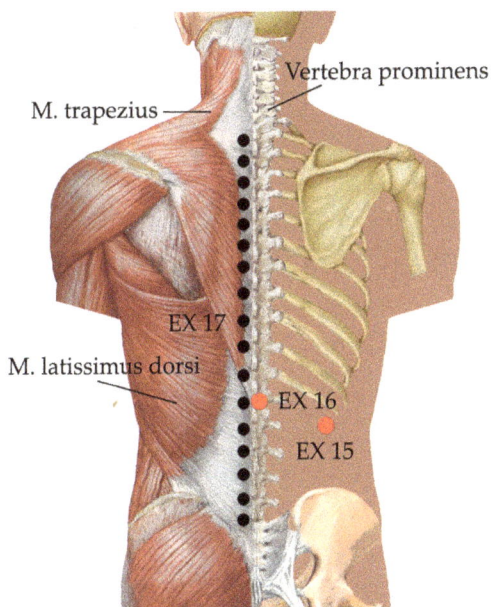

M. trapezius

Vertebra prominens

EX 17

M. latissimus dorsi

EX 16

EX 15

EX 18 – Sān Jiǎo Jiǔ

[Locating]	The point is located in the supine position, on the lower abdomen, forming an equilateral triangle with the umbilicus and two points inferior and lateral to the umbilicus, the length of the patient's mouth when relaxed.
[Regional Anatomy]	The needle passes through the skin and the subcutaneous tissues, penetrates the deep abdominal fascia, sheath of m. rectus abdominis and m. rectus abdominis.
[Acupuncture and Moxibustion]	Apply 5-10 moxa cones or place a moxa stick above the point for 20-30 minutes.
[Indications]	Hernia, pain around the umbilicus, and sensation of and sensation of gas in the stomach.

EX 19 – Lì Niào

[Locating]	The point is located in the supine position, at the midpoint of the line connecting the umbilicus to the upper border of the symphysis pubis.
[Regional Anatomy]	The needle passes through the skin and the subcutaneous tissues, penetrates the median umbilical fold.
[Acupuncture and Moxibustion]	Insert the needle perpendicularly 0.5-1.0 cun deep and stimulate until there is a numbing and distending sensation in the local area. This point can be moxibusted.
[Indications]	Urine retention, urinary system infection, and enuresis.

EX 20 – Zǐ Gōng

[Locating]	The point is located in the supine position, 3 cun lateral to the anterior midline, at the level with RN 3 (Zhōng Jí).
[Regional Anatomy]	The needle passes through the skin and the subcutaneous tissues, penetrates the m. obliquus externus abdominis and m. transversus abdominis.
[Acupuncture and Moxibustion]	Insert the needle perpendicularly 0.8-1.2 cun deep and stimulate until there is a sore and distending sensation in the local area radiating to the external genitalia.
[Indications]	Irregular menstruation, metrorrhagia, and infertility.

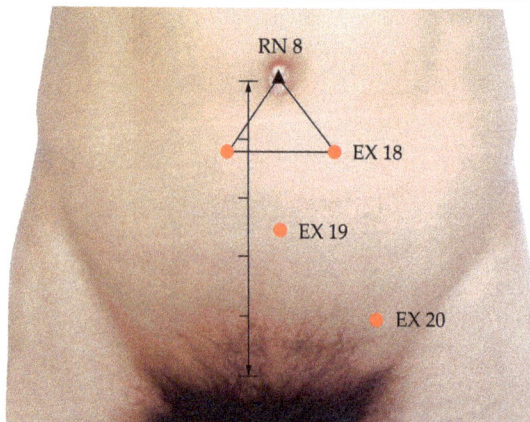

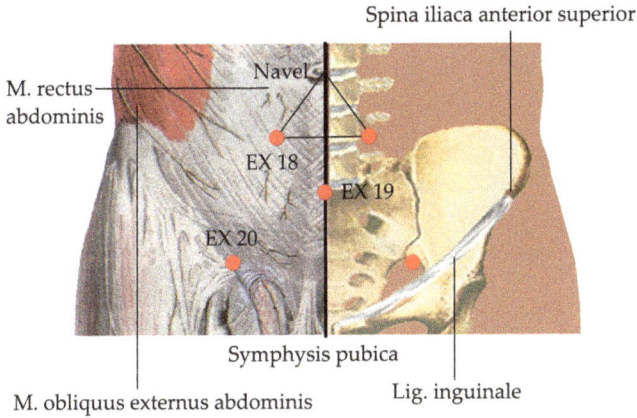

Spina iliaca anterior superior

M. rectus abdominis

Navel

EX 18

EX 19

EX 20

Symphysis pubica

Lig. inguinale

M. obliquus externus abdominis

EX 21 – Shí Xuān

[Locating]	The points are located when the palm is facing upward, in the center of the tip of the ten fingers, approximately 0.1 cun distal to the nails, a total of 10 points on both sides.
[Regional Anatomy]	The needle passes through the skin and the subcutaneous tissues.
[Acupuncture and Moxibustion]	① Insert the needle perpendicularly 0.1-0.2 cun deep and stimulate until there is a sore and heavy sensation in the local area. ② Prick with a three-edged needle to bleed. This point can be moxibusted.
[Indications]	Coma, acute tonsillitis, and hypertension.

EX 22 – Sì Fèng

[Locating]	The points are located when the palm is facing upward, on the palmar surface of the hand, in the midpoint of the transverse creases of the proximal interphalangeal joints of the index, middle, ring and little fingers. There are 4 points on one side and 8 points on both sides.
[Regional Anatomy]	The needle passes through the skin and the subcutaneous tissues, reaches tendo m. flexor digitorum profundus.

[Acupuncture and Moxibustion]	Prick with a three-edged needle 0.1-0.2 cun to bleed, or squeeze out a small amount of yellowish viscous fluid and stimulate until there is a sore and heavy sensation in the local area. Moxibustion is prohibited.
[Indications]	Malnutrition and indigestion in children.

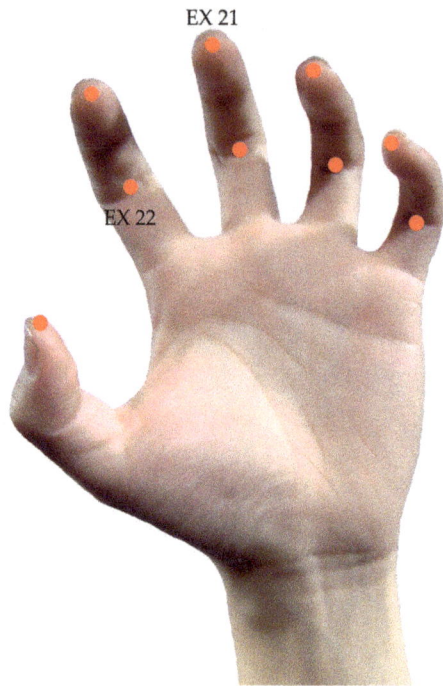

EX 21

EX 22

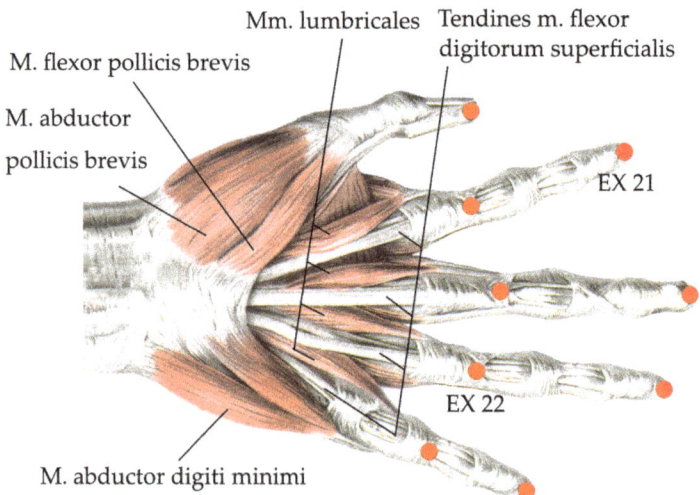

Mm. lumbricales

Tendines m. flexor digitorum superficialis

M. flexor pollicis brevis

M. abductor pollicis brevis

EX 21

EX 22

M. abductor digiti minimi

EX 23 – Bā Xié

[Locating]	The points are located on the dorsum of the hand, between the metacarpal bones, proximal to the web margins, at the junction of the red and white skin, a total of eight points on both sides.
[Regional Anatomy]	The needle passes through the skin and the subcutaneous tissues, reaches the interosseous muscles.
[Acupuncture and Moxibustion]	① Insert the needle obliquely 0.3-0.5 cun deep and stimulate until there is a sore and heavy sensation in the local area spreading to the tips of the fingers sometimes. ② Prick with a three-edged needle to bleed. This point can be moxibusted.
[Indications]	Finger numbness, headache, and sore throat.

EX 24 – Dà Gǔ Kōng

[Locating]	The point is located on the dorsal aspect of the hand, in the midpoint of the interphalangeal joint of the thumb.
[Regional Anatomy]	The needle passes through the skin and the subcutaneous tissues, penetrates the extensor pollicis longus muscle tendon.
[Acupuncture and Moxibustion]	This point can be moxibusted.
[Indications]	Conjunctivitis, cataract, and epistaxis.

EX 25 – Zhōng Kuí

[Locating]	The point is located on the dorsal aspect of the hand, at the midpoint of the proximal interphalangeal joint of the middle finger.
[Regional Anatomy]	The needle passes through the skin and the subcutaneous tissues, penetrates the dorsal digital aponeurosis and extensor tendon of finger.

[Acupuncture and Moxibustion]	This point can be moxibusted.
[Indications]	Stomach ache, vomiting, and hiccups.

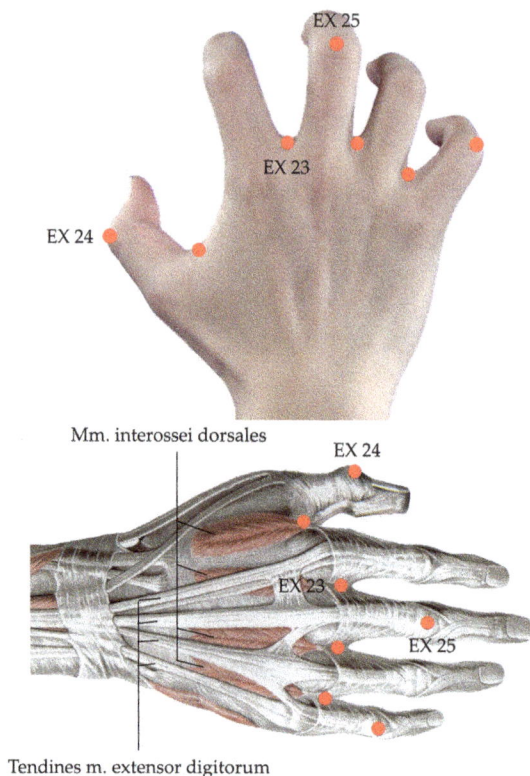

Mm. interossei dorsales

EX 25

EX 23

EX 24

EX 24

EX 23

EX 25

Tendines m. extensor digitorum

EX 26 – Xiǎo Gǔ Kōng

[Locating]	The point is located on the dorsal aspect of the hand, at the midpoint of the proximal interphalangeal joint of the little finger.
[Regional Anatomy]	The needle passes through the skin and the subcutaneous tissues, penetrates the dorsal digital aponeurosis and tendo m. extensor digiti minimi.
[Acupuncture and Moxibustion]	This point can be moxibusted.
[Indications]	Ophthalmic diseases and laryngalgia.

EX 27 – Wài Láo Gōng

[Locating]	The point is located on the dorsal aspect of the hand, between the second and third metacarpal bones, about 0.5 cun posterior to metacarpophalangeal joint.
[Regional Anatomy]	The needle passes through the skin and the subcutaneous tissues, penetrates the m. interossei dorsales II.
[Acupuncture and Moxibustion]	Insert the needle perpendicularly 0.3~0.5 cun deep and stimulate until there is a sore and heavy sensation in the local area spreading to the tips of the fingers. This point can be moxibusted.
[Indications]	Cervical spondylopathy, and neck stiffness.

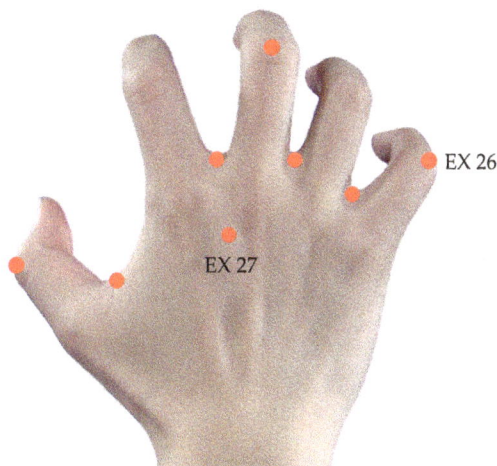

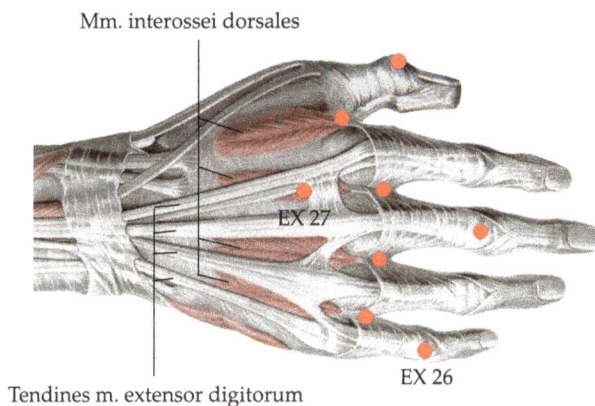

Mm. interossei dorsales

EX 27

Tendines m. extensor digitorum

EX 26

EX 28 – Yāo Tòng Diǎn

[Locating]	The points are located on the dorsal aspect of both hands, midway between the transverse wrist crease and metacarpophalangeal joint, between the second and third metacarpal bones, and between the fourth and fifth metacarpal bones, a group of 2 points on one sids.
[Regional Anatomy]	The needle passes through the skin and the subcutaneous tissues, penetrates the extensor digitorum tendon.
[Acupuncture and Moxibustion]	Insert the needle perpendicularly 0.5-1.0 cun deep and stimulate until there is a sore and heavy sensation in the local area spreading to the tips of the fingers. This point can be moxibusted.
[Indications]	Acute lumbar sprain.

EX 29 – Zhōng Quán

[Locating]	The point is located on the dorsal aspect of the hand, on the transverse wrist crease, in the depression on the radial side of the tendon of common extensor muscle of fingers.
[Regional Anatomy]	The needle passes through the skin and the subcutaneous tissues, passes between extensor tendon of finger and tendo m. extensor carpi radialis brevis.
[Acupuncture and Moxibustion]	Insert the needle perpendicularly 0.3~0.5 cun deep and stimulate until there is a sore and heavy sensation in the local area spreading to the tips of fingers and elbows.
[Indications]	Chest distention, gastric pain, cough and asthma.

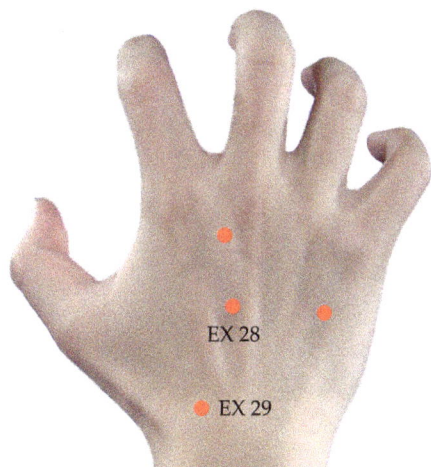

EX 28

EX 29

Mm. interossei dorsales

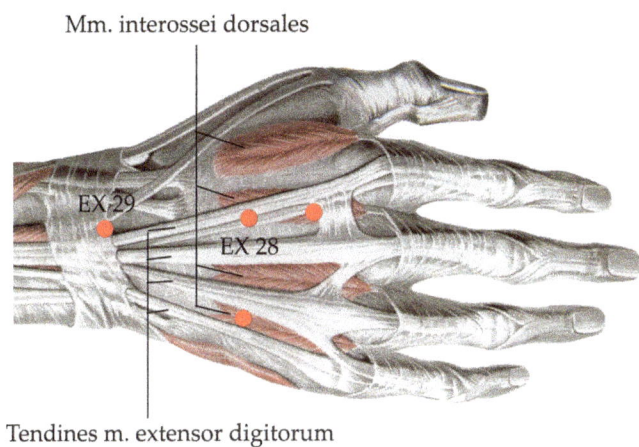

EX 29

EX 28

Tendines m. extensor digitorum

EX 30 – Èr Bái

[Locating]	The points are located on the medial aspect of the forearm, 4 cun superior to the transverse wrist crease, bilateral to the tendon of m. flexor carpi radialis, a group of 2 points on one side.
[Regional Anatomy]	The medial point is located near: The needle passes through the skin and the subcutaneous tissues, penetrates between the tendon of the m. palmaris longus and the m. flexor carpi radialis, m. flexor digitorum superficialis, n. medianus and m. flexor pollicis longus. The lateral point is located near: The needle passes through the skin and the subcutaneous tissues, penetrates between the m. flexor carpi radialis and tendon of the brachioradialis, m. flexor digitorum superficialis and m. flexor pollicis longus.
[Acupuncture and Moxibustion]	Insert the needle perpendicularly 0.5~0.8 cun deep and stimulate until there is a sore and heavy sensation in the local area spreading to the tips of fingers.
[Indications]	Hemorrhoids, and prolapse of the rectum.

EX 31 – Qì Duān

[Locating]	The points are located in the center of the tip of the ten toes, 0.1 cun distal to the nails, a total of 10 points on both sides.
[Regional Anatomy]	The needle passes through the skin and the subcutaneous tissues.
[Acupuncture and Moxibustion]	① Insert the needle perpendicularly 0.1~0.2 cun deep and stimulate until there is a sore and distending sensation in the local area. ② Prick with a three-edged needle to bleed. This point can be moxibusted.
[Indications]	Numbness of the toes, coma and shock.

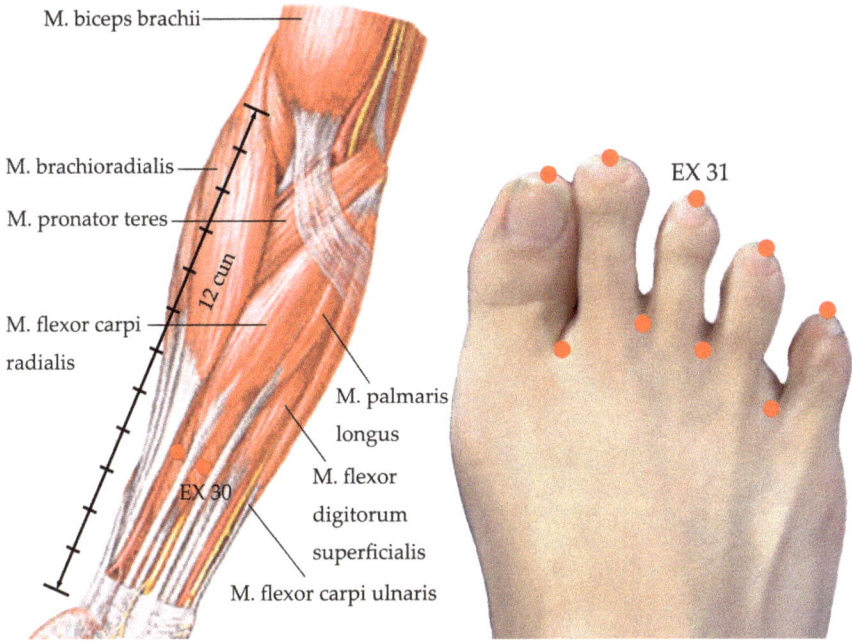

M. biceps brachii

M. brachioradialis

M. pronator teres

M. flexor carpi radialis

12 cun

M. palmaris longus

M. flexor digitorum superficialis

EX 30

M. flexor carpi ulnaris

EX 31

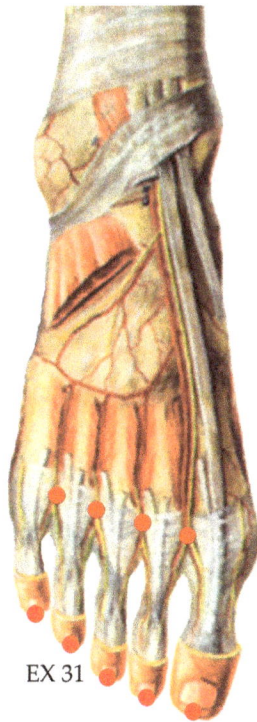

EX 31

EX 32 – Bā Fēng

[Locating]	The point is located in the sitting or prone position with the foot resting on the ground, in the depression between the first and the fifth toe, proximal to the margins of the webs, at the junction of the red and white skin. There are 4 points on one side and 8 points on both sides.
[Regional Anatomy]	The needle passes through the skin and the subcutaneous tissues, penetrates the extensor digitorum tendon.
[Acupuncture and Moxibustion]	① Insert the needle obliquely 0.5-0.8 cun deep and stimulate until there is a sore and heavy sensation in the local area spreading to the dorsum of the foot. ② Prick with a three-edged needle to bleed. This point can be moxibusted.
[Indications]	Headache, toothache, stomach ache, irregular menstruation, and numb toes.

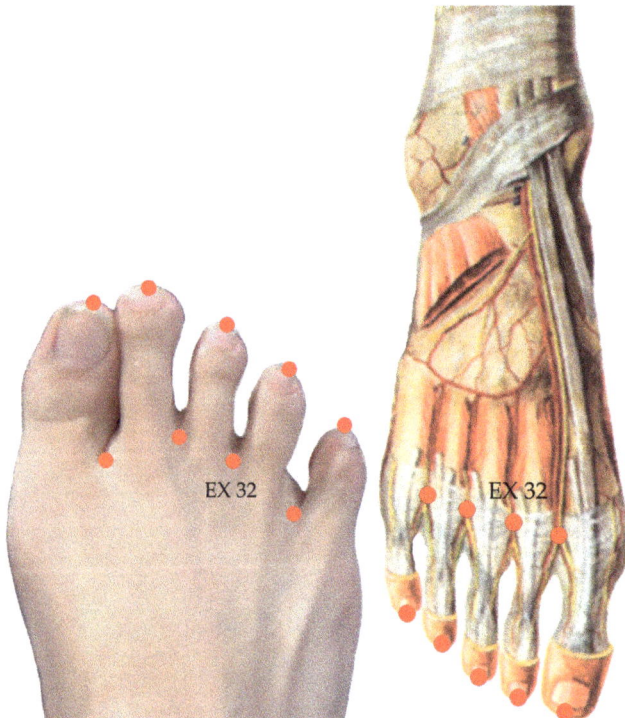

EX 32   EX 32

EX 33 - Dú Yīn

[Locating]	The points are located in the prone position on the sole of the foot, in the midpoint of the transverse creases of the distal interphalangeal joints of the second toe.
[Regional Anatomy]	The needle passes through the skin and the subcutaneous tissues, penetrates the flexor digitorum tendon.
[Acupuncture and Moxibustion]	Insert the needle perpendicularly 0.1-0.2 cun deep and stimulate until there is a sore and heavy sensation in the local area. This point can be moxibusted.
[Indications]	Angina pectoris, and irregular menstruation.

EX 34 - Lǐ Nèi Tíng

[Locating]	The points are located in the prone position on the sole of the foot, in the depression between the second and third toe, medial to the metatarsophalangeal joints, opposite with ST 44 (Nèi Tíng).
[Regional Anatomy]	The needle passes through the skin and the subcutaneous tissues, penetrates the m. plantar interosseous.
[Acupuncture and Moxibustion]	Insert the needle perpendicularly 0.3-0.5 cun deep and stimulate until there is a sore and heavy sensation in the local area. This point can be moxibusted.
[Indications]	Epilepsy, convulsion and spasm, stomach ache, and numb toes.

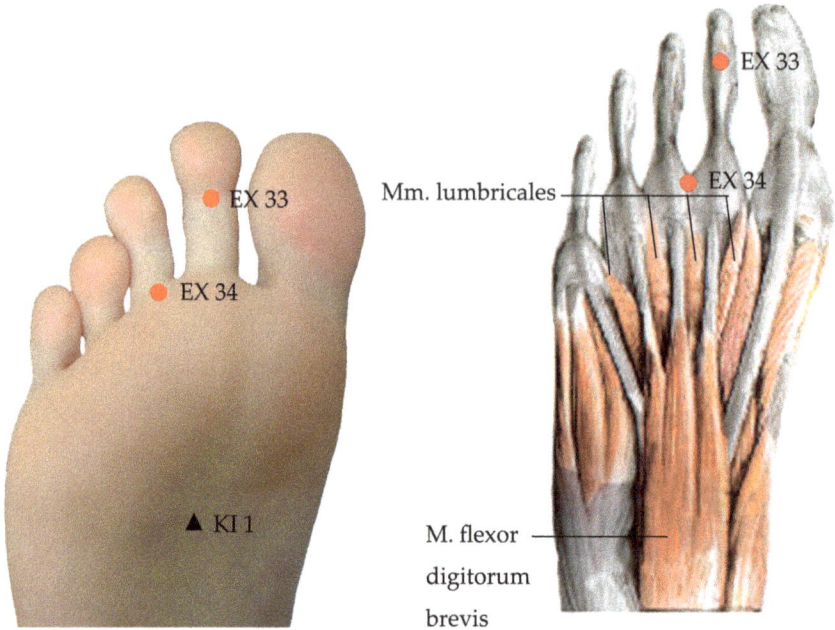

Mm. lumbricales

EX 33

EX 34

EX 33

EX 34

KI 1

M. flexor
digitorum
brevis

EX 35 – Dăn Náng Xuè

[Locating]	The point is located in the sitting or prone position when the knee is flexed, in the depression 2 cun inferior to GB 34 (Yáng Líng Quán).
[Regional Anatomy]	The needle passes through the skin and the subcutaneous tissues, penetrates the m. peroneus longus.
[Acupuncture and Moxibustion]	Insert the needle perpendicularly 1.0-1.5 cun deep and stimulate until there is a sore and heavy sensation in the local area radiating to the lower limbs. This point can be moxibusted.
[Indications]	Acute and chronic cholecystitis, and cholelithiasis and cholecystalgia.

EX 36 – Lán Wěi Xuè

[Locating]	The point is located in the sitting position when the knee is flexed, on the most obvious tenderness points between ST 36 (Zú Sān Lǐ) and ST 37 (Shàng Jù Xū), approximately 2 cun distal to ST 36 (Zú Sān Lǐ).
[Regional Anatomy]	The needle passes through the skin and the subcutaneous tissues, penetrates the m. tibialis anterior.
[Acupuncture and Moxibustion]	Insert the needle perpendicularly 0.5-1.0 cun deep and stimulate until there is a sore and heavy sensation in the local area radiating to the the dorsum of the foot. This point can be moxibusted.
[Indications]	Acute and chronic appendicitis, gastritis, and indigestion.

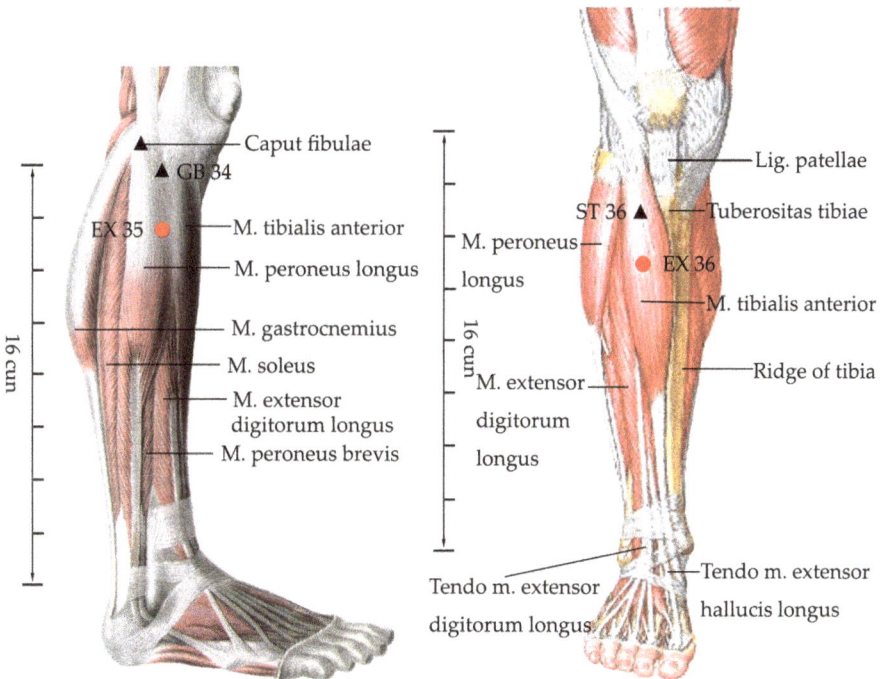

EX 37 – Xī Yǎn

[Locating]	The point is located in the sitting or prone position when the knee is flexed, in the depression on the medial and lateral aspect of the patellar ligament on the knee. On the medial is called Nèixīyǎn, on the lateral called Wàixīyǎn, ST 35 (Dú Bí).
[Regional Anatomy]	Nèi Xī Yǎn: The needle passes through the skin and the subcutaneous tissues, passes beside the patellar ligament and retinaculum patellae mediale, then reaches the capsule of knee joint. Wàixīyǎn is as same as ST 35 (Dú Bí).
[Acupuncture and Moxibustion]	Insert the needle obliquely 0.5-1.0 cun deep or penetrates the Nèixīyǎn and Wàixīyǎn opposite, stimulate until there is a sore and heavy sensation in the local area. This point can be moxibusted.
[Indications]	Knee pain.

EX 38 – Hè Dǐng

[Locating]	The point is located in the sitting or prone position when the knee is flexed, in the depression of the midpoint above the superior border of the patella.
[Regional Anatomy]	The needle passes through the skin and the subcutaneous tissues, penetrates the tendon of m. quadriceps femoris.
[Acupuncture and Moxibustion]	Insert the needle perpendicularly 0.5-0.8 cun deep and stimulate until there is a sore and heavy sensation in the local area. This point can be moxibusted.
[Indications]	Knee pain, and weakness and paralysis of the lower limbs.

EX 39 – Bǎi Chóng Wō

[Locating]	The point is located in the sitting or prone position when the knee is flexed, in the medial aspect of the thigh, 3 cun superior to the medial and superior border of the patella, 1 cun superior to SP 10 (Xuè Hǎi).
[Regional Anatomy]	The needle passes through the skin and the subcutaneous tissues, penetrates the m. vastus medialis.
[Acupuncture and Moxibustion]	Insert the needle perpendicularly 0.8-1.2 cun deep and stimulate until there is a sore and heavy sensation in the local area. This point can be moxibusted.
[Indications]	Rubella and eczema, urticaria, cutaneous pruritus, and gastrointestinal parasitic diseases.

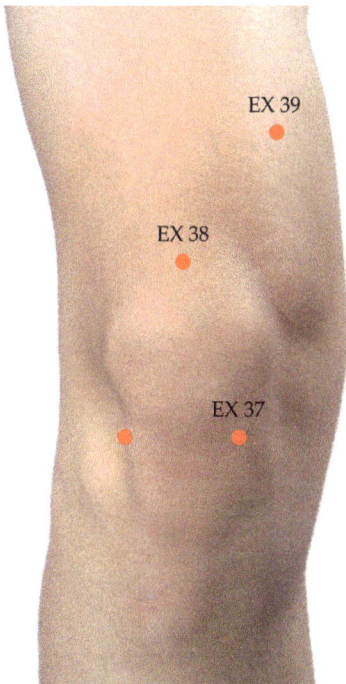

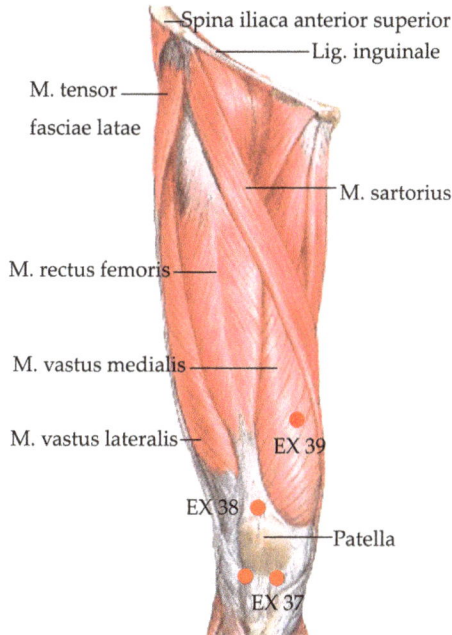

Introduction to Professor Yang Jiasan

Yang Jiasan (1919 -2001)

Yang Jiasan was born in Wujin County, Jiangsu Province in 1919. In 1932, he studied under Wu Bingsen as a teacher. In 1935, he studied under Chen Danan as a teacher and graduated from Wuxi China Acupuncture and moxibustion Special School. Then, he practiced under Hua Qingyun, who, is in fact, his father-in-law.

Yang Jiasan, is or has been; a professor of Nanjing Zhongmin School; director of acupuncture and moxibustion department of Beijing College of traditional Chinese Medicine; director of acupuncture department of affiliated hospital; director of acupuncture and moxibustion department of affiliated hospital; director of acupuncture and massage department of Beijing College of traditional Chinese Medicine; member, professor, doctoral supervisor of Beijing Institute of traditional Chinese Medicine; Director of the National Society of traditional Chinese Medicine; member of the standing Committee of the Acupuncture and Moxibustion Society; Technical adviser of the Acupuncture Branch of the Beijing Society of traditional Chinese Medicine; member of the Chinese Medicine Professional Group of the State Science and Technology Commission; Chairman of the Medical Science Committee of the Ministry of Health; academic Committee of the Institute of traditional Chinese Medicine Member of the Association; Vice Chairman of the academic Committee of the Beijing Institute of traditional Chinese Medicine; member of the editorial Committee of the Intermediate Medical Journal; member of the editorial and examination Committee of the National higher Medical Colleges and

Universities; consultant of the Guangming correspondence University; consultant of the School of Health Journalism; Honorary Professor of Zhongjingguo Medical University, member of the expert Committee of the Sino-Japanese Friendship Hospital; consultant of the Advisory Committee of the China Acupuncture and Moxibustion Association of Hong Kong.

He is particularly well respected at treating stroke, impotence, arthralgia, tremor paralysis, climacteric syndrome, diabetes mellitus, urolithiasis, as well as having expertise in many other complaints. He has practiced in; Indonesia, Sri Lanka, North Korea, Romania, the Philippines, France, where by, he has treated foreign heads of state and leaders. He has been invited to many countries to give academic lectures and exchanges. The film, *Acupuncture and Moxibustion taking points*, edited by the editor-in-chief, won the Class B Science and Technology Achievement Award of the Ministry of Health. His article, *Needle injection with one hand*, was appraised as an excellent paper by Beijing College of traditional Chinese Medicine. The main works are; *14 meridians, odd meridians eight pulse meridians wall chart, Acupuncture and moxibustion clinical acupoint selection diagram, Yang Jiasan acupoint selection experience*, (changed name in 1982), *Acupuncture and moxibustion acupoint selection method,* (Foreign language Publishing House translated into English, published and Spanish), *Acupoint Science, Pocket Point selection Picture*. Professor Yang has taught in Russia and run workshops in numerous countries, his students are spread all over the world. He has trained numerous master's degree students, and fifteen doctoral students, which in fact, are excellent successors for the cause of acupuncture and moxibustion in traditional Chinese medicine.

His original one-handed needle injection method (refer below) attributed the traditional "stab hand" and "escort hand" to one hand. According to the needle position, needle length and treatment, needs to be divided into air pressure type, angle pressure type, twisting type, continuous pressure type. His acupoint selection compatibility, in inheriting the previous sage experience of the basic soil, has a strong regularity, practicability, only taking the original acupoint application compatibility as an example, there are many methods, such as Zang-fu original point matching, original infusion matching, original collaterals matching, original matching and so on. Combined with anatomical knowledge, he put forward the "three sides, three middles" acupoint selection method, which has the characteristics of accurate acupoint selection, strong acupuncture feeling, safe and reliable acupuncture, and has been effectively applied in clinical teaching. His influence is extensive.

Clinical experience in acupuncture and moxibustion of Professor Yang Jiasan

Professor Yang Jiasan's experience in selecting acupoints

According to ancient records, clinical acupoint selection needs to have vertical and horizontal coordinate positioning. Longitudinal positioning is usually based on bone size, but it also needs transverse positioning, vertical and horizontal intersection in order to accurately locate. Professor Yang Jiasan summed up the law of horizontal positioning as "three sides" and "three middles". "Three sides", refering to the edge of the bone, the edge of the tendon, the edge of the flesh, the "three middles", refers to the bone, between the tendons, between the flesh, between the muscles and bones, between the tendons, and so on. This method is simple and easy to use, and the curative effect is reliable.

According to this law, combined with the anatomical knowledge of western medicine, and many years of clinical experience, the acupoint location analysis was carried out, one by one, and a unique acupoint selection experience was formed. The main points of acupoints selected from each meridian are as follows:

1. **Lung channel:** the radial edge of biceps brachii, the radial edge of biceps brachii tendon, the transverse stria of wrist, and the posterior part of metacarpophalangeal joint should be mastered.

2. **Large intestine channel:** mainly master the anatomical signs of the second metacarpophalangeal joint, between the metacarpal bones,

between muscles and bones, elbow flexion head, sternocleidomastoid muscle and larynx.

3. **Stomach channel:** Mainly master the anatomical marks of the straight line, mouth angle, mandibular angle, sidewall angle, zygomatic arch, sternocleidomastoid muscle, throat node, rib space, anterior superior iliac upper ratchet, external patella, external knee eye, tibial anterior crest, external ankle high point, second metatarsal toe joint and other anatomical signs.

4. **Spleen channel:** mainly master the first metatarsophalangeal joint before and after, the medial posterior edge of tibia, medial thigh muscle and other anatomical signs.

5. **Heart channel:** mainly master the fingernail root, metacarpophalangeal joint, ulna wrist flexor tendon, elbow transverse line, biceps brachii ulna lateral edge and other anatomical signs.

6. **Small intestine channel:** mainly master the nail root, the fifth metacarpophalangeal joint, the anterior and posterior deltoid bone, the lateral edge of ulna, the midpoint and ends of scapula, larynx, sternocleidomastoid muscle, mandibular angle and so on.

7. **Bladder channel:** mainly master the anatomical signs of medial canthus, eyebrow, hairline, spinal spinous process, gluteal transverse line, posterior median line of thigh, popliteal transverse line, sural muscle, lateral malleolus, metatarsophalangeal joint and so on.

8. **Kidney channel:** mainly master the anatomical signs of plantar, medial malleolus, Achilles tendon, semitendinosus muscle, semimembranous tendon, navel, ribs and so on.

9. **Pericardial channel:** mainly master the anatomical signs of nipple, biceps brachii, longus palmaris tendon and flexor Carpi radialis tendon, metacarpophalangeal joint, middle finger end and so on.

10. **Sanjiao channel:** mainly master the fourth and fifth metacarpal and phalangeal joints, total digital tendon, ulna, radius, ulna eagle mouth, shoulder peak, mandibular angle, sternocleidomastoid muscle, auricle and other anatomical signs.

11. **Gallbladder channel:** mainly master the anatomical signs of lateral canthus, auricle, mastoid, zygomatic arch, interhair, ribs, nipples, navel, greater trochanter of femur, anterior superior ilium spine, lateral median line of thigh, fibula, lateral malleolus, metatarsophalangeal joint and so on.

12. **Liver channel:** mainly master the first metatarsophalangeal joint, medial malleolus, medial side of tibia, flexion knee transverse head, nipple, ribs and other anatomical signs.

13. **Du vessel:** mainly master the tail sacral bone, spinal spinous process, hairline. Anatomical signs such as sulcus, ilium crest, inferior horn of scapula, scapula and so on.

14. **Ren vessel:** mainly master pubic symphysis, navel, sternal sword union, superior sternal fossa, larynx, chin-labial sulcus and other anatomical signs.

Familiar with these anatomical signs, according to the law of "three sides" and "three middles", combined with longitudinal bone size measurement, you can accurately select acupoints. According to the law of "three middles" and "three sides", it has the characteristics of "two easy and two less".

Two easy: first of all, it is easy to get the arrival of Qi. Acupuncture at the middle point, its gas operation, such as unhindered in the pathway, but piercing the muscles and joints, under the needle astringent and tight – this is not a comfortable feeling, it will be painful and uncomfortable. Whether the acupuncture feels Qi or not, is directly related to the effect of the acupuncture treatment.

According to this law, the acupoints taken are helpful to obtain the appropriate acupuncture feel and Qi.

Secondly, it is easy to exorcise bad energy. Acupoints are located in orifice, gap, because the muscle here is weak, most vulnerable to bad energy invasion. Set the acupoints here, stimulate the acupoints, adjust the meridian Qi, and make the evil Qi dispel from it.

Two less: first of all, there is less tissue damage. In the "three sides", "three middles" site acupoint, the tissue under the acupoint is relatively loose, the gap is large, which is not only convenient to exercise various manipulations, but also not easy to damage the tissue and cause pain during needle operation. Secondly, due to the less tissue damage, the discomfort after acupuncture will be reduced accordingly.

Professor Yang Jiasan's acupuncture manipulation experience

1. one hand needle

Professor Yang Jiasan summed up and formed a unique acupuncture method in clinical and teaching practice. Yang Jiasan felt that the traditional double-handed acupuncture method followed a feasible method of ancient experience, but it also had some shortcomings, such as slow speed, time-consuming and laborious, so he created an acupuncture method, which not only had the dual function of a "piercing hand" and "pressing hand", but also was simple and easy to do. The details are as follows:

Taking the right hand needle as an example, the thumb, index finger pinching needle handle (pinching needle body when using long needle), ring finger, small finger holding needle body, middle finger acting as "claw flipping and turning the needle". The formation of a unique single hand needle method, the left hand is liberated and can hold the needle with better control.

There are four kinds of needle feeding methods: hanging type (abbreviated as air pressure type), angle change type (referred to as angle pressure type), twisting type (referred to as twisting type), continuous pressure type. These four acupuncture methods can be selected arbitrarily according to the location of acupoints, the operational needs of clinical rehydration and so on – where each has formed an operating standard, which is characterized by less accuracy, pain, light and fast, standard and practical. This deft use of finger division of labor, finger force wrist force, distance, angle of the multi-element organic fusion of the needle into the way, suitable for the human body at various points, but also for any length of the needle.

The air pressure type is mainly suitable for most acupoints and various lengths of needle injection when the skin does not need gas. Acupoints with fat or flat muscles in the extremities and abdomen need to be used for direct or deep needling.

The angle pressure type is mainly suitable for the skin to get gas, can be used for all acupoints of the whole body needle, abdominal acupoints are especially suitable, generally using 1 inch to 1.5 inch length of needle for direct acupuncture.

The twisting type is suitable for the skin to get gas and twist to replenish and purge, the right twisting needle is the purging method, and the left twisting needle is the supplementary method.

Continuous compression is often used in very shallow parts of the skin of the head, as well as in a variety of diseases that require prickles and internal thorns.

2. pay attention to reinforcing and reducing

Acupuncture Reinforcing-reducing Methods have attached importance by doctors in the past dynasties. Yang Jiasan studied all schools , deleted and simplified, and formed his own acupuncture tonifying style. According to the standard, "you Fu" said, "move back the air rest, meet the right and cool; push the inside rub, with the left and warm up", the method and stimulation of the method and stimulation incisively summed up as "rub tight fixed plus vibration, push the left with supplementary work; move back to the right to welcome the diarrhea, wonderful stimulation in the strength of the strength." It means that on the basis of gaining Qi, the thumb is pressed forward, the needle turns left, to rub tight, and the method is to carefully guard the meridian Qi and push back as the supplement. On the basis of getting gas, the thumb is backward, the needle turns to the right to rub tight, to guard the meridian gas carefully, and then vibrate as the laxative method.
Yang Jiasan emphasizes the attention in the process of acupuncture, especially in the process of replenishing and reducing, we must without distraction in order to achieve the best effect of tonifying and reducing.

Yang Jiasan also has a unique view on the degree of stimulation: attention should be paid to light stimulation when needling every day, and the intensity of stimulation should be medium; when the needle is not angry, it should be strongly stimulated; if you want to be angry to the disease, you need to give strong stimulation; acute diseases should be given strong stimulation. At the same time, it should also be noted that there should be less acupoints used when strong stimulation is applied.

Yang Jiasan's prescription of acupoints experience

1. Five-Shu acupoints

Based on the in-depth study of the characteristics of the Five-Shu acupoints, Yang Jiasan holds that the points have obvious laws in the order of position distribution and the depth of pulse gas flow injection, and also have the same law in the main treatment. The main treatment characteristics of Wuliu point are as follows: the well point should be liver, regulate Qi, relieve depression and open orifice; Xing point should be heart, clear heart, purge heat and cool blood; infusion point should be spleen, invigorate spleen and stomach, transport water dampness; meridian point should be lung, Xuanfei scattered evil, stop cough and reduce Qi; the acupoint should be kidney, adjust kidney Qi, and stomach fall inverse. The main therapeutic effect of Wuyu point was unified with the pathogenesis of the five Zang organs. That is, under the guidance of the theory of meridians and collaterals, through the determination of its meridians, the second selection of its acupoints, and then the order of tonifying and reducing, the preliminary formation a method of diagnosis and treatment of "special disease, special meridians, special acupoints, special methods" has been worked out, and a set of complete and systematic application procedures for syndrome differentiation of five acupoints has been worked out. The details are as follows:

Based on the twelve meridians, we first determine where the lesions belong, and then further identify whether the lesions are external meridians or internal viscera lesions. For the treatment of external meridian diseases, Xing acupoints were treated with purging method and deficiency syndrome by filling points. Visceral lesions, the corresponding five losses. If in addition to the viscera lesions, but also other visceral lesions, add its corresponding five points.

Take the heart meridian as an example, the external meridian empirical Xiexing acupoint Shaofu, deficiency syndrome Bushu acupoint Shenmen. The syndrome of visceral disease was taken from the meridian point Lingdao. This diagnosis and treatment is characterized by the combination of the principle of acupoint selection and treatment of "meridians, main treatment" with the specific main therapeutic effect of the five acupoints, so as to locate the meridian syndrome longitudinally. The transverse orientation of the main treatment of the five acupoints expands the scope of the main treatment of the five points and improves the curative effect of acupuncture and moxibustion.

2. Head acupoints

Yang Jiasan is expert at using head acupoints and emphasizes the role of head acupoints in the treatment of cerebral diseases and facial diseases. According to the statistical analysis of clinical medical records, the main treatment laws of head acupoints are as follows: mental and mental diseases, taking Shenting, Benshen, SiShencong, combined with intradermic acupuncture, forming the effective "regulating spirit (energy) acupuncture method", which is widely used in seizures, schizophrenia, neuro-weakness, insomnia, forgetfulness and other diseases; wind syndrome takes Fengchi, Fengfu and other neck acupoints; the top acupoints of the head can be applied either exogenous or internal injury.

In the aspect of replenishment and diarrhea of head acupoints, Yang Jiasan believes that the first thing is that different acupoints have the effect of partial or partial diarrhea, and the skin meat of the acupoints in the head cover is shallow, so the tonifying and purging is different from the usual method, which means that the needle is pierced into the scalp without penetrating along the scalp about 15 °angle; the subcutaneous acupuncture is the cathartic method; that is, the needle is pricked between the scalp and the skull at the angle of 30° along the scalp. The acupoints in the head are relatively thick, and most of them are invaded by the evil of Fengyang, so Fengchi, Fengfu and other points should be pricked deeply. After gaining Qi, the method of lifting and twisting right is adopted, so that the bad Qi of Fengyang can disipate quickly. When Yang Jiasan applied to the head acupoints, he thought that first of all; the acupoint nature of different acupoints has the effect of partial or partial diarrhea, but supplement is as important as diarrhea. He believes that intradermic needling is a supplement and subcutaneous needling is diarrhea.

3. Compatibility of source acupoints

Through the study of Sanjiao, Yang Jiasan believes that the source acupoints, as the passage and retention of the original gas of the tricoke, not only has the function of regulating Qi and dispelling evil, but also has the function of tonifying deficiency and strengthening position. It is often used in combination with other specific acupoints in clinical syndrome. It can be summarised as the matching of the original points of the Zang-fu organs (the viscera, the viscera and the viscera), the matching of the original collaterals (the matching of the original collaterals between the subject and the guest, the matching of the original meridians), the matching of the original Shu, the matching of the original (lower), and the matching of the original recruitment, which has strong regularity and practicability.

As usual, Taiyuan permeates Jingqu, Daling passes through Neiguan, Taibai permeates Gongsun reduces Qi to treat persistent hiccups, and uses Taichong combined with valley to treat the hand and foot detention of the liver caused by depression, anger, anger and liver.

Tight or yin deficiency liver prosperity caused by dizziness and other syndromes. For the syndrome of deficiency of Zang-fu organs, the compatibility of original acupoints and Puyu acupoints was remarkable, and for the same disease of Zang-fu organs, the original acupoints of Yang meridians with Yin meridians or Xianhe acupoints has a good effect. Such as spleen and stomach discord and cause abdominal distension, vomiting and catharsis, can be treated via Taibai and Zusanli, invigorate the spleen and stomach, rise clear and reduce turbid; liver Qi invades stomach caused by stomach discomfort, chest and hypochial pain, irritable and can be used Taichong with Zusanli, soothing liver and regulating Qi, and stomach reverse.

Yang Jiasan's acupuncture and moxibustion treatment examples

1. Diabetes mellitus

Yang Jiasan believes that this disease is complex, and often accompanied by a variety of complications, not easy to cure. However, the symptoms can be alleviated and the development of complications can be controlled by treatment. The cause of diabetes mellitus is deficiency of spleen yin, deficiency of spleen yin is bound to cause hyperdryness of stomach yang, which affects the function of lung and kidney of the body, and the abnormal movement of body fluid leads to thirst, hunger and so on. Sugar in the body can not be absorbed and utilised normally, but can be excreted out of the body through urination, resulting in the loss of essence, loss of viscera and tissue, complicated with various organ diseases, such as encephalopathy, heart disease, kidney disease, pulse disease, peripheral neuropathy, fundus vascular disease, retinal disease, skin pruritus, skin infection and so on. In view of the inherent law of the development of this lesion, the method of tonifying spleen yin and clearing stomach dryness is emphasised in the treatment. According to the change of course of disease, acupuncture and moxibustion can control the condition and restore blood glucose by taking hand and foot Yangming meridians, foot Taiyin spleen meridians, hand sun small intestine meridians, as well as abdominal acupoints and back Shu points. On this basis, combined with disease differentiation and syndrome differentiation, it can also receive satisfactory curative effect.

2. Asthma

Elderly asthma is a common clinical refractory disease, the patient has difficulty breathing, sweating more, easy to catch a cold, especially in winter, it is difficult to heal, but for a long time it has emphysema and cor pulmonale. According to the law of Yang Jiasan's disease, and according to the characteristics of his deficiency and reality, Yang Jiasan adopted the methods of treating both its root and its standard, both its interior and its surface, paying attention to the treatment of the disease and adjusting it in good time according to the seasonal change. Acupuncture and moxibustion plus traditional

Chinese medicine decoction at the onset of the disease, the effect is very good; conditioning or single use of traditional Chinese medicine or alone acupuncture, pay attention to the curative effect, but also convenient for patients.

3. Tremor paralysis

Tremor paralysis in modern medicine mostly belongs to Parkinson's disease, with progressive movement slow, muscle rigidity and tremor as the main clinical characteristics. With the advancement of the disease it is difficult to walk, and self-care becomes dificult. Yang Jia-san believes that the disease is due to deficiency of liver and kidney yin, deficiency of Qi and blood, loss of brain marrow, loss of veins and nourishment. Treatment to tonify the liver and kidney, renourish the Qi and blood, fill essence and nourish marrow, phlegm and collaterals. Acupuncture and moxibustion points to head acupoints, and Ren du meridian, Yin and Yang stilts, foot Shaoyin temple points, the clinical effect is more significant.

4. Stroke

Yang Jiasan believes that the etiology and pathogenesis of apoplexy are deficiency of kidney yin, water does not contain wood, transversely invades spleen, dissipates wind and perturbed phlegm and blood stasis, and hinders cerebral collaterals. In the treatment of apoplexy, one disease can be divided into acute phase and convalescent stage.

In the acute stage, the method of clearing the heart and replenishing the liver was adopted, that is, the yang heat of clearing the heart and liver was mainly superior, and the yin of liver and kidney was adjusted. Acupuncture and moxibustion acupoints: head wind pool, Fengfu, Baihui, front top, back top, through the sky; upper limb Qu pool, branch ditch, column missing, Yanggu, eight evil; lower limbs take Zusanli, Sanyinjiao, Kunlun, Zhaohai, Bafeng. Acupuncture method: bilateral limbs were taken together, first on the healthy side, and then on the affected side. Fengchi, Fengfu catharsis method does not leave needles, Baihui, front top, back top, Tongtian skin internal needling method; Quchi, Yanggu, Zhigou, Kunlun, eight evil, eight wind purging method; lack, Zhaohai, Zusanli, Sanyin. It is characterized by the emphasis on purging fire to remove the wind, and To make up for the yin.

The treatment of convalescence period, to "complement the upper method" that is, to nourish the liver and kidney Yin in the lower, and to clear the heart and liver Yang in the upper. Acupuncture and moxibustion points: the head of the wind pool, Fengfu, Baihui, front top, back top, Tongtian; upper limb to take curved pool, Hegu, column missing, wrist bone; lower limb to take Zusanli, hanging bell, Taichong, Sanyinjiao, Kunlun. Acupuncture method: wind pond, fengfu diarrhea method without acupuncture, Baihui, front top, back top, all-day skin pricking method; quchi, hegu, kunlun with diarrhea method; column lack, carpal bone, shining sea, hanging bell, Zusanli, Sanyinjiao, Taichong with complement method.

Its combination of treatment, in the stage of syndrome differentiation flexible addition and subtraction. If it's a stroke. Then. In the above treatment, the method of tonifying acupuncture is reused, that is, Shenting, Benshen, SiShencong, Shenmen acupuncture.

According to the above treatment methods, the treatment characteristics are as follows: Yin meridians and yang meridians acupoints are selected at the same time. 2) pay attention to head acupoints, replenish and reduce at the same time. Different treatments are used at different stages of the disease. It embodies the theoretical essence of traditional Chinese medicine, such as syndrome differentiation and treatment, whole concept and so on. The acupoints of the shoulder and hip joint are not taken. Yang Jiasan believes that apoplexy is located in the head rather than in the limbs, so the limb acupoints can only be taken below the elbow and knee joint. Add and subtract at the same time, use acupoint essence, compatibility is flexible.

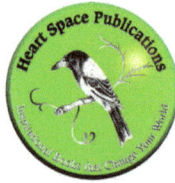

If you derived benefit from this manual,
please see the other three in the series of

Quick Reference Handbooks of Chinese Medicine

Acupuncture of Acupoint Combinations Quick Lookups

Illustrations of Special Effective Acupoints for common Diseases

Human Body Reflex Zone Quick Lookup, Bilingual
anatomical illustration of reflex zones (English
edition)

Quick Investigation On Acupunture Points – Selection of
Professor Yang Jiasan

Go to www.heartspacepublications.com

www.ingramcontent.com/pod-product-compliance
Lightning Source LLC
Chambersburg PA
CBHW052009030426
42334CB00029BA/3145